DOING RESEARCH WITH CHILDREN AND YOUNG PEOPLE

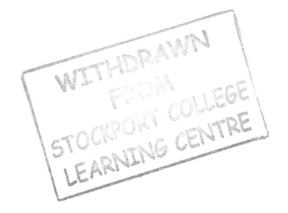

DOING RESEARCH WITH CHILDREN AND YOUNG PEOPLE

EDITED BY
Sandy Fraser
Vicky Lewis
Sharon Ding
Mary Kellett
Chris Robinson

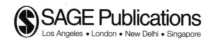

SAGE Publications
Los Angeles • London • New Delhi • Singapore

In association with

The Open University

First published 2004
Reprinted 2006, 2007

SAGE Publications Ltd
1 Oliver's Yard, 55 City Road
London, EC1Y 1SP

SAGE Publications Inc.
2455 Teller Road
Thousand Oaks, California 91320

SAGE Publications India Pvt Ltd
B 1/I 1 Mohan Cooperative Industrial Area
Mathura Road, New Delhi 110 044
India

SAGE Publications Asia-Pacific Pte Ltd
33 Pekin Street # 02-01
Far East Square
Singapore 048763

British Library Cataloguing in Publication data

A catalogue record for this book is available from
the British Library

ISBN-978-0-7619-4380-8 (hbk)
ISBN-978-0-7619-4381-5 (pbk)

Library of Congress Control Number: 2003109269

Typeset by C&M Digitals (P) Ltd., Chennai, India
Printed in Great Britain by The Cromwell Press Ltd, Trowbridge, Wiltshire

Contents

Contributor Affiliations

Lesley Abbott Professor, Early Childhood Education, Manchester Metropolitan University, England, UK.

Priscilla Alderson Professor of Childhood Studies, Social Science Research Unit, Institute of Education, University of London, England, UK.

Rachel Burr Lecturer in Childhood Studies, Faculty of Education and Language Studies, The Open University, England, UK.

Sharon Ding Staff Tutor, Centre for Childhood, Development and Learning, The Open University, England, UK.

Anne Edwards Professor of Pedagogic Practice, Centre for Sociocultural and Activity Theory Research, School of Education, University of Birmingham, England, UK.

Alan France Director of the Centre for the Study of Childhood and Youth, Department of Sociological Studies, University of Sheffield, England, UK.

Sandy Fraser Lecturer in the School of Health and Social Welfare, The Open University, England, UK.

Sandy Hobbs Leverhulme Emeritus Fellow, University of Paisley, Scotland, UK.

Adele Jones Lecturer, Department of Behavioural Sciences, The University of the West Indies, Saint Augustine, Republic of Trinidad and Tobago.

Mary Jane Kehily Lecturer, Centre for Childhood, Development and Learning, The Open University, England, UK.

Mary Kellett Lecturer, Centre for Childhood, Development and Learning, The Open University, England, UK.

Ann Langston Early Years Consultant, Manchester Metropolitan University, England, UK.

Vicky Lewis Professor, Centre for Childhood, Development and Learning, The Open University, England, UK.

Mani Maniam Associate Lecturer, The Open University, England, UK.

Judith Masson Professor of Law, Warwick University, England, UK.

Jim McKechnie Reader, Psychology Division, School of Social Sciences, University of Paisley, Scotland, UK.

Olga Nieuwenhuys Senior Research Fellow, Institute for Development Research, University of Amsterdam, Amsterdam, The Netherlands.

Vijay Patel Independent Researcher and Associate Lecturer, The Open University, England, UK.

Rob Pattman Thomas Coram Research Unit, Institute of Education, England, UK.

Helen Roberts Professor of Child Health, Child Health Research and Policy Unit, City University, London, England, UK.

Chris Robinson Senior Lecturer and Staff Tutor, School of Health and Social Welfare, The Open University, England, UK.

Satnam Singh Associate Lecturer, The Open University in Scotland, Scotland, UK.

Acknowledgements

A great many people contributed to this edited collection. Rachel Burr, Miriam David, Ginny Morrow and Nigel Thomas read and commented on drafts of all of the chapters. We are particularly grateful to them, especially since we were often asking for comments within very tight time scales. Their comments provided many valuable suggestions for ways to improve the chapters. We should also like to thank the contributors who also were often working to tight deadlines but nevertheless responded positively to feedback. A number of other people contributed to the production of this edited collection and we thank them all: Liz Benali, Louise Delaney, Maria Francis-Pitfield, Liz Freeman and colleagues in Co-publishing at the Open University, Chris Golding, Alison Poyner and colleagues at Sage Publications, Iris Rowbotham and Steph Withers.

The authors and publishers wish to thank the following for permission to use copyright material:

Chapter 11: Routledge for 'Example of a decision-making chart' and 'Example of a diamond ranking exercise' from O'Kane, C. (2000) 'The development of participatory techniques: facilitating children's views about decisions which affect them', in P.H. Christensen and A. James (eds) *Research with Children: Perspectives and Practices*, pp. 136–159.

Chapter 14: Enda Tiers-Monde for 'La priorisation: manque de structure de formation' from *Enfants en Recherche et en Action*. And Earthscan and UNICEF for 'Ladder of participation' from Hart, R. (1999) *Children's Participation, The Theory and Practice of Involving Young Citizens in Community Development and Environmental Care.*

Chapter 17: Organisation for Economic Community Development (OECD) for 'Implementation of policy' from OECD (2002) *Educational Research in England: Examiners' Report.*

1 Doing Research with Children and Young People: An Introduction
VICKY LEWIS

Research with children and young people is crucial. It can advance understanding of how they develop and live their lives, it can contribute to theoretical debates, and its outcomes can impact directly and indirectly on the lives of those researched and others in similar situations. However, if the research is to be in the best interests of the children and young people themselves, it is essential that researchers take heed of a number of critical issues which arise in the planning, carrying out and dissemination stages of research. Relevant issues include ethics, consent, the legal system, power relations, methodology and the dissemination process. It is also important when reading research papers to consider whether the various issues have been addressed appropriately, in order to evaluate the research and its contribution.

In this book we have brought together researchers who have expertise in a variety of different spheres and who are particularly well placed to iden-tify and reflect on some of the issues and questions which arise in research with children and young people. They differ from one another in many ways including the disciplines in which they work, the methodological approaches they favour, the groups of children and young people they research, and their primary interest – which for some is to understand children and young people better and for others is to improve the lives of children and young people. Despite these differences they share an interest in ensuring that research with children and young people is effective and appropriate. Although we invited particular researchers to reflect on specific topics there are a number of issues which appear in many of the chapters, such as access, consent, ethics and power relations. However, these are discussed by different authors from their different perspectives and often in relation to different groups of children and young people.

Not surprisingly, given their different backgrounds and experiences, the contributors express varied points of view and at times may even contradict one another in what they say. As editors we have not sought to ensure that a united picture is presented of how to tackle the different issues which are raised. This is because there is no single correct answer to each issue and it is important to acknowledge, debate and reflect on different views. Nevertheless, certain themes do emerge from many of the chapters. One recurring theme is that the theoretical and methodological approach that is taken influences the research outcome; another is that the power relations which exist between researcher and researched affect the process of research; a third is the positive shift towards children and young people participating actively in research, even to the point of carrying out research themselves.

There are also undoubtedly gaps, some of which will only become apparent in time. The contributors can only present an account of some of the issues which are uppermost on their research agendas at the time they are writing in the early part of the twenty-first century. Fashions and trends shift and change in research and while we may believe that we have identified and solved a problem once and for all it is a fact of research, as it is of life, that many of the problems we identify and views which we hold today will be challenged by future generations and surpassed as different questions and approaches to research emerge. We can only comment on issues and possible ways of dealing with them in the light of our existing knowledge and understanding. However, by bringing together contributors from varied backgrounds our hope is that the ensuing chapters will enrich and advance discussion rather than complicate it.

There are things which this book does not do. As already noted, the contributors are working within different disciplines and therefore utilise different methodological approaches in their own research. The contributors reflect the disciplines of Education, Health, Social Welfare, Psychology, Sociology, Childhood Studies, Youth Studies, and Law. What unites the contributors are the participants in their research, namely children and young people. Further, since the contributors are exploring questions which arise in research with children and young people, they do not describe different methodologies in any detail, although they do comment on methodological aspects to varying extents. So, if you are looking for a step by step guide through different methodological approaches to research with children and young people this is not an appropriate book. Nevertheless, many of the chapters do provide examples and suggestions for how research with children and young people can be carried out effectively. It is also important to note that the contributors are all based in and predominantly working in the minority or Western world, although research with children and young people in the majority or non-Western world is the topic of one of the chapters.

This edited collection was put together in conjunction with a companion volume, *The Reality of Research with Children and Young People* (Lewis, Kellett, Robinson, Fraser and Ding, 2004). *The Reality of Research...* includes published accounts of 13 research studies involving children and young people supplemented by commentaries written by the researchers. In these commentaries the researchers discuss how their research came about, describe difficulties they encountered during the research and how they overcame them (or not) and reflect back on the research after its completion. Many of the commentaries touch on questions which are covered in the present volume. Reflection is a vital part of the research process and is one way in which researchers can develop their expertise and advance their research. In the present book this is essentially what we have asked each contributor to do. We suggested a topic to each of them and asked them to reflect on the topic from their experience as a researcher. Self-reflection is a crucial part of the research process and we would encourage you to engage in this as you read each chapter in this book. As we have already pointed out, research fashions change over time, new issues arise and old issues may diminish in apparent importance, or resurface. Nevertheless, if research with children and young people is to result in better understanding and improved social conditions then we all need to stand back and take stock from time to time. We would not want this book to be seen as putting forward definitive answers to particular questions. Rather, it provides a starting point for us to reflect on a number of critical issues which every researcher working with children and young people should address.

In the remainder of this chapter I have provided an overview of the other chapters. The chapters are organised into four sections although, as you will discover, there is some degree of overlap between chapters within and across sections. The first section, 'Setting the Context', provides a background to research with children and young people from several different perspectives. The second section, 'Research Relations', explores the nature and influence on the research process of the varied relationships which arise between researchers and those who are researched. The third section, 'Diversity', examines a number of different populations who are often involved in research and draws out some of the implications of their diversity for research. The final section, 'Relevance, Evaluation and Dissemination', looks beyond the actual carrying out of research to what is done with the findings. Taken together, the chapters in this book provide an overview of research with children and young people.

In Chapter 2 'Situating Empirical Research', Sandy Fraser argues that for research to lead to better understanding of children and young people and to identify ways of improving their lives it is important to understand its limitations. He considers this in two parts. First he explores the characteristics of social and psychological research, such as discovery and engagement, and contrasts empirical research with other forms of knowledge such as may be gained through poetry and philosophy. He then addresses the question of why research should be *with* children and young people rather than *on* or *about* children and young people, arguing that for research to have positive benefits for their lives it is crucial that researchers engage with children and young people and negotiate the nature of the research with them. This argument is developed further in a number of chapters in later sections of the book and its importance is reflected in the use of the phrase research *with* in the book's title. Towards the end of this chapter Fraser mentions two crucial considerations which are also developed in more detail in later chapters, namely diversity and power relationships.

Fraser points out that historically developmental psychology led to children being viewed in particular ways, and briefly mentions how this view influenced research. This idea is developed further in Chapter 3, 'Images of Childhood'. In this chapter Mary Kellett, Chris Robinson and Rachel Burr provide an overview of different images that have been held of children and young people historically, culturally and within different disciplines. They give examples of how children have been portrayed in different ways at different times and in different places and how these images are affected by many factors. They demonstrate how research at a particular time or in a particular location can often be seen to reflect the ways in which children and young people are comprehended at that time and in that place. They show how different academic disciplines have influenced the images held of children and young people, looking at developmental psychology, anthropology and sociology in particular. They also consider the influence that economics, the media, language, religion, politics and culture have on how children and young people are viewed.

The legal system also impacts on how children and young people are viewed and Kellett, Robinson and Burr include examples of this. The current legal systems in England and Wales, Northern Ireland, and Scotland and their impact on research are examined in detail in Chapter 4, 'The Legal Context', by Judith Masson. Masson outlines the current legal rights of children and young people in the UK and points out that researchers must work within the relevant legal system. However, she makes the point that legal systems tend to set the minimum acceptable standard rather than specify good practice. It is therefore crucial that researchers address the ethical issues which arise in their research, a topic covered in greater detail in Chapter 7 and mentioned in other chapters. Interestingly, Masson points out that within the UK legally the term 'child' means anyone under the age of 18 years, which fails to acknowledge the clear differences between an infant and a young person. Like Fraser in Chapter 2, Masson also comments on the distinction between 'research on' and 'research with' children and young people and argues that it is important to include children in research, while ensuring that their rights are safeguarded. Masson deals with the important question of consent, describing the roles and responsibilities of gatekeepers and discussing the legal status of those with parental responsibility, as well as children's ability to consent. She contrasts the situation in Scotland with that existing in England, Wales and Northern Ireland and in clinical research as opposed to non-clinical research. Research confidentiality and the question of when researchers may disclose information are discussed in some detail. Likewise, the protection of data and of children and researchers are covered, as are the implications for involving children and young people as researchers. Many of these important points are also developed elsewhere in the book, in particular in Chapter 7 on 'Ethics' and in Chapter 12 'Young People'.

The final chapter in the first section, by Sandy Fraser and Chris Robinson, 'Paradigms and Philosophy', focuses on four paradigms used in social and psychological research and their philosophical underpinnings. The authors examine scientific, structuralist, interactionist and post-structuralist paradigms and point to the relevance of each for the sorts of research questions that researchers might want to ask. They deal with the scientific paradigm in some detail since this has impacted on the development of the other paradigms. They question whether social and psychological research can ever be scientific in the sense of being truly objective and point to the distinction between qualitative and quantitative research. In order to explore the background to this distinction, Fraser and Robinson examine three historical developments, namely positivism, falsification and Kuhn's view of paradigms. The structuralist paradigm is illustrated by reference to the views of Marx, Durkheim, Piaget, Chomsky and Lévi-Strauss, all of whom based their theories on the idea that there is some underlying objective structure that empirical research seeks to uncover. The interactionist paradigm sought to shift attention away from the facts of the scientific paradigm and towards the idea of individuals attributing meaning to events around them. Reference is made to the views of Robert E. Park, George Herbert Mead, Erving Goffman and Howard Becker. The final paradigm to be considered is the post-structuralist or social constructionist in which meaning and understanding are argued to be constructed through discourse.

The shift from research *on* children and young people to research *with* children and young people has a number of implications. One implication concerns the nature of the power relations between researchers, who are normally adults, and those who are researched, in this case children and young people. This topic is considered from a number of different perspectives in the second section, 'Research Relations'. In the first chapter in this section, Chapter 6, 'Power', Chris Robinson and Mary Kellett focus on power relationships between researchers and those who are researched in the minority world. They begin by examining the theoretical frameworks which have informed the concept of power, and the particular role of feminism. They explore the different ways in which children and young people may be viewed by researchers, from being seen as dependent and incompetent through to having an active participatory role in the research, and how this influences the research process as well as the power relationships. Robinson and Kellett argue that it is important to give children and young people an active participatory role in research and they provide several examples of how this can be achieved. They discuss the problems of the generation gap between adult researchers and child participants and the need for adult researchers to acknowledge the rights of children as citizens. In the final section of their chapter Robinson and Kellett consider particular questions to do with power which arise when carrying out research in schools, a point which Kellett and Ding develop further in Chapter 11.

Robinson and Kellett point out that discussion of the power relations arising in research with children and young people raises questions about ethics. This is the focus of the second chapter in this section, 'Ethics', by Priscilla Alderson. Importantly, Masson in Chapter 4 and France in Chapter 12 comment that not everything that is legal is ethical and researchers must ensure that not only are they working within the relevant legal system but that their research meets appropriate ethical standards. Alderson begins by providing the historical context for research ethics, particularly within medicine. She discusses the importance of ethics and how careful consideration of ethical issues can make a useful contribution when any piece of research is being planned. In this context she comments on a number of existing formal ethical guidelines. Throughout her chapter Alderson provides examples of how researchers can address some of the ethical questions which arise when research is carried out with children and young people, such as designing information leaflets which are appropriate for children, and watching out for indications that children and young people might prefer to withdraw from the research despite the fact that they may not express this desire verbally. She points out a number of things that researchers should avoid doing. In her conclusion Alderson returns to her earlier point that addressing ethical issues can benefit research in often surprising ways.

In both Chapter 6 and Chapter 7 reference is made to different ways in which children and young people can be involved in research and in Chapter 2 Fraser argues for the importance of this, hence 'research *with...*' rather than 'research *on...*' One way that children and young people can be involved is as active participants, which can sometimes lead to the children and young people actually carrying out the research, for example interviewing other children or young people. As Robinson and Kellett point out, when children and young people become co-researchers in a project this can be genuinely empowering. The topic of children and young people as co-researchers is the particular focus of Chapter 8, 'Involving Children and Young People as Researchers', by Adele Jones. Although this is more participatory and consequently empowering than many other approaches, Jones points out that when children and young people act as co-researchers the research is usually initiated and guided by adults. Involving children and young people as co-researchers raises additional issues, such as ensuring that the research activities and arrangements are appropriate for the child-researchers and considering the consequences for the children when they cease being researchers. Jones addresses the issues she raises by describing how children and young people can be involved as researchers at all stages of the research process from design through to dissemination. She illustrates her argument by describing three projects in which children and young people were involved at different stages: design and data collection, interpretation and finally dissemination.

The final chapter on 'Research Relations' addresses the topic of gender. In their chapter, 'Gender', Rob Pattman and Mary Jane Kehily focus on the ways in which gender, both of the researcher and the participant, can influence the form an interview takes. There is an interesting link between this chapter and Chapter 6 by Robinson and Kellett. Robinson and Kellett examine some of the questions which arise when research is based in schools, arguing that the power relations which exist in schools have specific implications, such as making it difficult for children and young people to refuse to be involved in a piece of research. Pattman and Kehily argue that the very structure of schools can directly influence the gendered development of children and young people. They make the important point that it is the participants in the research, in this case children and young people, who are the experts and therefore it is essential when carrying out research with children and young people to find ways of enabling them to share their experiences. Pattman and Kehily provide an insight into how this can be achieved, focusing on male and female interviewers talking with both boys and girls individually and together. Although Pattman and Kehily discuss the role of gender in the particular context of interviewing, it is important to remember that the genders of both researchers and the children and young people involved can influence the research process and the outcomes, whatever methodology is used.

Pattman and Kehily's chapter reminds us of the diversity of the children and young people who may take part in research and that it is essential that researchers think carefully about the suitability of their methodological approach, given the participants. Some of the implications of researching with different participant groups are the focus of the third section in this book, 'Diversity'. A number of themes recur throughout the chapters in this section. These include the contributions of different disciplines to our beliefs about the competence of children and young people and how these affect research, questions of power relations, and who should provide consent.

The first chapter in this section, 'Early Childhood', is by Ann Langston, Lesley Abbott, Vicky Lewis and Mary Kellett and considers research with children from birth to five years. Langston, Abbott, Lewis and Kellett begin by discussing how, although researchers have portrayed pre-school children as relatively incompetent in the past, this has not accorded with how these children have been viewed by the largely female workforce who care for them and they question why this has been the case. They examine the status of early childhood research in terms of who carried it out. In the remainder of their chapter they discuss a number of methodological issues which arise with this age group: who carries out the research, access, consent, the context in which the research is carried out, appropriate methods and interpreting findings. These and other issues are all important ones to consider when carrying out research with young children. Langston and her co-authors conclude by arguing that research in which early childhood practitioners and academics collaborate is crucial in order to gain as full an understanding of young children's development and lives as possible.

Langston, Abbott, Lewis and Kellett are justifiably critical of research which fails to take account of the social contexts of young children's lives. Often such research has been the domain of developmental psychologists who may study young children in unfamiliar situations using materials which may have little meaning or relevance to the children involved. This criticism is not just relevant to studies of pre-school children but is also evident in research with older children. This is the starting point for Mary Kellett and Sharon Ding's chapter, 'Middle Childhood'. After exploring the influence of developmental psychology, in particular the Piagetian account, Kellett and Ding examine some of the methodological challenges facing researchers studying children in the middle years of childhood. They discuss the nature of competence and argue that it is up to researchers to identify methodologies which enable children to demonstrate their competence. They delve into one methodology, that of interviewing, in some detail and indicate a number of aspects which any researcher planning to interview children in middle childhood should consider, including gender, a topic which is covered more fully in Chapter 9. Kellett and Ding also consider a number of non-verbal ways in which children's views can be sought effectively. They conclude by emphasising one of the themes that runs through many chapters in this book, that of enabling children and young people to participate as fully as possible in all aspects of the research process.

Chapter 12 considers 'Young People'. As the title suggests the focus is the period between being a child and becoming an adult, although as Masson points out in Chapter 4, and Alan France does in this chapter, within the UK legal system the term child includes anyone below 18 years of age. France begins by reviewing how concern with the problems often seen to be the province of young people has motivated researchers both historically and currently. France, like other contributors, also points to the relatively recent move towards research *with* as opposed to research *on* young people, and how this change in approach has led to changes in how young people are viewed. Some of the issues raised by Pattman and Kehily in their chapter are also mentioned by France, as is the importance of social context for making sense of any situation. Two issues are dealt with in some detail by France, namely consent and protection. France, like Masson, comments that the law is not always ethical, and illustrates this with respect to obtaining consent for young people to be involved in research, pointing out that how researchers go about this says something about how young people are viewed. He also raises the question of whether competence should influence decisions on who is included or excluded from research. While debating these questions France provides a number of useful pointers to ways in which the focus can be on the young people themselves providing informed consent. France then considers the second key issue of protecting young people from harm, discussing where the research takes place, the impact that the research might have on young people emotionally, protection from harm by adults and questions of confidentiality.

In Chapter 11 Kellett and Ding raise the question of competence and argue that rather than seeing children as incompetent, researchers must adopt approaches which are inclusive rather than exclusive. Interestingly, in Chapter 12, France comments that incompetence should not be a reason for exclusion from research and describes the insights he gained from including, against the advice of the teachers, a young person with learning difficulties. The issues arising in research with disabled children and young people are the focus of Chapter 13, 'Disability', by Vicky Lewis and Mary Kellett. They begin by discussing how the ways in which disabled children and young people are referred to can have implications for how they are perceived. They consider some of the issues which arise when researchers study the development of disabled children and young people, such as the heterogeneity of children and young people who are described as having the same disability, and the problem of comparison groups. They examine the implications of research with children with severe learning difficulties and provide several examples of ways in which such children have been involved successfully in research studies, pointing out that an inclusive approach increases the social validity and real world relevance of research. They argue that a reflexive and flexible approach is essential, and point out that researchers need to question assumptions of apparent incompetence. They end by raising a key question in the shift towards increased participatory research, that of whether able-bodied people should research disability.

An especially prominent theme throughout this book is of children and young people participating actively in the research process. This is brought to the fore once again in Chapter 14, 'Participatory Action Research in the Majority World' by Olga Nieuwenhuys, who describes the use of the Participatory Action Research (PAR) approach with children in the majority world. She begins by contrasting childhoods in the minority and majority worlds and points to the implications of the differences for research in the majority world. She then outlines the philosophy behind PAR and its aims of empowering those involved and of carrying out research of direct relevance to their lives. She addresses a number of questions, or dilemmas as she refers to them, which arise in PAR with children: the balance between children's active role and their dependency on adults; the role of the researcher as a facilitator while also ensuring that the children and young people participate; making sure that research findings actively benefit the children and young people involved rather than being used in ways which might not be in their best interests. She illustrates each dilemma with numerous examples from research with children and young people in the majority world.

The focus of the final chapter in this section, 'Race and Ethnicity', by Mani Maniam, Vijay Patel, Satnam Singh and Chris Robinson, is on issues of race and ethnicity in research within the British context. After clarifying some of the terms used in this area, Maniam, Patel, Singh and Robinson explore some of the issues for research by discussing different approaches to race and ethnicity since the 1960s. They begin by taking a critical look at early studies of race and ethnicity. They then explore some of the problems of the multi-cultural approach which replaced the earlier assimilationist approach. They point out that multi-culturalism failed to take issues of power into account and they examine the anti-racist approach which focused on racial oppression and questions of power. Throughout their chapter these authors refer to a range of qualitative and quantitative research methods. In their final section they examine ethnographic approaches to research into race and ethnicity. They discuss the importance of research taking account of the experiences of black and ethnic minority children and young people. Although they do not provide specific suggestions for how to carry out research in this area, by appraising different research approaches Maniam, Patel, Singh and Robinson raise a number of key issues which researchers need to take into account.

The final section in the book, 'Relevance, Evaluation and Dissemination', considers issues which arise when a particular piece of research has been completed. Three areas of research are covered: health and social care, education, and childhood. Not all research has implications for policy and practice but one area that often does is research in health and social care. In Chapter 16, 'Health and Social Care', Helen Roberts focuses on issues which arise in making sure that the voices of children and young people are heard and responded to in these fields. Roberts begins by discussing the extent to which the usefulness of research is on the agendas of the main agents influencing the dissemination of research, namely the United Nations *Convention on the Rights of the Child*, the Research Assessment Exercise within UK Universities, and the organisations who fund research. She provides a number of examples of how various factors can affect dissemination, ranging from pressure groups to researchers not believing what research participants tell them. In order to illustrate some of the questions which arise during the dissemination phase of research, Roberts describes three pieces of research and how their findings were disseminated. She then considers the important stage of evaluating the impact of research and suggests a number of factors which contribute to successful dissemination. Finally, Roberts explores how researchers can increase the likelihood of their research findings having an impact on policy and practice.

In Chapter 17, 'Education', Anne Edwards takes this further when she considers the dissemination of educational research findings. She begins by contrasting the practices of teaching and research and argues that for research to impact on practice, dissemination strategies must be thought through at the beginning of any research project rather than being left to the end. She contrasts a linear view of the relationship between educational research, policy and practice with a model in which research, policy and practice mutually interact and influence each other. In order to develop her argument for a mutually reciprocal model she explores how communities, such as early years teachers, produce and apply knowledge. She follows this through by illustrating how involving educational practitioners in the design of a research study can increase the likely benefit of the research for the end users. Thus, Edwards argues for a participatory type of research, in which the practitioners contribute to the planning and analysis of the research. However, such an approach depends on effective and ongoing communication between researchers and practitioners which extends beyond the end of the research, even to the generation of further research questions. She concludes by identifying several ways in which educational research is moving and which should inform both practice and research.

The final chapter in the book, 'Childhood Studies', by Jim McKechnie and Sandy Hobbs, examines academic research on childhood and asks whether this has had any impact on policy. They begin by taking a look back in time and examine the impact on policy and practice of John Bowlby's research on maternal deprivation. Through this historical account they emphasise the role of the context in which Bowlby was working on the impact that his research had. They then discuss different ways in which research may influence policy and practice and examine two current research areas focusing on childhood – bullying and child employment – and their rather different impacts on policy and practice. They use these two examples to illustrate a number of more general issues associated with dissemination and the effect of research: the way in which research influences policy; the need to disseminate research in a range of different ways depending on the audience; and the increasing influence of funding bodies in setting the research agenda. They end by reflecting on how research can influence policy by leading to shifts in how issues are conceptualised. As an example they discuss a theme which is evident in many of the chapters in this book, that of listening to what children and young people have to say.

As this introduction has hopefully demonstrated, the chapters in this edited collection make an important contribution to discussion and debate about research with children and young people. They cover a number of underlying themes and concerns and make a number of suggestions for how to address the issues. However, despite offering various practical suggestions, it is also clear that addressing the questions which are raised and discussed at some length by the contributors is not straightforward. There is no single solution to each question. Rather, it is up to individual researchers to reflect with great care on the many and varied issues which may arise in their research and to think creatively about ways to address them at all stages of the research process, from the initial design and choice of methodology through to dissemination.

Reference

Lewis, V., Kellett, M., Robinson, C., Fraser, S. and Ding, S. (eds) (2004) *The Reality of Research with Children and Young People*, London, Sage.

SECTION 1 SETTING THE CONTEXT

2 Situating Empirical Research
SANDY FRASER

Social and psychological researchers conduct empirical research concerning children and young people because they hope that their work will result in real and measurable benefits for children and young people. Benefit might be in terms of an explanation or understanding of children. It might also have specific benefits in particular contexts: in their relations with parents or caregivers; how they learn in schools; changes in how they are Looked After away from home or how their health could be improved. However, we should understand that the promise and delivery of these beneficial effects is based upon claims about the status of knowledge produced by research. Knowledge based on research tends to assert a significance that other forms of knowledge e.g. 'practice wisdom', 'common sense', 'intuition', etc., do not share. It is therefore important to identify and understand: What is research with children and young people? There are two aspects to this question. The first concerns the general nature of empirical research. The second aspect concerns the use of the phrase: *with* children and young people.

The first aspect concerns empirical research in general. We will not discuss the different theories, paradigms and disciplinary nature of social and psychological research. Such issues are discussed in Chapter 5. This chapter focuses on the commonalities that arise in discussing the *empirical* nature of social and psychological research. Research creates knowledge by setting questions that explore issues through actively engaging with the participants of research and other stakeholders in the research process. Often this involves setting questions which otherwise would not have been asked. We begin by giving positive illustrations of what this means. We then examine what distinguishes empirical social and psychological research from 'speculative research' and other empirically based activities. We subsequently discuss potential rival claims to significant truth – poetry, prose, drama and philosophy. The second aspect of the question concerns why we use the phrase research *with* and not *about* or *on* children and young people. We also consider the question of whether research with children and young people is different from research with adults.

What is research?

Research is discovery either because 'no one has been there before' or because someone predicts what it is like there even though no one has been there. Research can confirm or upset expectations. For example, one long-held view of social and psychological researchers has been that young children are not competent to describe or understand their own world. On occasions children have been valued and understood in terms of being 'a work in progress' towards adulthood, concerning what they might become and not who they presently are: 'children [are] often denied the right to speak for themselves either because they are held incompetent in making judgements or because they are thought of as unreliable witnesses about their own lives' (Qvortrup et al., 1994: 2). This can undermine the status of the research. If children are not listened to and if children are competent in a way that has previously been ignored, then our education and social policies will not be grounded in reality.

One example of exploratory research that maps out and 'discovers' young children is the Mosaic approach used by Alison Clark and Peter Moss of the Institute of Education at the University of London. This research 'discovers' the relatively uncharted world of young children on the assumption that young children are 'experts in their own lives' (Clark, 2004).

> Surveys and audits, questionnaires and interviews are all excellent techniques to record information, but sometimes they are not appropriate to explore the subtle and hidden feelings that connect us with a place. They do not reveal the experiences and memories of childhood and youth that contribute to creating a sense of place. (Adams and Ingham, 1998: 149)

The Mosaic approach used a number of standard research techniques, like observation and interview but in addition 2–4-year-old children participated in the research by using a disposable camera to photograph what was important to them in their nursery setting. The children were invited to take the researcher on 'tours' of the nursery, providing a 'running commentary' on their routine activities, on whom they typically met and where they met them, which rooms they had access to or not as the case might be. The children were in charge of the tour and how it was recorded: by photograph, tape recorder, drawings, etc. Not only did this process of discovery lead to tangible and immediate benefits for the children, it also led to insights at the institutional level. The research discovered the importance of the children's private spaces within the nursery as well as the need to involve the children in planning the use of external play areas.

Inclusion of and engagement with the perspectives of research participants can enhance the claims of empirical research. Such engagement may require that 'older' methods of data collection that perhaps depended on a rigid separation between 'fact' and 'value' have to be adapted to become more inclusive of children and young people. Engagement between researchers, participants and stakeholders is a crucial part of the research process.

The majority of children and young people in the world grow up in circumstances and expectations that are quite different from those of their counterparts in the European Union, Japan, the USA, and other affluent countries. South African children and young people find themselves placed between the affluence of Western European countries and the uncertainty of living in post-colonial, post-apartheid circumstances. Many adults have grown up under apartheid and their children have had to experience the prospect of sudden moves of accommodation as a result of unplanned urbanisation. Like many other people throughout the majority world, moves thought to aid progress towards greater affluence often result in poor housing or housing which is swept away. In 'Children in South Africa can make a difference', Dev Griesel, Jill Swart-Kruger and Louise Chawla report on an evaluation of an ongoing action-research project which involves 10–15-year-olds from low-income areas in 'documenting their own perspectives on the places where they live and in developing ideas for community improvements', as the following excerpt shows (Griesel et al. 2002: 83).

the project goal of child and youth participation in improving the urban environment coincides with the nation's urgent need to build a post-Apartheid civil society as well as address a legacy of poverty and housing shortages in the context of a rapidly changing urban population.

Fifteen girls and boys aged between 10 and 14 years took part in the full range of GUIC activities at [Canaansland]. Because the activities took place during a series of Saturday morning workshops, the children quickly named the sessions 'Saturday school'. In addition to making drawings of their homes and neighbourhood, answering interview questions, taking the researchers on walks to show important places in daily life, role playing, and doing group activities to identify problems, envisage a better place to live and suggest changes to improve Canaansland, the children also took part in songs and games and shared refreshments. When these activities were completed, Mayor Isaac Mogase, of the Greater Johannesburg Metropolitan Council, hosted a one-day workshop at which the children presented the results of their work to the mayor, four regional mayors, city planners, representatives of donor agencies and young members of the city's Mini and Junior Councils. Following these presentations, the members of the audience drafted action plans to respond to the children's needs and the needs of squatter families as well as to urban children in greater Johannesburg as a whole.

Distinguishing different types of research

This section attempts to demarcate 'empirical research' from other apparently similar activities and this introduces the core ideas of empirical research: that it should involve *a systematic investigation of experience*, that it should be *sceptical* and that it should be *ethical* (Robson, 2002). However, we exclude from our discussion certain types of research. For example, market research shares many of the qualities of empirical research but is distinguished by its primary purpose of obtaining information that is intended to lead to profit maximisation. The research we discuss here tends not to have the search for profit as its goal. Neither do we discuss in depth any empirical research in the disciplines of economics, politics or history.

Answering questions, discovery, creating knowledge, engaging with people – all these things can be 'research', but none of them necessarily requires methods that are exclusive to social and psychological research. For example, good journalists or barristers might similarly be involved in asking questions, discovering things, creating new knowledge and engaging with people but their knowledge is widely deemed to be different from that of a researcher. Moreover there are people who are designated as 'researchers' who might not have a full claim to that title in the sense that we want to use it. For example, we often see in the credits rolling up after a TV programme the job title of 'researcher'. In the field of politics, Members of Parliament some-times recruit staff designated as 'researchers'. Parents might 'research' which school or teaching technique is likely to be best for their child. In each of these three fields, TV, politics and parental responsibilities, the common link is that someone is finding things out – often by going to the primary empiri-cal research on the topic. And journalists, barristers or parents – whatever truths they discover – often turn to researchers to describe, understand or explain things. Therefore, we might say that there is something special about primary empirical research that gives it this status as containing a 'better sort of truth'. How did this view of empirical research emerge?

Empirical research emerged from philosophical or *speculative* research during the late Middle Ages. Initially university-based research concerned the rediscovery of ancient knowledge, e.g. the philosophies of Aristotle and Plato. Philosophical or speculative research concerned thinking about logic, morality and metaphysics (metaphysics derives from a Greek phrase mean-ing beyond or after matter, i.e. physical reality). This involved reflective speculation about the nature of the human mind, on our being and how we know things about ourselves and the world in which we live. There was a belief that by simply thinking 'logically' about things we could arrive at definite truths about the world. This idea proved unsatisfactory. Logic chopping, however useful for clarifying concepts, turned out to be quite stale and perhaps misleading. Finding things out and working out if some-thing was true or false required another element. Two of the leading pro-ponents of this new way of thinking were the Englishmen Francis Bacon (1561–1626) and John Locke (1632–1704). They proposed that empirical research was required. If research is empirical, it means that any knowledge that is derived has been developed not merely from thinking or theory but from observation or experiment which requires us to accept sensory expe-rience as valid. Empirical research can be distinguished from speculative or philosophical research because it accepts our experience of the world as a valid way of deriving new knowledge.

This leads directly to a problem. We all experience the world in different ways. We have different perspectives and we disagree about what is true in our different experiences. How do we manage to establish the truth between different and often conflicting experiences? Empirical researchers have been trying to answer this question at least since the Enlightenment. Whether or not empirical social and psychological research should be 'scientific' and whether it can be 'objective' is something that is dealt with in Chapter 5. Yet we can certainly say that empirical research should have the general qualities of being a *systematic investigation of experience*, which is *sceptical* about existing claims (made by ourselves or others) about what is true. Even commonplace assumptions, perhaps widely regarded as 'common sense', have to be treated with doubt. Every claim that something is true should be treated as requiring some sort of test to determine whether or not it is true or if apparently true then how far the claim is true. Moreover, any research activity has to be *ethical*. Ethical research involves having a regard and concern for the interests and needs of participants and those upon whom the findings of the research might have an impact. That is, in doing research we have to be frank and critical about what, how and why our research is taking place. We should make our observations accurately and clearly, whether or not such observations accord with our previous assumptions. We have to describe the circumstances in which an observation or measurement was made and who made the observation. We have to explain how children and/or young people were involved in the research and how the research process was explained to them. This is because empirical researchers should expect their methods and findings to be open to scrutiny. We should expect our claims to be doubted and examined by others (Robson, 2002).

There are different ways of systematically investigating experience. All investigations are coloured by the philosophical and theoretical predisposition of researchers, and these are directly discussed in Chapter 5. However, mention should be made here of the distinction between quantitative and qualitative research approaches. 'Quantitative research is empirical research where the data are in the form of numbers. Qualitative research is empirical research where the data are not in the form of numbers' (Punch, 1998: 4). The form that the data take is dependent upon the kind of question or hypothesis posed and the underlying research paradigm. Systematic investigation of experience need not always involve the counting of properties attached to a child or young person. It can also involve systematically understanding perceptions directly through what children and young people say, draw, sing, wear, etc. It can involve both approaches. At one time quantitative approaches in social and psychological research were completely dominant. A range of paradigms that used qualitative approaches successfully challenged this. During the latter part of the twentieth century 'either/or' debates raged but more recently there have been many examples which seek to combine qualitative and quantitative approaches. We should avoid sanctimonious-sounding prescriptions regarding 'quantitative' or 'qualitative' approaches; rather we should clarify what kind of research question or hypothesis we are posing and match the approach to the data required to answer the question.

This concern to be consistently systematic, sceptical and ethical about the observation and testing of social and psychological experience is what distinguishes empirical research from other ways of creating knowledge that a journalist, barrister, TV or political researcher might take part in. What the latter types of research have in common (quite openly at times) is that they use research in order to advocate and represent a view. They deliberately create evidence and argument to support their own existing view rather than doubting or challenging their own view. This does not mean their view or position is false but it could mean that they fail to acknowledge when their view is or might be false. A prosecutor or defence barrister summing up his or her case in a courtroom would be unlikely to seriously invite a jury to doubt the evidence he or she has just presented to them. In any evaluation of empirical research then, whenever the research appears only to follow on with its own theories or views without opening itself to scrutiny and test, then the research becomes less trustworthy. This does not mean to say that such findings are fraudulent or untrue: only that we have less means of knowing whether the findings are likely to be true.

Rivals and allies of empirical research

The results of empirical research can inform people about the lives of children and young people, and can provide this information in a way that is relevant to the services that children and young people receive. However, this information is often disputed. Empirical knowledge may allow further understanding but settles few fundamental arguments. This section further distinguishes empirical research from other forms of knowledge such as poetry and prose, religion and philosophy, which do not directly rely on an empirical element. It is suggested that other forms of knowledge may equally inform our judgement and appreciation of any given topic, including what is 'true' about children and young people. These forms of knowledge can be regarded either as alternatives or as companions to empirical research.

Poetry, prose and drama can often convey in a sentence or a mood the 'truth' of a situation that an empirical researcher would take years of tedious but very worthy research to demonstrate. Our language is replete with phrases and aphorisms from Shakespeare that express this kind of truth. For example at the outset of *A Midsummer Night's Dream*, set in Shakespeare's ancient Athens, Egeus comes to Theseus (the ruler of Athens) to complain of his daughter's choice of fiancé. Egeus enlists Theseus to persuade his daughter, Hermia, to change her mind. Theseus' clinching argument to her is: 'To you, your father should be as a god' (Act I, scene i). Shakespeare renders the truth of some kinds of relationships between father and daughter, conceivably of ancient Athens, probably of Elizabethan England and possibly of contemporary society. And this type of relationship need not only apply to daughters; it finds some reflection in the recent movie *The Road to Perdition*, in which Tom Hanks plays a father who, for his son, has a godlike quality. Poetry and prose contain many truths that are not easily verifiable or falsifiable. Books like *The Color Purple* by Alice Walker or *Empire of the Sun* by J.G. Ballard offer us accessible insight and truth about children who have been abused or maltreated which in contrast make some empirical studies of the same subject obscure and opaque. Alice Walker's *The Color Purple*, first published in 1982, tells the story of Celie, a Black woman from one of the southern states of the USA. J.G. Ballard first published *Empire of the Sun* in 1984. The novel concerns Japanese-occupied Shanghai after 1941 and follows events through the eyes of a young boy called Jim, who has until then lived with his British parents in the European Settlement area of Shanghai. We relate to this kind of 'truth' without needing to empirically verify its existence. Empathy with either Celie or Jim provides ample enough information. We might experience, understand and apply such 'truth' in a multitude of ways. We share such knowledge but there is no obvious way of accessing this knowledge on a 'level playing field'. And there is no obvious way of subjecting this 'truth' to a scepticism that is not more than a form of aesthetics. Arguably there is 'taste' but no test. Religious knowledge too can carry 'truths' which people use as either an alternative or a companion to knowledge gained by empirical research: 'Do not judge, and you will not be judged; do not condemn, and you will not be condemned; forgive, and you will be forgiven…because the standard you use will be the standard used for you' (Luke 6: 37–38).

Truth or trust can be empirically researched, but empirical research can never tell us exactly what trust is. Though it is possible to observe or measure (subject to an 'operational definition' – Punch, 1998: 47) people being 'truthful' or 'trustworthy' this might not clarify what these properties are; still more for concepts like 'informed consent'. Empirical research cannot determine what informed consent is, although it might be able to evaluate the use of different models of informed consent in practice. For example, empirical research could measure the relative impact each model has upon a child or young person. But would that kind of research be ethical? By its very nature the research would impose a differential and unpredictable impact upon the children involved. So in what way would the research participants be 'informed' when that fact would offer no protection against possible harm? In these muddy waters we must seek clarification through a return to speculative research and philosophy; we have to examine the concepts we use in order to ensure that our approach is reasoned and reasonable. The type of discussion required arose in the 2002 'Reith Lectures' given by Onora O'Neill, Principal of Newnham College, Cambridge. She has chaired the Nuffield Council on Bioethics and the Human Genetics Advisory Commission, and she is currently chair of the Nuffield

Foundation. She has been President of the Aristotelian Society, and a member of the Animal Procedures (Scientific) Committee.

Excerpt from Reith Lecture 5 (2002)
Informed Consent and Trust

Informed consent is one hallmark of trust between strangers…We give informed consent in face-to-face transactions too, though we barely notice it. We buy apples in the market, we exchange addresses with acquaintances, we sit down for a haircut. It sounds pompous to speak of these daily transactions as based on *informed consent*: yet in each we assume that the other party is neither deceiving nor coercing. We withdraw our trust *very* fast if we are sold rotten apples, or deliberately given a false address, or forcibly subjected to a Mohican haircut. So everyday trust is utterly undermined by coercion and deception.

Informed consent is supposed to guarantee individual *autonomy* or *independence*. But I think this popular thought is pretty obscure, because so many views of autonomy are in play. Some people identify *individual autonomy* with *spontaneous choosing*. A New York student of mine once decided that she would strip and streak across Broadway with a group of male students, and so convinced herself that she was *autonomous*. She had at least shown that she could act in defiance of convention, and probably of her parents, but hardly of her male contemporaries. Her eccentric choice was harmless enough, but in other cases *spontaneous choosing* can be harmful or disastrous. Other people identify individual autonomy not with *spontaneous,* but with *deliberate choosing*. But deliberate choosing doesn't guarantee that much either. The real importance of informed consent, I think, has little to do with *how* we choose. Informed consent is every bit as important when we make conventional and timid choices, or thoughtless and unreflective choices, as it is when we choose deliberately and independently. Informed consent matters simply because it shows that a transaction was not based on deception or coercion.

Informed consent is therefore always important, but it isn't the basis of trust. On the contrary, it *presupposes* and *expresses* trust, which we must already place to assess the information we're given. Should I have a proposed operation? [*Should I participate in this research*?]* Should I buy this car or that computer? Is this Internet bargain genuine? In each case I need to assess what is offered, but may be unable to judge the information for myself. Others' expert judgement may fill the gap: I may rely on the surgeon who explains the operation, or on a colleague who knows about cars or computers or Internet shopping. But in relying on others I already place trust in my adviser: as Francis Bacon noted, 'the greatest trust between man and man is the trust of giving counsel'. When we draw on friendly – or on expert – help we ultimately have to *judge for ourselves where to place our trust.* To do this we need to find trustworthy information. This can be dauntingly hard in a world of one-way communication.

*Inserted by current author

The lecture can be downloaded on portable document format from http://www.bbc.co.uk/radio4/reith2002/lecture5_text.shtml (last accessed 20.05.03)

The kind of discussion that Onora O'Neill engages in does not depend upon reference to empirical knowledge but relies on clarifying and relating concepts to each other. For example, we may think that informed consent is the basis of trust. Onora O'Neill argues against this, suggesting that informed consent presupposes trust. For the moment we need not enter into that particular debate. The point is, just like Shakespeare or *The Color Purple*, philosophy can establish a kind of truth that is different from knowledge derived from empirical research.

Empirical research *with* children and young people

We have discussed the general nature of research, albeit without discussing a more detailed philosophy of research, and we have left aside issues like 'objectivity' and 'science'. That discussion can be found in Chapter 5. But what we do need to do is to look at why this chapter, and indeed other chapters in this book, concerns research *with* children and young people as opposed to research *about* or *on* children and young people. We can be convinced by empirical research because we understand that its inquiries are systematic, sceptical and ethical. However, empirical researchers can be empirical without being 'empiricist'. The latter term applies to a philosophy that regards all ideas, theories, etc. as secondary to sensory experience. Consequently, only a dispassionate and disinterested inquiry that sets aside ideas and theories in favour of collecting 'facts' about a topic will yield significant and unbiased knowledge. Empiricism would tend to eschew one of the factors that we have cited as characteristic of research – engagement.

Engagement has different dimensions. The term 'child-centred' or 'young person-centred' can be used in different ways; for example, it could mean that the researcher – for the purposes of the research – only relates to a child in a way which the 'stages' of developmental psychology predict. This is perhaps a little unfair to developmental psychology. The point is that any theoretical framework which makes predictions and which lies outside the direct experience of the child may be imposed. Much of the recent literature on research with children and young people argues against the objectification of children that is implied by some types of developmental psychology. The work of Piaget (1896–1980) came in for significant criticism by Margaret Donaldson (1978) and others. Donaldson's work tended to show that younger children were capable of the logical reasoning that Piaget asserted occurred at a much later stage. Consequently Woodhead and Faulkner argue that Donaldson's studies 'helped developmental psychologists recognise that children's true competencies are revealed *only in situations which make sense to them*' (Woodhead and Faulkner, 2000: 24, emphasis added).

Alternatively, 'child-centred' could mean that research attempts to negotiate an understanding of research aims in a situation and in terms that 'make sense' to the children and young people concerned. The crucial equipment for any negotiation is comprehension of a range of relevant vocabulary. This is true for adults too. There is no *necessary* reason why an adult should have a more adept vocabulary for research than a child or young person. However, it is arguable that an adult will have a greater 'stock of experience' to draw upon which could provide relevant conceptions for empirical research – but this is not an issue of cognitive stage. And it is possible that some children or young people will have had a more diverse stock of experiences and a greater facility with different languages than some adults.

I take 'make sense' to mean that a child or young person must have a vocabulary and conceptions that are capable of relating to the context of a researcher's concerns. Equally, a researcher must have a vocabulary and conceptions that relate to the child's conception of their world. Such vocabularies and conceptions emerge *in situ with* the child or young person and need to be negotiated with as few preconceptions as possible. Researchers may lack specific knowledge of the concepts used by children and young people. Neither the child's nor the researcher's lack of vocabulary implies a lack in reasoning powers. It may well be predictable that by virtue of extent of experience a young child's vocabulary is different from that of a 15-year-old or of a 43-year-old researcher. Crucially the nature of vocabulary is a function of culture, not 'age or stage' (Dunn, 1988: 189).

> The child does not enter the life of his or her group as a private and autistic sport of primary process, but rather as a participant in a larger public process in which public meanings are negotiated. (Bruner, 1990: 13)

Negotiation may lead to particular types of 'child-friendly' data collection methods: drawings, photography, diaries, and other innovative techniques that have not yet been conceived. These methods are not 'friendly' because they are relevant to developmental stage but because they have been negotiated between the researcher and the researched. Their reliability and validity as methods will be related to the degree of shared understanding of the aims of research. This implies something else: the way in which research can be negotiated with children and young people will differ according to habits and mores which the child or young person has learned. Moreover this involves a degree of acceptance of the power relationships to which the child or young person is already subject. Necessarily this means there will be great diversity in negotiated research relationships – a quality also found in research with adults because, like 'adults', 'children and young people' are not a homogeneous mass. Like adults, children and young people are diverse in their competencies. Their competencies or lack of them may not necessarily imply a definite generalised cognitive 'stage'. This means that on occasion children and young people could well be 'equal partners' in all parts of the research process; arguably there is no 'developmental' reason why this cannot occur. Yet negotiating the 'research space' on the basis of a shared vocabulary might be practically difficult to do.

Part of the practical difficulties may involve the political context; i.e. the network of power relationships that a child or young person is already part of before any research begins. This can be in terms of the pattern of peer relations, family relationships or institutional relationships for example being in school, etc. Moreover, the research may concern children and young people but it would be unusual if they were the only stakeholders involved. This may restrain a researcher's ambition to achieve equal partnership. Yet children and young people can never be the sole voice that is heard within any piece of research; other stakeholders should have a voice too.

Research with children and young people is therefore different from research with adults but not necessarily because of any inherent cognitive deficit of children as compared to adults. Samantha Punch (2002) argues that there are clear differences between research with children and young people as compared to research with adults. She suggests that in the critique of developmental psychology by the new sociology of childhood: 'There has been a tendency to perceive research with children as one of two extremes: just the same or entirely different from adults.' Elsewhere she notes:

> It is somewhat paradoxical that within the new sociology of childhood many of those who call for the use of innovative or adapted research techniques with children, are also those who emphasise the competence of children. If children are competent social actors, why are special 'child-friendly' methods needed to communicate with them? (Punch, 2002: 322 and 321)

My answer to Punch's question is that 'child-friendly' methods are negotiated compromises that allow communication between the different conceptual outlooks of children and young people on the one hand, and those of researchers on the other. Child-friendly data collection techniques have no permanent 'objective' status because they will be used and understood differently according to context. There is nothing inherently or essentially 'child-friendly' about such techniques; they are all contingent to the frames of cultural reference of researchers and participants. Such techniques are 'participant-friendly' rather than 'child-friendly'.

Finally, there is a context in which research can be *about* children and young people with no necessary loss of credibility. There can be research about services for children and young people that does not directly involve children and young people; e.g. comparing different systems of financial accounting of school budgets; studying management structures of social services teams that make assessments of need; making comparisons of the numbers of health visitors and midwives in rural areas of the United Kingdom. Research in these areas genuinely relates to childhood and youth but does not directly involve research with children and young people.

Concluding remarks

In this chapter we have looked at two aspects of research with children and young people. What is *research* with children and young people? And, what is research *with* children and young people? Both have simple and complex answers. Firstly, research can help us to understand childhood and children, it can show us how in various contexts their experiences can be enriched and strengthened. However, for this to be done we must understand what research is and what it is not and what research can and cannot do. Empirical research can provide information to help us answer fundamental questions but not solve them. The heightened standing of empirical research has to be based upon a rigorous use of a method of systematic inquiry that is open to scrutiny and is ethical. We have also come to understand that a positive engagement with children and young people is not only desirable it is also necessary to improve the credibility of the knowledge we derive from research.

References

Adams, E. and Ingham, S. (1998) *Changing places: Children's Participation in Environmental Planning*, London, Children's Society.

Bacon, Francis (2002) *Essays XX, Of Counsel*, Oxford, Oxford University Press. First published 1625. Bacon's essays are downloadable from http://www.shu.ac.uk/emls/iemls/resour/mirrors/rbear/bacon.html

Ballard, J.G. (1994) *Empire of the Sun*, London, Flamingo. First published 1984.

Bruner, J. (1990) *Acts of Meaning*, Cambridge, MA: Harvard University Press.

Clark, A. (2001) 'How to listen to very young children: the Mosaic approach', *Child Care in Practice*, 7(4): 333–341.

Clark, A. (2004) 'The Mosaic Approach and research with young children', in Vicky Lewis, Mary Kellett, Christine Robinson, Sandy Fraser and Sharon Ding (eds) *The Reality of Research with Children and Young People*, London, Sage.

Donaldson, M. (1978) *Children's Minds*, London, Fontana.

Dunn, J. (1988) *The Beginnings of Social Understanding*, Oxford, Blackwell.

Griesel, R.D., Swart-Kruger, Jill and Chawla, Louise (2002) 'Children in South Africa can make a difference: an Assessment of Growing Up in Cities in Johannesburg', *Childhood*, 9(1). [Also in Lewis et al. (2004) *The Reality of Research with Children and Young People*, London, Sage, the companion volume to the present book.

Punch, K.F. (1998) *Introduction to Social Research: Quantitative and Qualitative Approaches*, London, Sage.

Punch, S. (2002) 'Research with children: the same or different from research with adults?' *Childhood*, 9(3): 321–341.

Qvortrup, J., Bardy, M., Sgritta, G. and Wintersberger, H. (eds) (1994) *Childhood Matters*, Vienna, Europe Centre.

Robson, C. (2002) *Real World Research*, Oxford, Blackwell.

Takei, W. (2001) 'How do deaf infants attain first signs?' *Developmental Science*, 4(1): 71–78.

Walker, A. (2001) *The Color Purple*, London, The Women's Press. First published 1982.

Woodhead, M. and Faulkner, D. (2000) '*Subjects, objects or participants? Dilemmas of psychological research with children*', in P. Christensen and A. James (eds), *Research with Children: Perspectives and Practices*, London, Routledge Falmer.

3 Images of Childhood
MARY KELLETT, CHRIS ROBINSON AND RACHEL BURR

Was there ever a time when the concept of childhood did not exist? Do children have an exclusive identity or is this merely subsumed within adult apprenticeship? Can children ever just 'be' or are they always in a state of 'becoming'? These are some of the questions that have shaped images of childhood over time, constructed from a variety of conceptions and assumptions about what it is to be a child. In this chapter we outline how some of these images have come about and how they vary within socio-cultural groups and across historical and disciplinary perspectives. We examine disparate images informed by religion, culture, politics, economics and the media and explore the impact these have on the approach to research with children and young people. The aim of this chapter is to introduce and overview these issues and therefore it is not possible to cover these topics in detail. We refer interested readers to the cited references and signposts to other chapters in this book where some of the topics are addressed more fully.

Historical overview

There are many excellent texts that chart the history of childhood and it is not our intention to reproduce such chronologies here (see e.g. Heywood, 2001). However, since history has had a significant part to play in the construction of childhood images it is appropriate to acknowledge these principal sources of influence at the outset.

How far back we go in history to find the first conceptualisation of childhood has been a matter of some debate. One of the most well known and most debated writers on childhood was the French historian Ariès. In his book *Centuries of Childhood* (1962) he claimed that the Middle Ages had no understanding of the child as anything other than an 'adult in waiting' and that there was no perception of a transitional period between infancy and adulthood. Using images of children from this historical period as the basis of his work he argued that, once weaned, children were in effect adults. In his opinion it was not until the fifteenth century onwards that children were gradually separated from adult life, a process culminating in entry into education outside the home in the late nineteenth century. Ariès' work fuelled lengthy debates about whether the medieval period really did have any appreciation of childhood, about when childhood was 'discovered' and about the nature of parent–child relations. Cunningham (1991) points to medical treatises on the subject of childhood diseases and Shahar (1990) to literature where childhood is divided into 'sub-periods' as evidence to refute Ariès' claims. Pollock (1983) studied extensive primary sources between 1500 and 1900 and concluded that even if children were regarded differently from present times they could still have been regarded as children. Ariès has also been criticised for an overemphasis on middle- and upper-class children, taking no account of the importance of social class and gender in determining the nature of childhood. Nevertheless, his work did challenge the notion of childhood as universal for all societies in all times in history. He showed how conceptions of childhood change and are rooted in their own times and cultures. Childhood continues to be robustly debated. Today, in our own 'period of history', some are suggesting that children are growing up more quickly and childhood as a separate entity is again diminishing.

There is more of a consensus amongst historians that the origins of a recognised 'theoretical' conceptualisation of childhood are generally attributed to the early seventeenth century (Hendrick, 1997). This more theoretically oriented discourse on childhood originated in religious thinking of this time, when images of childhood came to be dominated by Puritan dogma. It was epitomised by the belief that children were innately evil, born with 'original sin' that must be purged from them. The Puritans maintained that children could only be enlightened through education, strict discipline and control. Sayings such as 'spare the rod and spoil the child' and 'only fire can straighten crooked wood' originate from this time and aptly illustrate the harsh images that prevailed.

Later in the seventeenth century John Locke (1632–1704) challenged the idea that children were innately evil, or innately anything for that matter, arguing they were merely a product of their environment. He posited the image of the child as 'a blank slate' capable of being shaped by environment and experiences. With the right environment and education this blank slate child could become a responsible adult. Developing logic and reasoning were key elements of this process. He recognised that children had specific needs of their own but the emphasis was still on the importance of 'becoming' rather than 'being'.

By the eighteenth century secular discourse had replaced religious dogma. Instead of 'evil' children who must be saved from corruption and moulded into responsible adults came a new notion of childhood innocence. Children were born pure and naturally good and any wrongdoing could be attributed to the corrupting influence of adult society. One of the principal proponents of this discourse was Jean-Jacques Rousseau. In his book, *Emile, or On Education* (1762) he expounded his theories on how he thought children should be educated. He argued that they needed a natural environment where they could develop at their own pace. Rousseau's construction fostered an idyllic image of childhood. Children were commonly portrayed in angelic garb surrounded by the beauties of Nature. Poets exalted their natural wisdom and spiritual vision. Becoming adult represented a process of steady decline from innocence to corruption.

By the beginning of the nineteenth century this idealised, romantic construction of childhood was solidly rooted amongst wealthy middle class families with a consensus that childhood was something to be enjoyed and protected. It was a different picture for poorer, working class families where children as young as five might be put to work on the street or in factories. Harsh economic reality put paid to any notions of childhood innocence or the preservation of a special child identity. With industrialisation, women and children could now undertake work that had previously required the strength of an adult male. Indeed, some of the early spinning machines in cotton factories were designed to suit the smaller fingers – and cheaper wages – of children. In this social sphere children were an important economic commodity and the survival of many families depended on them. Such conditions did not favour the spread of idealised images of childhood. 'Childhood', as we understand it in modern terms, was delayed for the poorer classes until social reforms later in the century began to have a real impact on the lives of children. The 1842 Mines Act, which banned employment of those under 10, significantly reduced the number of young working children. The introduction of half-time working for school age children in the 1844 Factory Act caused numbers to dwindle further and to all but disappear when compulsory schooling became a reality in 1880.

Urbanisation brought large numbers of children together in classrooms, playgrounds and after-school associations. Childrearing was glorified as a mother's most important occupation. Published child observation studies became very popular with mothers, educators and welfare workers who were motivated by the belief that their teaching and parenting would be more effective if it were geared to the child's level of development. The American psychologist, Stanley Hall actively campaigned for the establishment of child study associations, convinced that scientific child study was the only rational basis for work with children and that teachers and parents should be introduced to the facts of development through first hand study of the child. The child study movement spread rapidly and soon had an international network of training centres and journals (see Donzelot, 1977).

Extensive social reform and subsequent child labour legislation brought significant changes in the construction of modern childhood. Children were no longer important in the workplace. Zelizer (1985) argued that childhood assumed an 'economically worthless' but 'emotionally priceless' image. She claimed that by the second half of the nineteenth century most urban middle classes had accepted this view of childhood although poorer, working class families continued to rely on whatever wages children could earn until legislation and compulsory schooling finally put an end to this in the first part of the twentieth century. It prompted a 'sacralization' of childhood (Heywood, 2001) among some American reformers, who asserted that to profit from children's labour was a profanity. This led to a more sentimental attitude towards children being adopted. In the aftermath of the First World War there was a reappraisal of childhood and its importance. Children were now seen as the 'future of the nation', as valuable commodities to be emotionally prized and preserved at all costs. They had a singular identity with physical, mental and emotional needs to be satisfied. Research began to focus on improving the health and welfare of children and enhancing their mental prowess. This era of preserving and protecting children harvested research in areas of nutrition, health and preventative medicine such as childhood vaccination. This had many positive benefits, including a measurable fall in the rate of infant mortality. Comparative studies of children's physical well-being and mortality rates also exposed inequalities amongst the different social class structures and heralded a new wave of research spearheaded by politicians and welfare reformers.

The rise of the Welfare State brought with it an increasing interference in the childrearing practices of the nation. Reformers tried to impose middle class values on working class families, eschewing many of their more flexible, traditional practices in favour of rigid rules such as advice on breast-feeding on demand that took no account of mothers who needed to work. The number of child guidance clinics grew rapidly and with it a new impetus for childhood research.

> The significance of the clinics was that they took 'nervous', 'maladjusted' and delinquent children and 'treated' them, producing as they did a new perspective on the nature of childhood. (Hendrick, 1997: 53)

The twentieth-century school was an important focal point for this research. Previously children (apart from those of the upper classes) had been educated through apprenticeships and charity schools and parents had managed to retain a modicum of control and influence. For the majority of children control passed into the hands of the state, which seized the moral and spiritual high ground. Local authorities decided what was taught, how it was taught and for how long. With the emphasis on educational reform, research started to focus on child development. Compulsory schooling presented new opportunities for the study of childhood with ready-made, convenient samples of participants. Thus the first half of the twentieth century witnessed a mushrooming of child research dominated by developmental psychologists. It is these influences that we turn to next.

Influences of developmental psychology

Early developmental psychology fostered images of the child as an incomplete, malleable organism developing differently in response to different stimuli. 'The child is portrayed, like the laboratory rat, as being at the mercy of external stimuli: passive and conforming' (James and Prout, 1997: 13). Childhood was once again viewed in terms of a preparation for adulthood but now it was 'theorised' and divided into age-graded developmental stages. Schools and nurseries provided ideal opportunities to observe large numbers of children of the same age at the same time and under 'controlled' conditions. This made it possible to analyse average ability and arrive at standard definitions of what constituted 'normal'. One of the tools for establishing what was 'normal' was the intelligence test. Psychologists produced a range of different tests for measuring mental processes. This led to the 'labelling' of children and segregation according to their IQ. Whilst research of this nature added to the body of knowledge about cognitive development it also produced some negative outcomes, particularly for those children who were assigned to 'mentally defective institutions' on the basis of their IQ scores. Furthermore, researchers such as Louis Terman (1877–1956) (who regarded IQ as genetically and racially determined) opened the door to abusive practices of eugenic social control and the promotion of the image of the white child as superior.

Jean Piaget's (1896–1980)work has been pivotal within developmental psychology (also see Chapters 7 and 11 for discussions of Piaget). His work outlined clearly defined stages of cognitive growth from the *sensory-motor* stage of infancy through *pre-conceptual*, *intuitive* and *concrete* to the *formal operations* of adolescence and adulthood. Movement from one stage to the next was argued to be dependent on achievement of a specific 'schema' of physical and mental actions and a gradual process of 'de-centring'. He maintained that all normally developing children pass through these stages, if not at the same rate, then certainly in the same sequence.

However, much of Piaget's work has been misunderstood and there is often a failure to credit him with emphasising a child's active role in his or her cognitive development, as Woodhead and Faulkner (2000: 23) point out.

What such critiques fail to acknowledge is that Piaget had a deep respect for children. He listened to them closely and did not belittle their explanations as examples of inferior (non-adult) ways of thinking.

The hierarchical continuum that is implied in the linear nature of developmentalism (infant sensory-motor intelligence at the lowest end and adult formal operative intelligence at the highest) is open to criticism. If mature, rational adult thought is judged to be the ultimate, highly prized goal then the corollary is that child thought can have little intrinsic value, hence notions of childhood as separate and special must necessarily be devalued along with the integrity of the child. A paradox exists here. More and more child research was being undertaken which implied there was more and more interest in children and childhood, but the focus of this new research was increasingly oriented to cognitive development and the process of 'becoming adult'.

Another powerful critique of developmentalism was that it took no account of socio-cultural differences (Richards and Light, 1986; Burman, 1994a;

Woodhead, 1999). Lev Vygotsky (1896–1934) is credited with first premising a social constructivist model and its emphasis on the socially interactive nature of learning. The social constructivist standpoint is to dispense with assumptions about social structures that define childhood and go back to original consciousness in order to show how it has built up. Within a socially constructed world, therefore, there are no constraints and childhood is not viewed in any precise, identifiable form (for a more detailed exposition of the social constructivist position see James, Jenks and Prout, 1998).

Influences of anthropology

Anthropology emerged as a discipline because of a desire to understand other people's social processes. Its origins date from the end of the nineteenth century, a period when interest focused on discovering, and in some cases conquering, unfamiliar corners of the globe. Bronislaw Malinowski (1884–1942) is regarded as a founder of the discipline and the first researcher to establish 'ethnographic research', which entails the researcher being immersed in fieldwork living among the subjects of his or her research for an extended period of at least a year but often for longer. This approach, which involves taking part in their daily lives, often learning their language and practising their customs, is termed 'participant observation'. While completing this type of research anthropologists may keep diaries, use video to record what they observe and do extended interviews among members of the community.

Traditional anthropology has been criticised for rarely examining children in their own right. In the 1920s Margaret Mead was among the first anthropologists to complete work on children. Her ethnographic studies, *Coming of Age in Samoa* (1928) and *Growing up in New Guinea* (1930) give us insight into the lifestyles of Samoan and New Guinea children and young people. However, her interest was prompted not by a desire to understand local children so much as to finalise the running debate over whether nature or nurture determined human behaviour. She set out to discover whether biology or socialisation shaped adolescent behaviour but has since been criticised for using as her theoretical base Western developmental theory.

Later anthropologists shifted away from using Western theory about childhood as a starting point for learning about the lives of children in other societies. In the 1950s Jean Briggs (1970) lived among the Inuit people of Qipsia on Baffin Island in the Arctic. Her ethnography questioned the relevance of Western developmental theory outside the West. She found that children behaved and were treated differently because of environmental factors. For example, she describes her distress at seeing a three-year-old girl sobbing and being left without comfort once her younger sibling was born.

It seemed that overnight she was expected to defer to the needs of the baby. As a result she learned not to cry, but to withdraw into herself silently when she became upset: in this way silence rather than crying was an indication of distress among children just out of babyhood. This ethnography demonstrates that culture shapes behaviour. As the anthropologist Jean La Fontaine (1986) argues: 'The immaturity of children is a biological fact of life but the way in which this immaturity is understood and made meaningful is a fact of culture' (quoted in James and Prout, 1990: 7).

Anthropological research has led the field in questioning many of the dominant Western-led ideas about childhood, in which childhood is seen as a period of preparation and socialisation. Anthropologists' approach differs from that of sociologists in a number of respects: first the fieldwork process is wedded to participant observation and secondly anthropologists have a tradition of examining the lives of children outside their own culture. Most significantly, anthropologists do not assume children have an individual sense of the self. It is the autonomous self that is at the heart of Western thinking and because both psychology and sociology are grounded in Western philosophy it is the child as the individual self that informs both disciplines. Anthropologists' ethnographic findings from around the world remind us that this view of childhood is a minority viewpoint. Their ethnographies show us that in many parts of the world people consider the greater collective of the family above and beyond the rights of each individual. Findings such as these raise questions for contemporary anthropologists about the extent to which the child rights movement – which is grounded in Western ideas about giving individual children rights rather than treating the child as part of a larger collective – can be universally applicable.

Influences of sociology

The influence of sociological thinking to our understanding of childhood is complex and cannot be encompassed within this short section, but we will be able to glimpse some core themes relating to research with children and young people which are developed elsewhere within this book. Sociology has been preoccupied with power relations in society and in questioning the taken for granted ways in which roles and relationships within societies are understood. Sociology by its very subject matter raises political and ethical issues. In its 200-year existence it has developed a wide range of theoretical approaches from those that consider the economic and social structure of whole societies to approaches which study the minutiae of day to day interactions between people (Giddens, 1995). Despite a substantial focus on the 'family', and within the feminist tradition on the roles of women, children in their own right have remained largely invisible until recently. Sociological approaches to crime and deviance have been concerned with teenagers. Standard texts on introductory sociology often do not have a separate section devoted to children or childhood.

The study of the sociology of childhood as a distinct topic has grown and developed. A number of approaches contributed to this development, for example the work of Denzin (1977) who reacted against the structuralist perspective in his development of alternative approaches to the concept of socialisation. Denzin's work was concerned to examine how participants socially construct meanings and, together with other trends in reviewing the historical development of childhood discussed earlier, a new paradigm for understanding childhood began to emerge. James and Prout (1997: 4) noted that:

> The traditional consignment of childhood to the margins of social sciences...is beginning to change...it is now much more common to find acknowledgement that childhood should be regarded as part of society and culture rather than a precursor to it; and that children should be seen as already social actors not beings in the process of becoming such.

James, Jenks and Prout (1998) introduced the notion of 'presociological' and 'sociological' models of childhood.

Frones, Jensen and Solberg (1990) have warned against the collectivisation of childhood, stressing the importance of divisions of race, gender, class, disability and religion. As we have seen already, much research into the lives and behaviour of children in the twentieth century has been undertaken within the parameters of psychology. In the late 1960s the impact of the sociological interpretivists led to criticisms of the individualism of the approach and this led to calls for greater recognition of the social construction and social context of childhood (Prout and James, 2000: 15). The work of Prout and James has been significant in influencing the direction of research with children and young people and is recognised elsewhere in this book.

Another important image that sociologists bring to the table is that of children as social actors with an active role in the construction and determination of their own social lives. This widening of the scope of childhood to a societal level is spawning an interest in research that gives voice to an agenda of children's rights and to an increased focus on childhood as a social category and children as a distinct population group. This has led to developments relating to the ways in which children should be involved in research, with a growing recognition of the value of ethnography and a resulting convergence of sociology and anthropology in the grounded study of childhood.

Contemporary images of childhood

A contemporary view of childhood acknowledges that it is both biological and social. There are complexities inherent in this image. For example the cultural differences that abound with regard to how much physical work children are expected to do may conflict with biological acceptance of children as physically smaller and weaker than adults. At what point does the biological argument persuade us that the cultural practice may be exploitative? This brings us to a consideration of some of the dominant images of contemporary childhood – those rooted in civil rights set out by the United Nations *Convention on the Rights of the Child* (1989) and adopted by all countries except Somalia and the USA (although the USA has signed up to some of the clauses relating to child labour). Whatever the complexities and controversies of this document it signals that a clear, discursive space has been delineated for children. They have an autonomy that exists outside family, school and institutions and a voice conditioned neither by competence nor chronological age.

It is worth reflecting at this point on whether contemporary discourse is moving towards a global image. Minority world images of childhood as a special time of innocence and of children as individuals with rights and needs who must be protected from the harshness of the adult world are being persuasively propelled into the majority world. To this end there have been many interventions by global institutions and charities, particularly in relation to child labour issues and other so-called 'oppressive' practices. Such interventions, whilst well intentioned, are frequently counterproductive. It is well documented (Burman, 1994b) that when pressure is exerted to end exploitative (as perceived through minority world eyes) child labour markets the result often leads to child labour going underground and children engaging in even more hazardous occupations to avoid destitution.

Influences of economics

Child labour is often seen as an emotive topic: the mention of the term may conjure up images of small children making carpets for 14 hours a day in India. Considering the involvement of children within the labour market of their society can contribute to our understanding of the ways in which children are perceived and how that perception can impact upon their needs for care and protection. The involvement of children in the economy of their society, especially when it is in the public sphere of the street, can contribute to their marginalisation and victimisation. There is a literature on street children in Brazil being routinely murdered by the police: in 1994 the *Guardian* newspaper reported that between 1988 and 1991 an estimated 5,000 children were murdered on the streets of Brazil. There is a stark contrast with the public outcry and concern about the death of children in Western society, for example the murder of 16 children and their teacher in Dunblane in Scotland in 1996 led to worldwide media coverage and the changing of the gun laws in the United Kingdom.

Children's participation in the economy is common throughout the world but takes different forms and is portrayed in different ways. Much child 'labour' is hidden, particularly that undertaken in the home and often by girls. Labour by boys features much more frequently in the public sphere of life, whether in Belfast (Leonard, 1999) or Bogota (Connolly, 1990). However, there are also differences between rural and urban children's experience of labour. Examining child labour also enhances our under-standing of the position of children within their society, by serving to illus-trate the control of social space. Access and control of space is greater for males than females and increases with age (Katz and Monk, 1993). Katz in her study of children in rural Sudan found that labour outside the home enabled boys to have greater control and access to social space than girls of the same age.

There is growing evidence from research that the majority of British children have some experience of working before they leave school (Leonard, 1999). Hobbs and McKechnie (1997) found that children's involvement in work increases as they grow older. Research undertaken in majority world countries has for some years examined the role of children in the economy of their societies, for example work on street children. Most academic work on street children has originated in South America; for example, Agnelli, 1986; Connolly, 1990; Glauser, 1990 and Lusk, Peralta and Vest, 1989.

In many affluent societies children work for spending money; in poorer countries they work for the survival of themselves and/or their families. The impact of working on children is an under-researched area but the research which has been done indicates that children who work are at greater risk of harm wherever they may be in the world. In Britain, Hobbs and McKechnie (1997) found that children who worked were more prone to accidents and Leonard (1999: 198) also found in her research that one in four children who worked had experienced an accident. The figure rose to one in two for children who delivered newspapers.

Despite similar themes relating to child labour between the minority and majority worlds, there are major differences in their image, which has sig-nificant implications for their care and protection. Most street children are between 10 and 14 years. As they become older they are able to take on other tasks and when begging are less attractive. 'When street children reach puberty, they become street people' (Aptekar, 1989: 793). The age profile of street children is a function of the demands of their existence. UNICEF (1995) found that the average age 'of street life' is 11 years of age.

Another area in which children and young people are part of the eco-nomic life of their country is through being 'carers'. The concept of 'carer' is still alien to most of the majority world where it is often taken for granted that care will be provided from within the family and that children will play a part from an early age. Majority world children who care for others in their families do not have the image of being gallant and courageous but merely that of leading their daily lives. In the minority world the concept of being a 'carer' and thereby relieving the state of the cost of care of an older or disabled relative is quite recent, and together with its development has come the recognition of young carers, who are frequently portrayed as 'heroic' and selfless. Research with young carers (e.g. Grady, 2001) found that many young people disliked this image and felt it isolated them from their peers; however, the media persistently regards them as 'children of courage' to be treated as separate from children and young people who lead 'ordinary lives'.

Influences of advertising and the media

It is difficult to escape the influence of advertising in contemporary Western society with the prevalence of television, magazine culture and the Internet. Advertisements commonly portray children in adult garb and adult poses – sometimes pseudo-sexual. Toy manufacturers bombard young children with cosmetic kits and beauty sets that transcend the 'dressing up' world of children. Conventional notions of childhood such as innocence and purity are juxtaposed with adult commercial products in order to sell them. Such has been the influence of advertising that it has led to claims that childhood as a separate entity is disappearing (Postman, 1983). The boundaries between childhood and adulthood are becoming increasingly blurred.

> These new forms of media are now systematically undermining that distinction between child and adult due to an indifference to difference...a child subject to a diet of violence, sexuality, exploitation and a persistent invitation to consume cannot sustain an autonomous realm of being. Thus the new media conveys and creates the message that childhood is no more. (Jenks, 1996: 117)

Advertisements frequently adopt stereotypical images of children to promote their products. How often is the 'intelligent child' portrayed as white, bespectacled and middle class? Gender stereotyping is also commonplace. Adverts for the latest designer football boots are unlikely to be fronted by a girl, and however amazing the new look-a-like baby doll might be there will be no boy cooing lovingly over it. The inclusion of children from minority ethnic communities in advertising is increasing, but disabled children are very rarely used in advertising, which tends to have an underlying discourse of 'perfection'. Clothing for children is now big business in richer countries and children may be concerned about their own image as fashionable and up to date. Bondine has suggested that 'children's clothing serves as a screen on which are projected all kinds of beliefs and aspirations about children' (2003: 46).

Not all advertisements aim to sell a product. Some target our conscience and our emotions. Pictures in the media that portray children of the majority world in harrowing poses with skeletal frames and fly-infested, lethargic bodies are intended to arouse our emotions and tweak our consciences so that we dig deep into our pockets. Well-intentioned as they may be, such images reinforce stereotypical expectations that majority world people are poor, helpless and incompetent. It suggests that they cannot care for their own children and that the only solution to their problem is money to 'buy' them a childhood closer to the minority world model.

Influences of language

Language use has had a powerful influence on childhood imagery. Over the centuries pithy sayings have been coined that mirrored prevailing images of the time. Sometimes termed 'proverbs', they provide a linguistic kaleido-scope of childhood images that have successfully migrated across global, cultural and historical boundaries. Like musical jingles and advertising slogans, they 'fix' an impression in our minds. Some examples below illus-trate how these may, at different times, endorse, refute and ridicule many of the images already described in this chapter.

> An inch of a lad is better than a foot of a girl
>
> There is no light in the house where there are no children
>
> Blood is thicker than water
>
> Eagles do not breed doves
>
> Many a good cow has an evil calf
>
> The child who is always led will never walk alone
>
> He that does not beat his own child will later beat his own breast
>
> Soft wax will take any impression
>
> (abridged from Palacios, 1996)

Cultural diversity and different parenting practices produce choices of language that evoke contrasting images of childhood. For example words like 'assertive' and 'spirited' to describe girls are viewed favourably by parents in some cultures but not in other cultures. In the Indian sub-continent, for example, parents of girls are likely to favour terms such as 'modest' and 'hospitable' (Harkness, 1996: 43).

There are a plethora of terms used to describe children in different circumstances. They can be minors, pupils, patients, subjects, infants, babies, toddlers, kids, juniors, seniors, teenagers, adolescents, young people and no doubt a host of other things too. And within each of these categories exists a myriad of depersonalising labels that repackage them further and serve to reinforce adult control over their place in society. Educational labels such as PMLD (Profound and Multiple Learning Difficulties) and medical labels from only a generation ago such as 'idiot', 'imbecile' and 'mental defective' create images that spotlight membership of abnormal categories ahead of membership of childhood. These issues are discussed further in Chapter 13.

Influences of religion, politics and culture

> The caretakers of young children of all societies do have goals that are universal (e.g. protection, socialisation), there are societal differences in the behaviors of caretakers that are related to the community's ecology, basic economy, social organisation, and value systems. (Whiting and Edwards, 1988: 8)

The meanings of religion, politics and culture are themselves complex. Culture and race are often used synonymously but there is an important conceptual distinction (Owusu-Bempah and Howitt, 2000: 85). Phinney (1996: 167) describes ethnicity as 'a multidimensional construct consisting of cultural norms and values…and the experiences and attitudes associated with a given group'.

There are debates in the literature (e.g. Markus and Kitayama, 1991) about the classification of cultures in terms of whether they are group or individually oriented.

Owusu-Bempah and Howitt (2000) have argued that generally speaking Western cultures are individualist whereas most other cultures are collectivist. However, they go on to suggest that it is more helpful to avoid dichotomising cultures and see cultures as occupying a place along a continuum between autonomy and interdependence. This notion can help us in thinking about research with children and young people.

Research into the religious beliefs of children is a sensitive topic. Renezetti and Lee (1993) discuss sensitive areas in research generally and identify religion as an area potentially sacred to those being studied. Geaves (1998) has pointed out that the concept of religion is not straightforward: children may have parents with different religions and there are many variations in the way religious beliefs are expressed.

Researching children's views and experience of religion can help to challenge critically stereotypes of their experience, e.g. child brides, arranged marriages, and ways in which they may discriminate against other children from a different religious group. There are complex relationships therefore between the impact of religion, politics and culture on the images of children. They have been seen as needing control, understanding and care but, as discussed earlier, there are worldwide differences in the images of children relating to the economic and political context in which they are living. We find many paradoxes when we begin to examine the images of children: they can be innocent choir boys and girls pictured on the front of a CD cover in one context, aggressive beggars in another society who are moved on and in some contexts exterminated by the local police. The children's rights movement has flourished since the Second World War, but its implementation around the world has been patchy. Images of children as a threat to adult values and order is a powerful factor in how societies respond to their poorest children. Hendrick (1997) wrote persuasively about images that delineate the child as threat and the child as victim.

Implications and future directions of child research

Images such as children as victims, consumers, active agents in their societies, young criminals and threats to established order have impacted upon research into their lives in different ways. Some research, e.g. that of Griesel et al. (2004), specifically sets out to measure how children can be empowered to bring about change in their own communities. The child as a 'consumer' has led increasingly to research which talks and listens directly to children and young people, involving them in the process. For example in the majority world the Child to Child movement sees children as active promoters not just the receivers of health. One of the most comprehensive evaluations, by the Aga Khan Foundation in India, found that the programme was effective in bringing positive health messages to children (Pridmore and Stevens, 2000).

How will images and constructs of childhood affect the future directions of child research? Will the increasing focus on children as social actors and capable agents foster more research by children themselves? Will children, as a distinct population group, armed with a rights agenda, succeed in carving out a niche for themselves in adult-centred social research where their contributions have traditionally been ignored? If 'childhood is the life-space which our culture limits it to be' (Qvortrup et al., 1994: 3), then perhaps future images of childhood will be fashioned from emancipatory rhetoric that challenges the extent of those limits.

References

Agnelli, S. (1986) *Street Children: A Growing Urban Tragedy*, London, Weidenfeld and Nicolson.

Aptekar, L. (1989) 'Colombian street children: gamines and chupagruesos', *Adolescence*, 24(96): 783–794.

Aptekar, L. and Behailu, A. (1997) 'Conflict in the neighbourhood: street and working children in public space,' *Childhood*, 4(4): 447–490.

Ariès, P. (1962) *Centuries of Childhood*, London, Cape.

Bondine, A. (2003) 'School uniforms and discourse of childhood', *Childhood*, 10: 43–60.

Briggs, J.L. (1970) *Never in Anger: Portrait of an Eskimo Family*, Cambridge, MA, Harvard University Press.

Burman, E. (1994a) *Deconstructing Developmental Psychology*, London, Routledge.

Burman, E. (1994b) 'Poor children: charity appeals and ideologies of childhood', *Changes*, 12(1): 29–36.

Connolly, M. (1990) 'Adrift in the city: a comparative study of street children in Bogota, Colombia and Guatamala City', *Child and Youth Services*, 14: 129–149.

Connolly, M. and Ennew, J. (eds) (1996) 'Introduction', *Childhood* ('Children Out of Place': special issue on working and street children) 3(2): 131–145.

Cunningham, H. (1991) *The Children of the Poor*, Oxford, Blackwell.

Cunningham, H. (1996) 'The history of childhood', in C.P. Hwang, M.E. Lamb and I.E. Sigel (eds), *Images of Childhood*, Hillsdale, NJ, Lawrence Erlbaum Associates, pp. 27–35.

Denzin, N.K. (1977) *Childhood Socialisation*, San Francisco, Jossey-Bass.

Donzelot, J. (1977) *The Policing of Families*, Baltimore, Johns Hopkins University Press.

Frones, I., Jensen, A. and Solberg, A. (1990) *Childhood as a Social Phenomenon: Implications for Future Social Policy*, Vienna, Eurosocial Report no 36/1.

Geaves, R. (1998) 'The borders between religions: a challenge to world religions' approach to religious education', *British Journal of Religious Education*, 21(1): 20–31.

Giddens, A. (1995) *Sociology*, Cambridge, Polity Press.

Glauser, B. (1990) 'Street children: deconstructing a construct', in A. James and A. Prout (eds), *Constructing and Reconstructing Childhood*, Basingstoke, Falmer Press, pp. 145–164.

Grady, L. (2001) 'Young carers', MSc Thesis, Glasgow Caledonian University, Glasgow.

Griesel, D., Swart-Kruger, J. and Chawla, L. (2004) 'Children in South Africa can make a difference: an assessment of "growing up in cities" in Johannesburg', in V. Lewis, M. Kellett, C. Robinson, S. Fraser and S. Ding (eds), *The Reality of Research with Children and Young People*, London, Sage Publications, pp. 277–294

Guardian (1994) 'Child killings', *Guardian*, 14/05/94.

Harkness, S. (1996) 'Anthropological images of childhood', in C.P. Hwang, M.E. Lamb and I.E. Sigel (eds), *Images of Childhood*, Hillsdale, NJ, Lawrence Erlbaum Associates, pp. 36–46.

Hendrick, H. (1997) 'Constructions and reconstructions of British childhood: an interpretive survey, 1800 to present', in A. James and A. Prout (eds), *Constructing and Reconstructing Childhood*, 2nd edn, Basingstoke, Falmer Press.

Heywood, C. (2001) *A History of Childhood*, Oxford, Blackwell.

Hobbs, S. and McKechnie, J. (1997) *Child Employment in Britain: A Social and Psychological Analysis*, Edinburg, The Stationery Office.

Hutz, C. and Koller, S.H. (1999) 'Methodological and ethical issues in research with street children', in M.Raffaeli and R. Larson (eds), *Developmental Issues among Homeless and Working Street Youth*, San Francisco, Jossey-Bass, pp. 59–70.

James, A. and Prout, A. (eds) (1990) *Constructing and Reconstructing Childhood*, London, Routledge.

James, A. and Prout, A. (eds) (1997) *Constructing and Reconstructing Childhood*, 2nd edn, Basingstoke, Falmer Press.

James, A., Jenks, C. and Prout, A. (1998) *Theorizing Childhood*, Cambridge, Polity Press.

Jenks, C. (1996) *Childhood*, London, Routledge.

Katz, C. and Monk, J. (eds) (1993) *Full Circles: Geographies of Women over the Life Course*, London, Routledge.

La Fontaine, J. (1986) 'An anthropological perspective on children in social worlds', in M. Richards and P. Light (eds), *Children of Social Worlds*, Cambridge, Polity Press.

Leonard, M. (1999) *Playfair with Working Children: A Report on Working Children in Belfast*, Belfast, Save the Children Fund.

Lusk, M., Peralta, F. and Vest, G. (1989) 'Street children of Juarez: a field study', *The British Journal of Social Work*, 32: 289–302.

Malinowski, B. (1932) *The Sexual Lives of Savages*, London, Routledge and Kegan Paul.

Markus, H.R. and Kitayama, S. (1991) 'Culture and self: implications for cognition, emotion and motivation', *Psychological Review*, 98: 224–253.

Mead, M. (1930) *Growing up in New Guinea*, New York, Morrow Quill Paperbacks.

Mead, M. (1928) *Coming of Age in Samoa: A Psychological Study of Primitive Youth for Western Civilisation*, New York, Dell.

Owusu-Bempah, K. and Howitt, D. (2000) *Psychology beyond Western Perspectives*, Leicester: British Psychological Society.

Palacios, J. (1996) 'Proverbs as images of children and childrearing', in C.P. Hwang, M.E. Lamb and I.E. Sigel (eds), *Images of Childhood*, Hillsdale, NJ, Lawrence Erlbaum Associates, pp. 75–98.

Phinney, J.S. (1996) 'The multigroup ethnic identity measure: a new scale for use with diverse groups', *Journal of Adolescent Research*, 7(2): 156–176.

Pollock, L. (1983) *Forgotten Children: Parent–Child Relations from 1500 to 1900*, Cambridge, Cambridge University Press.

Postman, N. (1983) *The Disappearance of Childhood*, London, W.H. Allen.

Pridmore, P. and Stevens, D. (2000) *Children as Partners for Health*, London, Zed Books.

Prout, A. and James, A. (2000) 'New paradigm for the sociology of childhood', in A. James and A. Prout (eds), *Constructing andf Reconstructing Childhood*, Basingstoke, Falmer Press, pp. 145–164.

Qvortrup, J., Bardy, M., Sgritta, G. and Wintersberger, H. (eds) (1994) *Childhood Matters, Social Theory, Practice and Politics*, Aldershot, Avebury.

Renezetti, C. and Lee, R. (1993) *Researching Sensitive Topics*, London, Sage.

Richards, M. and Light, P. (eds) (1986) *Children of Social Worlds*, Cambridge, Polity Press.

Rousseau, J. (1991) *Emile, or On Education*, trans. Allan Bloom, Harmondsworth, Penguin. First published 1762.

Shahar, S. (1990) *Childhood in the Middle Ages*, London, Routledge.

Taylor, A. (1998) 'Hostages to fortune: the abuse of children in care', in G. Hunt (ed.), *Whistleblowing in the Social Services*, London, Arnold, pp. 41–64.

Terman, L. (1906) *Stanford Revision of the Binet-Simon Scale*, Stanford, CA, Stanford University Press.

United Nations International Children's Emergency Fund (1995) *The State of the World's Children*, New York, UNICEF.

Whiting, B.B. and Edwards, C.P. (1988) *Children of Different Worlds: The Formation of Social Behavior*, Cambridge, MA, Harvard University Press.

Whiting, B.B. and Whiting, J.W.M. (1975) *Children of Six Cultures: A Psychocultural Analysis*, Cambridge, MA, Harvard University Press.

Woodhead, M. (1999) 'Reconstructing developmental psychology – some first steps', *Children and Society*, 13(1): 3–19.

Woodhead, M. and Faulkner, D. (2000) 'Subjects, objects or participants? Dilemmas of psychological research with children', in P. Christensen and A. James (eds), *Research with Children*, London, Routledge Falmer.

Zelizer, V. (1985) *Pricing the Priceless Child*, New Haven, Yale University Press.

4 The Legal Context
JUDITH MASSON

Including child participants in research, as respondents or interviewers, raises ethical and legal dilemmas about children's rights and the obligations of researchers. This chapter explores the legal dimensions of children's involvement in research in the three separate jurisdictions which make up the UK – England and Wales, Northern Ireland, and Scotland. Although each country has its own statutory codes of law relating to children, there are many similarities. Each draws on the common law; the Children (Northern Ireland) Order 1995 is based on the Children Act 1989 and the Children (Scotland) Act 1995 applies many similar concepts; also European Law applies equally throughout the UK. Those researching in other Common Law countries, for example, the USA, Canada, Australia or New Zealand, will also find that similar concepts have taken root; elsewhere differences are likely to be greater. Wherever the research is to be conducted, the researcher must seek to be informed about law, custom and good practice.

There is a close relationship between law and ethics but not everything that is legal is ethical. Frequently law, when used as a tool of regulation, attempts only to set the minimum acceptable standard. The aspirations of ethical practice are higher. Having clarified in their own minds that what they propose is legal, researchers should also consider how it measures up against the ethical standards of their own professional body, of the funding organisation and of any other body which is involved in facilitating the research. It can never be appropriate to defend proposed practice solely on the basis that it is legal. But nor can it be assumed that those who question the approach taken know or understand the relevant legal or ethical issues.

Within the UK the term 'child' means anyone below the age of 18 years, which is the voting age throughout the country. The use of the same word for infants and those on the verge of adulthood may appear to emphasise lack of capacity but the law treats young people differently, according to their age, stage of development and the attitudes prevailing when it was enacted. Despite differences in societal attitudes to appropriate behaviour by and towards young men and young women, the law generally makes no gendered distinctions about their rights. In this chapter, rather than stress family relationships or assumed limitations, I have preferred to use the phrase *children and young people* in an attempt to recognise the capacities and wisdom of those who are not adults.

Children and young people are not powerless, nor without legal rights. Various statutes recognise children's rights to make specific decisions at particular ages (Hamilton and Fiddly, 2001) and under Scots law full legal capacity is acquired at age 16 (Age of Legal Capacity (Scotland) Act 1991). All persons in the UK, whatever their age, have the protection of the European Convention of Human Rights which is incorporated into UK law by the Human Rights Act 1998. Amongst other things the Convention guarantees the right to respect for private and family life (art. 8) and thus supports provision for research access based on the participant's or (sometimes) their parent's consent. In practice, those over 16 are regarded as autonomous in most areas of life and subject to parental control only in limited circumstances. Under Scots law, parental rights cease when the child reaches age 16 (s.2(7)). And throughout the UK much younger people may make decisions for themselves where they have the legal, emotional and intellectual capacity to do so (see the discussion of capacity to consent, below).

This account of the legal context of research with children and young people outlines the obligations of researchers and the rights of children, their parents and carers in these three jurisdictions. It focuses on key aspects of the research relationship – consent and confidentiality – which are relevant to all research settings, and explores legal issues which arise in particular forms of research such as clinical trials and research into legal proceedings. It also considers wider issues such as researchers' responsibilities towards children and young people participating in research, whether as research subjects or as investigators and interviewers.

Involving children and young people in research

Involving children and young people in research is a relatively modern phenomenon that recognises that they have an important contribution to make. In the past, much research was conducted *on* children but relatively little *with* them. Researchers in the fields of education and health relied on the consent of teachers or parents to gain access to children but rarely sought to explain to children or young people the purpose of their studies, or tried to reflect their concerns or give them the option of not taking part. In contrast, those working in sociology, social policy and law tended to ignore children on the basis that their (in)competence, (un)reliability and need for protection made them inappropriate or too problematic as subjects for research. Both these approaches compromise research legally, ethically and in terms of research findings.

Without children's perspectives there cannot be a complete account of schooling, paediatric care or child protection services. It is increasingly accepted that children's perceptions provide a crucial and often distinct dimension in examining the wide range of services for families. Being able to see an arrangement from a child's point of view quite simply changes everything (Smart et al. 2001: 156). But researchers cannot simply focus on researching children and young people who can be readily contacted and are articulate. Children's perspectives are particular to the childhood they experience; the challenge for researchers is to be inclusive. Researchers need to develop ways of engaging children in a wide range of different circumstances, including those with special educational needs and disabilities, in order to obtain high quality information that is not otherwise available. While doing this they must also satisfy those who care for or work with children that their rights are not undermined and children's rights are safeguarded.

The law should not be seen as a barrier to participation in research by children and young people who are competent and willing to do so. To interpret the law in such a restrictive way undermines the rights that it enshrines. Although parents have rights because they are parents, there is no recognised tort of interference with parental rights (*F. v. Wirral MBC* 1991). This means that parents cannot claim damages from a person who has done something with their child of which they do not approve. Penalties could of course follow if the activity was against the criminal law, but this would be the case even if the parents' consent had been obtained. The capacity of children and young persons to consent to research may not be clear cut, but depends on the researcher's assessment of their understanding. A researcher who wrongly considered that consent had been given may be acting unethically but their decisions could only be challenged by a child or young person who had been harmed by the research.

Researchers may owe a duty of care to all those they involve in their research and could thus be liable for foreseeable injuries which befall participants in the course of the research. Particular care should always be taken with the practical arrangements for interviews or tests. The interviewee who fell when their chair broke could have a claim. The law makes allowances for children and young people being less careful than adults, so the responsibilities for young participants can be greater than for adults. But researchers are not at risk of legal proceedings merely through involving children or young people in social research. Indeed, unless research is a cover for malign activity, it is difficult to see what proceedings could be brought, or who could bring proceedings, against someone who spoke or corresponded with a consenting child. Involving those under the age of 16 years as interviewers is more problematic in that it raises questions about youth employment and the special care that should be taken of young employees, but many of the precautions which should be taken are relevant to the safety of all interviewees.

'Gatekeepers'

The nature of children and young persons' lives in families, schools, day care and institutions means that they are rarely entirely free to decide for themselves whether or not to participate in research. They are surrounded by adults who act as 'gatekeepers', controlling researchers' access and children's and young persons' opportunities to express their views. Even though they may have no legal rights in respect of the child's decision to participate in research, they generally control the places – homes and schools – which provide the safest and most suitable venues for interviews. Their position as parents, employees or carers includes legal responsibilities for children's well-being. Outside the family, carers and professionals are generally subject to managerial control that means they may not be able to agree to requests. Although they have direct, personal responsibility for the welfare of the children in their care, they must comply with their employers' directions and codes of practice. They may face disciplinary action, even dismissal, if they fail to meet the standards expected of them.

Gatekeepers have a positive function in ensuring that children are protected from potential harm. Researchers should expect gatekeepers to test their motives for wanting access, and to act as a barrier to poorly thought out or potentially damaging research. Researchers should be able to explain why children's participation is so important, the steps they have taken to maximise the benefits of their study and how they have minimised its risks and inconveniences. Positive support from gatekeepers can be very helpful. The gatekeeper may support a request for access to their organisation. Also, an introduction from a known person means the researcher ceases to be a complete stranger. However, gatekeepers can also use their power to censor children and young people. Researchers need to be sensitive to the gatekeeper's position and to understand the source and limits of their power. This information can assist them to negotiate opportunities to allow children and young people choice in whether or not to take part in their research.

Parental responsibility

Young children are subject to the control of those who have 'parental responsibility' for them but the law acknowledges that as children mature, parental control diminishes. In England, Wales and Northern Ireland there is no clear statutory definition of parental responsibility (see Children Act 1989, s.3(1); Children (Northern Ireland Order 1995, art. 6(1)). Rather it is necessary to turn to case law to understand what decisions those with parental responsibility can make. The Court of Appeal has held that providing confidential information about a child's medical treatment or education to a third party – a company making a documentary about the child's treatment at an educational institute – was an exercise of parental responsibility (*Re Z.* 1996). By analogy parental responsibility also includes the right to provide information to a researcher, or to consent to participation by children who are unable to consent for themselves.

Under Scots law parents have statutory responsibilities to safeguard their child's health, development and welfare and are given rights so that they can do this. Parents have the right to 'control, direct or guide, in a manner appropriate to the stage of development of the child, the child's upbringing' (Children (Scotland) Act 1995, ss. 1(1)(a), 2(1)(b)) and this similarly gives parents the power to decide whether their child should participate in research but only where this control is appropriate. In addition, Scottish parents are under a duty to consult their children before exercising their powers (s.6). In the case of more mature children, the parents' power is limited to providing guidance but this does not give them rights to information from third parties who have a confidential relationship with their child.

The law relating to who holds parental responsibility is very similar throughout the UK. Parental responsibility is not held exclusively by parents, and most fathers who have not married the child's mother have not acquired it. Amendments in the Adoption and Children Act 2002 will give parental responsibility to unmarried fathers who jointly register their children's birth. It will only apply to births registered after its implementation. It is not clear when this Act will be implemented, however October 2004 is a likely date. Parental responsibility is held by all mothers, by fathers married to the mother and by those with parental responsibility orders or agreements. In addition, guardians, anyone who has a residence or special guardianship order, a parental responsibility order or a parental responsibility agreement has parental responsibility. In most cases, the people the child or young person lives with have parental responsibility, but this is not the case where children are in state care. Except in Scotland, the local authority will have parental responsibility if there is a care order, but the foster carers or residential home staff will not have it, although they may have the power to make some day to day decisions delegated to them.

Researchers who wish to include young children who are not mature enough to decide about participation for themselves must obtain the agreement of at least one person who has parental responsibility for the child. In the absence of court orders to the contrary the law recognises that each parent has equal power to consent (Children Act 1989, s.2(8); Children (Northern Ireland) Order 1995, art. 5(6); Children (Scotland) Act 1995, s.2(2)). However, it may not be ethical to privilege the view of a parent who is less involved in the child's day to day care. Researchers should engage with parents and provide them with the information that allows them to decide whether to permit their child's involvement. Where one parent agrees, the other could apply to the court for an order to prevent this. If the court accepted that participation would not be in the child's best interests it would have to veto it. This has occurred, albeit in circumstances where the parents had already engaged in acrimonious litigation and in relation to a television documentary about the child's upbringing rather than anonymous research. The father obtained a court order to override the mother's consent (*Re Z.* 1996). Those working in sensitive areas such as children's contact after parental separation should consider whether to seek consent from both separated parents, bearing in mind that this may exclude research with children whose parents cannot co-operate with each other.

Children's capacity to consent

In England, Wales and Northern Ireland, children's capacity to consent to participate in research depends on the Common Law. In the leading case, *Gillick v. W. Norfolk and Wisbech A.H.A.*, decided in 1985, the House of Lords held that a child who has sufficient understanding could consent to medical treatment, and that a parent of such a child has no right to override the child's consent. This decision is taken as applying to decisions about all other matters unless a specific provision in statute operates, and therefore applies to decisions about research participation, except 'clinical trials'. Parents may override a mature child's refusal of medical treatment (see below) but this decision is limited to necessary medical treatment and would not allow a parent to make their child participate in social research.

What amounts to sufficient understanding depends on the particular circumstances and is determined by the person who will act on the child's behalf. Those working with children are likely to make different decisions about a child's capacity dependent not only on their assessment of the child but also on their attitudes to childhood and to treating children as autonomous. Where information about research in general and the particular study can be given clearly and simply, quite young children are able to consent to taking part. In order to give a valid consent, a child needs to understand the nature of his or her engagement with the researcher, and that it differs from that of other adults who may seek information in order to take decisions about or for the child. A child must be able to understand that information is collected only so that the researcher and other people can understand the particular topic better. No one will take decisions about the child because of what he or she has told the researcher; and importantly, the researcher cannot take any action that makes a difference to the child's life. The research may be intended to improve provision for children but no researcher can offer this in return for consent. If improvements are made, ethically these should be provided to all, not just those who agreed to participate.

In Scotland the position is somewhat different. Parental rights and responsibilities are set out in statute and the analogous Common Law rights no longer apply. The Children (Scotland) Act 1995, section 2(1) gives the parents the right 'to control, direct or guide, in a manner appropriate to the stage of development of the child, the child's upbringing' up to the age of 16 years. This enables a parent to agree to a young child participating in research but does not preclude an older and more mature young person making his or her own decision without involving a parent. A parent who acts on behalf of their child should have regard to the child's views; a child aged 12 or over is presumed to have the maturity to form a view (s.6(1)). A researcher who relied on parental consent would not be acting illegally because the parent had not consulted their child (s.6(2)), but there are circumstances where failing to check a child's willingness to participate could undermine the research process and others where it would be unethical.

Under the Age of Legal Capacity (Scotland) Act 1991, section 1, children over the age of 16 years can enter into any 'transaction' but younger children have no legal capacity to enter any 'transaction' unless this is provided by statute. Under the Act, 'transaction' means 'a transaction having legal effect' (s.9) and this would include some but not all arrangements for research. Where consent is required for legal rather than ethical reasons, the process of giving consent amounts to a 'transaction'. For example, medical research which involves an examination could amount to an assault without the consent of the patient. In such cases, the child's parents (or other person with parental rights and responsibilities) as the child's 'legal representative', generally has the right to consent for the child (Children (Scotland) Act 1995, s.2 (1)(d)). In contrast, research based on observing children's activities at school or at play does not involve any 'transaction' by any child for which legal capacity is required. This is so even if a child is engaged in making and recording the observations.

In Scotland, a child or young person below the age of 16 does have legal capacity 'to enter into any transaction of a kind commonly entered into by persons of his age and circumstances, and on terms which are not unreasonable' (s.2 (1)). This provision was specifically designed to ensure that the law continued to reflect social developments in childhood (Scottish Law Commission, 1987). The increasing emphasis on obtaining children's views as service users and citizens may create a case that children themselves have capacity to consent to participation in some studies where consent is a legal requirement. Also, children with sufficient understanding have the capacity to consent to medical procedures and treatment (s. 2(4)). Taken together, these provisions allow research (but not clinical trials – see below) into use of oral contraceptives by girls under 16. Comparable research could also take place with boys. Indeed, because of young patients' rights to confidentiality, such research could only ethically be conducted with their consent and without informing any parent or other person with parental responsibility.

Overall, the Age of Legal Capacity (Scotland) Act 1991 may not have much impact on research with children and young people. However, researchers must consider whether their study requires children to enter 'transactions' as defined in the Act, and if so, whether these are of a kind commonly entered into by children. Where payment would be provided for adult participation, it is fair to value children's time and inconvenience in a similar way. To seek children's involvement without some form of compensation (which need not be notified in advance) could be taken as imposing unreasonable terms and precludes a valid consent from a child.

Consenting to research

Having identified who must consent, consideration must be given to the nature of that consent. As far as medical practice is concerned, a concept of 'informed consent' has been developed in a number of countries. Where informed consent is required, only the consent of someone who was *fully* informed of *all* the relevant issues before they gave their consent is valid. The courts in the UK have repeatedly refused to accept the need for informed consent for medical treatment, preferring to accept doctors' views about what patients need to be told. This approach leaves medical staff with considerable scope and frees them from the possibility of facing an action for assault on the basis that the patient's consent was obtained without disclosure of every possible risk.

On this basis there is no legal requirement for informed consent for research participation. However, ethics may impose higher standards. Researchers neither face the risks that informed consent would impose on doctors nor can they claim that their actions are designed and intended to benefit those from whom they seek co-operation. The fundamental importance of consent, freely given, to research participation reinforces the view that the research should always explain fully the purpose, process and intended outcomes of research and seek consent on that basis. Where general consents have already been given, for example as part of the arrangements for a child's care or education, these may not be adequate when judged against high ethical standards. At the very least, consideration should be given to the possible advantages to both researcher and participant of approaching each new study on the basis that fully informed consent should be obtained.

Requiring high levels of understanding for a valid consent could operate to exclude research with children unless an adult has consented on their behalf. Where children can understand enough to distinguish research from other interventions, and to understand the impact on them of participating, it may be more ethical to act on their consent than to require the fully informed consent of a parent. Such an approach gives children the maximum opportunity to have their views and experiences recorded and avoids the exclusion of children whose parents would not respond to a request or would wish to control whom their child speaks to.

If consent is to be freely given, care also needs to be taken that children (or other potential respondents) do not feel obliged to participate. Where the person seeking children's participation is in a powerful position over them, as in the case of a teacher or carer, children may feel that they have to agree or, worse still, that they will be penalised if they do not.

Researchers need to be alert to such possibilities, particularly where their access is arranged by those who provide services for children.

Clinical research on children

Special rules apply to some forms of medical research conducted anywhere in the European Union (EU). The Directive on Good Practice in Clinical Trials (Directive 2001/20/EC), which will come into force in 2004, sets obligatory standards for clinical trials. Further steps are required to implement the Directive in the UK. The Department of Health is currently preparing the necessary regulations and these will be incorporated into the Department of Health's research governance framework. Further details can be found on the Medical Controls Agency website (www.mca.gov.uk/index.htm last accessed 23.5.03). The Directive covers all 'clinical trials' of 'medicinal products' but does not apply to 'non-intervention studies' – that is research into the effects of products which are prescribed in the usual manner and which relies on epidemiology rather than additional tests on the patient for the analysis of the data. All clinical trials require 'informed consent', a risk/benefit analysis and Ethics Committee approval. The person giving consent must have received a properly documented account of the nature, significance, implications and risks of the study. Their consent should be written and signed; exceptionally, a witnessed oral consent will suffice. In addition, clinical trials involving minors (those under the age of 18 years) are subject to further controls under article 4 of the Directive. These are similar to those applying in Europe under internationally agreed guidance (Clinical Investigation of Medicinal Products in the Paediatric Population – CPMP/ICH/2711/99).

Clinical research on children can only be undertaken where research has already been conducted without involving children, where research on minors is essential and where the patients concerned will derive a benefit. The interests of the child patient must always prevail over any other interests, and inducements may not be given to secure children's participation. Where minors are to be involved in clinical trials in England, Wales or Northern Ireland, the informed consent of a parent or some other person with parental responsibility must be obtained. This consent is additional to the child's and may be withdrawn at any time. In Scotland, the consent of a parent or legal representative is not required for anyone aged 16 years or older, unless they lack the mental capacity to make decisions (Age of Legal Capacity (Scotland) Act 1991, s.1 (3)(b)). In the case of younger children the person giving consent (usually a parent) must have regard to the child's views (Children (Scotland) Act 1995, s.6 (1)). All children must be given appropriate information about the risks and benefits of the trial. A decision by a '*Gillick* competent' child to refuse to participate or to withdraw from the trial must be considered by the investigator but does not appear to be decisive.

This is in line with court decisions which allow parents to override a mature child's refusal of medical treatment (*Re W*. [1993]).

Confidentiality

The notion of confidentiality has a very particular meaning amongst researchers which needs to be explained and agreed with those participating. Research confidentiality usually entails taking considerable care not to pass information to those connected in any way with the respondent and disclosing information only in ways which protect the identity of those who provided it. The location where the research took place is generally not identified, individuals are anonymised, or given pseudonyms, and some facts, which might otherwise identify them, are changed or omitted. All research participants, including children and young people, need careful explanations of research confidentiality when (or before) their consent to participate is sought. Again, those undertaking research with children should ensure they can give clear explanations.

Where children are competent to make decisions, the law allows them the associated confidentiality which it would allow an adult. The confidentiality of younger children, who lack the capacity to consent, also needs to be considered. Although these children may keep secrets from their parents they are not entitled to confidential relationships automatically. Where arrangements for children's participation have been made with parents or other 'gatekeepers', these people will of course know that an individual child has taken part, and what the focus of the research is. Natural curiosity and concern for their child may lead them to question the child or the researcher about what was said. This can put pressure on the child. Researchers should consider this when negotiating access or consent for interviews with children and young people. Where parental consent is needed, it can be sought on the understanding that what the child says will not be passed to parents (Hamilton and Hopegood, 1997). In such cases, parents may need to be reassured that certain types of information would be passed to them, and where this is the case children should know that this will happen and what parents will be told. Some children may want to give the account of the interview but others may prefer the researcher to explain on their behalf.

There are ethical considerations in research (and other work) with children which may mean that the same degree of confidentiality cannot be guaranteed to a child as would be given to an adult. There are two areas of particular concern: where a child discloses that he or she is being seriously harmed or ill-treated, and where the researcher identifies a condition, for example a medical condition or learning difficulty about which the parents could take action. Failure of the researcher to take appropriate action might not only lead to criticism on ethical grounds, in some limited circumstances it could also give rise to legal liability.

In the United Kingdom, those who suspect that a child is being ill-treated are not generally under a legal duty to report this fact to social services or the police. The Education Act 2002 contains a provision for regulations to impose a reporting law on those working in education in England and Wales. No regulations have yet been drafted. Yet a wide range of professionals may be obliged by (a) local authority child protection procedures and/or (b) their respective professional codes of conduct to report suspicions of abuse. If it is subsequently shown that a professional had knowledge of abuse but failed to comply with relevant procedures or codes then disciplinary action or termination of employment is the likely outcome. In some other countries, e.g. certain states of the USA and Australia, mandatory 'Reporting laws' commonly exist. This means that specific persons, professionals or otherwise, are required by law to report any suspicions of child abuse. Any failure to report when it can be shown that a person knew of child abuse is a criminal offence. However, when a client discloses to their lawyer that he or she has ill-treated a child, the lawyer is usually excepted from mandatory reporting but will be subject to the ethical code of their profession. In the UK, guidance to both doctors (Department of Health, 1999) and lawyers (Solicitors' Family Law Association, 2000) advises that the confidential nature of the relationship with the patient or client does not justify failing to pass on information when children are being abused. Moreover, gatekeepers, particularly those who have legal obligations to children and young people, such as education and care authorities, may make it a condition of permitting access that specific information is passed to them.

Researchers should be mindful that the promise of confidentiality may have encouraged a child to discuss their dreadful circumstances, and the child may feel betrayed if information is passed on without his/her knowledge. Researchers should be aware of local child protection procedures. If a child or young person does suggest that they or someone they know has been abused or ill-treated, the researcher should be sensitive to their needs but should not further investigate, probe or interrogate the child or young person. Researchers should listen carefully and record any information from the child or young person. Researchers should be aware that their conversation could later be used as testimony in a court setting. Researchers may feel that they ought to offer further support to the child but care should be taken not to overstep the professional boundaries of being a researcher. The ethical complexities of these issues should be considered in any research where children have the opportunity to talk about themselves and their lives. Being a researcher does not qualify a person to offer support. It is not acceptable for a researcher to adopt another role, e.g. counsellor, mediator, social worker, etc. This is true even if he or she has qualifications or is motivated by the wish to help. Providing accurate information about agencies or groups who exist to support young people in a leaflet about the research can provide those interviewed with a way of obtaining support if they choose. In such cases interviewers may also need support. Employers of researchers could even be liable for trauma suffered by interviewers whom they knowingly required to conduct distressing interviews.

There will some be studies, particularly those involving the use of diagnostic instruments, where the researcher may obtain information about individual children which would be useful to children or their parents. In addition to any ethical duty to disclose this information, there could be a legal duty to do so, particularly for anyone conducting the research in the course of employment to provide services for children, for example a doctor or an educational psychologist. It is well accepted that doctors owe a duty of care to their patients; a similar duty has been held to apply to educational psychologists carrying out assessments of, or providing advice about, individual children (*Christmas v. Hampshire* CC; *Keating v. Bromley LBC* 1995). Although it would be more difficult to establish that a researcher who was not otherwise providing a service owed a duty of care, an education authority which employed the researcher or permitted the research to take place might be held liable. Consequently, researchers need to consider whether and how to provide information about identifiable children. Where young people could take the necessary steps themselves, information should be provided to them directly but the researcher should consider whether they have the necessary maturity to handle it. In the case of younger children parents should be given the information; they too may need help to know what steps to take.

Research confidentiality and legal proceedings

Where there are legal proceedings, the law places the interests of justice above the confidentiality of research. Children who participate in a study related to the issue before the court, for example the incident which led to their being a witness in a criminal trial or their relationship with a parent who was disputing custody, cannot be offered confidentiality because the researcher can be required by the court to disclose any record of their interview. This material might then be used to undermine any evidence the child gives.

Those conducting research on children need to be sure that they cannot be thought to have impacted on their ability to be witnesses. Providing a child with an opportunity to give an account of what happened to them could be viewed as rehearsing their evidence. Similarly, research on facial recognition could impact on evidence if identification were crucial. Where a child had been abused, the exclusion of their evidence could prevent the successful prosecution of the perpetrator and have a very damaging effect on the child, and leave other children at risk. However, these concerns should not be taken to preclude any research with children involved in proceedings. Researchers must consider whether their study could be thought to impact on evidence, and whether it should only take place after proceedings have ended.

Complying with the Data Protection Act 1998

The Data Protection Act also derives from EU law and applies throughout the UK. It sets out principles for data processing (which includes storage, use or disclosure) to protect the rights of individuals to privacy and fair treatment. Generally, data can only be processed for a specified purpose and, in many cases, with the consent of the data subject, or in the case of young children, someone with parental responsibility. Children who are '*Gillick* competent' can consent; this also applies in Scotland where under section 66(2) children aged 12 are presumed to have sufficient understanding. There are some exemptions where data are used for 'research purposes', but this cannot include any work which leads to decisions about particular individuals, as may occur in clinical research (s. 33). Researchers must also ensure that any findings do not identify the individuals (s.33(4)(a)). Where the research exemption applies, data may be used in research even though not originally supplied for this purpose (s.33(2)). However, where a project includes both direct contact with individuals and use of records about them the Information Commissioner expects researchers to seek consent before accessing records (Information Commissioner, 2002). Organisations which regularly undertake research using clients' records generally obtain agreement to this when clients first access their service. Where they do not, researchers must consider whether they can obtain consent and, if not, whether their proposed study is lawful. Guidance is available from the Information Commissioner's website www.dataprotection.gov.uk (last accessed 23.5.03) and in relation to social services records from the Department of Health (Department of Health, 2001).

Protecting children participating in research

Current concerns about the victimisation of children by those who have gained access to them through employment in schools or care homes or through organising leisure activities, have drawn attention to child sexual abuse occurring outside the home. Although children are generally at far greater risk of abuse within their families, no one who plans activities involving children and adults can disregard the dangers that some adults pose. Registers are kept of those considered unsuitable to work with children (Protection of Children Act 1999) and some employers are required to check these before engaging individuals, including volunteers, to work with children. Childcare organisations as defined in s.12(1); similar provisions relate to the employment of teachers (Education Reform Act 1988) and carers of vulnerable adults (Care Standards Act 2000).

Research organisations do not routinely have access to enhanced Criminal Records Bureau checks although it may be possible for this to be arranged where the research is being conducted in partnership with social services, childcare charities or schools. Alternatively, researchers could recruit sessional interviewers who work in jobs that require checks. However, an absence of convictions is not a sufficient basis for determining the suitability of an interviewer or the safety of children. Both detection and conviction for offences against children remain extremely low. Far greater care is necessary in recruitment to ensure the protection of children.

The arrangements for interviews also need to be considered. Both children and interviewers must feel and be safe during the research. Children may feel more comfortable if they can bring a friend or parent to an interview but this may also inhibit what they say and can make concentration difficult. There are cases where it will be appropriate for the researcher to arrange for chaperons, particularly where the research involves the child travelling to a facility where the research will be conducted. Particular care must be taken both in selection and training if the chaperon is not someone already known to the child. Using large public rooms or corridors allows the interview to be observed but not overheard but may not be practicable. Where children are interviewed at home interviewers often have little choice about where they see a child. It may be difficult to get a sufficiently quiet place in living areas without disrupting family activities. Bedrooms are not usually the places where children see strangers alone, although they may like to show them to visitors. The garden or the stairs can in some cases provide the most suitable place for an interview.

Children as researchers

More attention has been given recently to involving children in the research process either as part of advisory groups helping to design and direct studies about things which concern them or as interviewers of other children (Ward, 1997). These initiatives raise further legal concerns about children's status and their safety. Children who are engaged as interviewers are working for the researcher and should be accorded no less consideration than adult interviewers. Even though under minimum wage legislation it is legal to pay those aged under 21 years less than the adult minimum wage, ethical researchers will not rely on this to exploit young people who work with them. Children possess special skills, such as the ability to get good rapport with other children, and this should be recognised in the rate of pay as it would be for an adult. The strict regulation of children's work requires additional safeguards to be provided. Interviewers are often not regarded as employees but as sessional workers. However, where there is control over whom they interview and the contents of the interview, as would be the case where children are carrying out fieldwork, it is difficult to argue that they are not employees.

Directive 94/33/EC on the Protection of Young People at Work imposes major limitations on the employment of young people under the age of

16 years throughout the United Kingdom. Those below the age of 14 years may generally not be employed. Working hours are restricted; those under 15 years may not work for more than two hours on any school day or Sunday, or five hours on a Saturday. They cannot work for more than 25 hours a week in the school holidays. The Health and Safety (Young Persons) Regulations 1997 impose further safeguards for young people (those under the age of 18 years) and children (those below the school leaving age). Before employing anyone below the age of 18 years employers must assess the risks posed by the work, taking account, amongst other things, of the immaturity and inexperience of young people. All employees have to be given 'comprehensible and relevant information' about risks and protective measures; where children are employed this information must also be given to a parent.

The concerns about the vulnerability of children being interviewed also apply where children or young people are interviewers. Interviewees are at risk as they travel to interviews; where interviews will take place in private homes they may also be at risk from other household members, about whom little may be known. Those planning the research need to consider these risks with interviewers. Chaperon/drivers who wait outside provide a way of protecting interviewers both on the way to and during an interview, but other arrangements such as pairs of interviewers will be more suitable for some studies. As well as physical risks attention also needs to be given to the potential psychological harm caused by hearing disturbing accounts from other children. Young interviewers may well need more training and support than adults; under the regulations this is a legal requirement not just a professional issue.

Conclusion

The law provides only a general framework for research and this is largely derived from other areas of children's lives. The ethical researcher will use this as a base from which to develop an approach that respects the individuality and personhood of young research subjects and seeks to enable them to exercise rights to participate. In doing so, the researcher must be responsive to the pressures on young people which arise from their dependency on adults and the social contexts in which they live, study and play. It is not enough to treat children and young people as adults: research must be designed and conducted to give children and young people real choices about participation, and to ensure that their views and understandings are properly captured. In doing this researchers must be prepared to face some antagonism from adults who continue to view children as objects for concern and protection, rather than as individuals who have the right to be heard.

References

Department of Health (1999) *Working Together to Safeguard Children*, London, The Stationery Office.
Department of Health (2001) *The Data Protection Act 1998: Guidance for Local Authorities* London, Department of Health.
Hamilton, C. and Fiddly, A. (2001) 'At what age can I?' *Childright*, 180: 9.
Hamilton, C. and Hopegood, L. (1997) 'Offering children confidentiality: law and guidance', *Childright*, 140: 1–8.
Information Commissioner (2002) *Use and Disclosure of Health Data*, Wilmslow, Information Commissioner. www.dataprotection.gov.uk.
Scottish Law Commission (1987) *Legal Capacity and Responsibility of Minors and Pupils* (Scot. Law Com. 110) London, HMSO.
Smart, C., Neale, B. and Wade, A. (2001) *The Changing Experience of Childhood*, Cambridge, Polity Press.
Solicitors' Family Law Association (2000) *Code of Practice and Guidance Notes on Good Practice on Acting for Children*, Orpington, SFLA.
Ward, L. (1997) *Seen and Heard*, York, YPS.

Case list

Christmas v. Hampshire CC; Keating v. Bromley LBC [1995] 2 F.L.R. 276
F. v. Wirral MBC [1991] Fam 69
Gillick v. W. Norfolk and Wisbech A.H.A. [1985] A.C. 112
Re W. [1993] Fam 64
Re Z. (a minor) (freedom of publication) [1996] 1 F.L.R. 191

Directives

The Directive on Good Practice in Clinical Trials (Directive 2001/20/EC) http://europa.int/eur-lex/en/index.html accessed on 27.05.03.
Clinical Investigation of Medicinal Products in the Paediatric Population (CPMP/ICH/2711/99) http://europa.int/eur-lex/en/index.html.
The Directive on the Protection of Young People at Work (Directive 94/33/EC) http://europa.int/eur-lex/en/index.html.

Paradigms and Philosophy
SANDY FRASER AND CHRIS ROBINSON

In Chapter 2 we introduced the idea of what empirical research is and suggested that it concerned the systematic investigation of experience. This chapter takes a more detailed look at different types of 'systematic investigation'. It combines philosophical considerations of empirical research with an examination of its different paradigms. A paradigm is a set of beliefs about the way in which particular problems exist and a set of agreements on how such problems can be investigated. Empirical research can be conducted without detailed knowledge of its philosophy or awareness of the different paradigms it operates under. Nevertheless, any approach to empirical research will rest upon a particular paradigm and philosophical outlook even if unconsciously held. Considering paradigms and philosophies of research enables an overview and assessment of the general strengths and weaknesses of different assumptions about how we know what we know. Philosophical consideration is useful in the preparatory stages of research in helping us to focus on the right kinds of research question to ask. It is also helpful at the end of a period of research. No piece of empirical research is perfect and when doubts arise about the approach that was taken we can use philosophy reflectively, to justify or change future strategy.

The main organising principle of this chapter is to give an overview of paradigms of social and psychological research. It is not an exhaustive account. Readers who find themselves interested by one or another account will need to follow reading this chapter by looking at the original sources. We will look at four paradigms: (1) the scientific paradigm; (2) the structuralist paradigm(s); (3) the interactionist paradigm and (4) the post-structuralist and social constructionist paradigm. Feminism has been an important influence on empirical research methods over the last 20–30 years. This is discussed in Chapter 6.

It is important to understand that simply because a philosophical idea is old does not mean it lacks contemporary purchase. Some recent paradigms are resonant of older ideas, with a gloss of contemporary language and expression. Many of the ideas presented below, e.g. 'empiricism', 'inductivism', 'falsificationism', 'structuralism', are presented in a way which highlights their main features. However, contemporary exponents of these paradigms may regard these examples as too limited or naïve. Certainly, there have been significant responses to the critiques of the various positions that we describe but there is no space here to detail adequately the various claims and counter-claims of each position. What we intend is a brief introduction to the main paradigms which have informed methods of empirical research. We begin by looking at the 'scientific paradigm'. Many other paradigms have come into existence or have been influenced by reactions to the scientific paradigm and to understand them we need to understand the assumptions made by 'science' at various points. As a result, our discussion of the scientific paradigm will be slightly longer than discussion of other paradigms

The scientific paradigm

> We can no longer think about society, about human behaviour, as if the natural sciences had never existed. This is true not only of sociology, of course, but of economics, psychology, political science, anthropology and even history. Indeed, most of these disciplines – the exception being history, but even this was not immune from the ensuing debates – owe their origins to the desire to create *sciences* of human behaviour. That is not to say that these disciplines have slavishly followed the method of natural sciences; far from it. It is simply to point out that they have the natural sciences as an inevitable feature of their intellectual background and one to which they feel it necessary to respond either by rejection of the natural science model or by embracing it. Neutrality is not, seemingly, an option. (Hughes, 1990: 2)

Science can be regarded as a complex paradigm that emerged from the European Renaissance (fifteenth and sixteenth centuries) and the Enlightenment (eighteenth century) developing further in the nineteenth and twentieth centuries. 'Science' as popularly understood concerns natural phenomena. Can science be applied to social and psychological phenomena? Atoms and molecules are unlike humans, they do not 'talk back'. Observation or experiment in physics has never required an atomic particle to give a verbal account of its trajectory. By contrast social and psychological phenomena carry meaning, opinion and point of view. In any systematic study, the empirical researcher's viewpoint will colour and be coloured by what he or she studies. We might consider that an atom 'objectively' exists, that is, exists independently of our perception or consciousness of it. An atom may exist beyond our 'opinion' of it. But can we say the same for social and psychological phenomena? Is 'poverty' or 'attachment' real in the same way that atoms and molecules are popularly understood to be real? Does 'childhood' objectively exist or is it only a figment of our 'Western' cultural imagination? Even if a chemist studies a molecule with her/his opinions of it, a test can be developed to distinguish between that opinion and 'resisting reality' (Popper, 1979). Yet in the investigation of people and their society the very existence and definition of the objects of study, e.g. poverty, childhood, attachment or disability, could be a matter of opinion and not part of the objective world.

   In grappling with this type of issue the scientific paradigm tends to assert a philosophical distinction between two classes of assertions about the world; on the one hand 'facts' and on other 'values'. Facts describe what exists, what *is*; and values describe what *ought* to be. The latter kind of assertion is moral and the former is not. To say that water heated to boiling point creates steam is to assert no moral point of view. It implies no value. It is simply a 'fact'. The scientific paradigm asserts that great care should be taken to separate fact from value: science should be 'value-free'. Moreover, whatever can be discovered by science about what causes a phenomenon to exist cannot logically be taken to imply what human action ought to occur as a consequence. *An 'is' does not imply an 'ought'*. The role of science is to provide *factual* information which is not 'loaded' with value. Science *describes* and *explains* by counting the *quantity* of facts; we *discover* that a species is endangered because we counted and noted a decline in its quantity over successive years. Also by monitoring a range of quantities of fact we can note that increases or decreases in one fact seem to coincide with increases or decreases of quantity in one or many other facts. Science has developed means of disentangling relationships between different quantities of facts to explain if and how such facts interact with each other. For example, how fact A might always be associated with, and always occur prior to, fact B (Punch, 1998: 111–134).

   The idea of cause and effect is prominent in science and empirical research. Research begins with a problem, such as 'What causes apples to fall down and not up?' 'What are the causes of poverty?' 'What causes young people to take drugs?' One idea about causality is that cause and effect are objectively discrete. There is no inherent purpose to apples falling down or to the existence of poverty or to the tendency to take drugs. If person A inhabits a particular set of circumstances B then there will be a definite outcome C. If there is water in the kettle and an electrical current of 240V and 15amps is applied then the water will boil. Here 'cause' occurs without a 'reason'. An alternative view, whose origins are often attributed to Aristotle (384–322BC), is that all effects are caused for a reason. Effects have a meaning. It is the *meaning* and purpose of an interaction between two objects which is primary. There is a purpose, design or meaning to apples falling down or why people are poor or why drugs are taken. The technical term for this is *teleological explanation*.

   Prior to Darwin (1809–82) it was commonly thought that the natural world had been designed by God. Darwin inserted natural selection in place of God's design. Plants and animals had not been *designed* to fill niches within nature. Rather, the interactions between climate, geography, specific interactions between species and opportunity had, via an incredibly long process, developed inherent physical and social attributes in plants and animals to enable them to survive by adaptation or otherwise perish. The beauty of plants and animals did not offer any evidence of God's care or design – nature had no inherent purpose. However, even if the issue of God's design is left to one side some contemporary biologists still refer to the way in which a cheetah is 'designed' to run fast, or a cactus is 'designed' to limit its transpiration of water. In other words, explanation of what a cheetah is, is related to its goals and purposes – to eat swift-footed food. Event C happens because it *means* something to animal/person D. Here the empirical researcher starts with the end of a process, explaining prior events in terms of that goal. This means that different facts have different *qualities* and these qualities may be more significant than their quantities (Punch, 1998: 139–168).

This distinction is important in research with children and young people. During the nineteenth century the German historians/philosophers Johann Gustav Droysen (1808–84) and Wilhelm Dilthey (1833–1911) sought to make a distinction between *Erklärung* (Explanation) and *Verstehen* (Understanding). They argued that the former was relevant to natural science and the latter to the study of history. Social and psychological phenomena could not be explained by the notions of causality as referred to in the example of the water boiling. Events had to be *understood* rather than merely explained. History in Dilthey's view was the reconstruction of the past by *intellectual empathy (Einfühlung)* (von Wright, 1971).

This nineteenth century discussion clearly relates to any current discussion of the differences between quantitative and qualitative research. The goals of empirical research can differ. We can ask questions in which children and young people are seen as discrete groups whose lives are impacted upon or determined by other discrete groups or conditions. Our task is then to identify these groups and their properties and quantify them and explain (*erklären*) the extent of their influence. This is largely the concern of quantitative research. Alternatively, empirical researchers can seek to establish *intellectual empathy* to understand (*Verstehen*) the experience of children and young people. This is largely the concern of qualitative research. In the former, we may be considering empirical research without any attempt at explaining the intentions and motivations of the subjects of the research, whereas in the latter this would be essential. If both processes in empirical research are valid then it will result in different types of 'truth'. For many scientists this is problematic.

> When you take a 747 to an international convention of sociologists, the reason that you arrive in one piece is that a lot of western trained scientists and engineers got their sums right. If it gives you satisfaction to say that the theory of aerodynamics is a social construct that is your privilege, but why then do you entrust your plans to a Boeing rather than a magic carpet?…show me a cultural relativist at 30,000 feet and I will show you a hypocrite. (Dawkins, 1994)

To wrestle with this problem many *social scientists* have used arguments which have underpinned developments in natural science e.g. physics, chemistry, biology. In the following sections we draw attention to three strands of argument in order of their historical appearance: (1) empiricism and inductivism, (2) falsificationism; and (3) Kuhn's idea of paradigm. The first two are often conflated and described as *positivist*. Some empirical researchers are critical of positivism but its assumptions are still widespread in social and psychological research.

Empiricism and inductivism

John Locke (1632–1704) asserted that it is 'when he first has any sensation' that 'a man begins to have any ideas' (Locke *Essays* Book 2:1:23 in Fraser, 1959: 141). He suggests that we can only create ideas from the information gained from our senses. This philosophical outlook is called empiricism. There are no innate ideas. All our knowledge and ideas develop from the inundation of experience. We should be clear about what our senses are telling us and we should not let ideas of what we think we are observing interfere with or clutter our sensations. This is the origin of the modern idea of 'objectivity'. Objectivity excludes preconceptions, whether theoretical or moral, from the act of observing what our senses are telling us. This has led over time to the construction of 'protocol language' in empirical/scientific research: 'the physicist does not deal with billiard balls, falling feathers, crashing cars, boiling water, but with bodies of a particular shape, size, mass, motion, wavelength' (Hughes, 1990: 39). By controlling the language used and making it uniform between empirical researchers 'superfluous' associations and qualities that might be implied by common terms can be ruled out.

We should only establish an idea of what is occurring *after* we have collected the facts of our experience. Once collected, known facts of a given problem could be demonstrated to others in proof of observations; such demonstrations became known as experiments. Modern usage of the word 'experiment' has a slightly different but not inconsistent meaning – see falsificationism below. The methodical organisation of observed experience that *verified* facts and *proved* the relationship between facts allowed generalisations to be made via *inductive logic* and these were described as natural laws (Chalmers, 1978: 1; 1999: 5). Inductive logic is a method of reasoning by which a general law is inferred from observations of particular instances; we might note that each and every time we observe a swan it is white in colour, generating a law: 'all swans are white'. Such a conclusion is reached by inductive logic (but see below for the 'problem of induction').

The Renaissance and Enlightenment encouraged the 'scientific' exploration of nature. The success of this project in the late eighteenth and early nineteenth centuries, together with the impact of social and political revolutions in America and France, encouraged the idea that people could be empirically/'scientifically' understood. Auguste Comte (1798–1857) in *Cours de philosophie positive* traced the development of human thought from theology, metaphysics and superstition to knowledge in its so-called *positive* stage. This had led to the term 'positivism', by which it is meant that we make positive or definitive statements about nature or society. Facts derived from observation and experiments were seen as providing positive proof of something that was *true*. Repetition of observations yielding the same or similar results *verified* the truth of such observations. In the social sciences this inspired Comte but also later writers like Marx, Spencer, Durkheim and also many others. They wanted to make observations of social and economic facts by which social laws, like natural laws could be discovered.

Falsificationism

Developments in science and its philosophy undermined the notion of verification, proof and the certainty implied by natural law. Researchers began to generate ideas and theories that could not be supported by direct observation. When the idea of the atom as the fundamental particle in nature began to emerge in the nineteenth century it could not be directly observed but its existence could be *deduced*. Facts had to be interpreted.

More significantly still, Albert Einstein (1879–1955) successfully developed theories which disrupted the view that observation and experiment were simple matters requiring only technical refinement and language which excluded speculation. Contradicting the physics of Sir Isaac Newton, Einstein successfully suggested that the position of the observer in relation to an observed event determined what it was possible for the observer to 'see'. These considerations disrupted the certainties of early empiricism. Karl Popper (1902–94) suggested that it was impossible to say that a statement was positively true. Further research might via exception disprove it. This is known as *the problem of induction*. Even if all our experience suggests that event A always follows event B, it is theoretically possible that event B could occur without event A, for example as occurred when the first Australian Black swans were discovered; all swans are not white. Thus, empirical research cannot demonstrate absolute or eternal truths. However, Popper suggested that statements about the natural or social world could not be *verified* as true but they could be determined to be false.

Popper asserted that philosophers like Immanuel Kant (1724–1804) were right in

> insisting that all knowledge, and the growth of knowledge…stems from ourselves, and that without these self-begotten ideas there would be no knowledge…Thus Kant was right that it is our intellect which imposes its laws – its ideas, its rules – upon the inarticulate mass of our 'sensations' and thereby brings order to them. Where he was wrong is that he did not see that we rarely succeed with our imposition, that we try and err again and again, and that the result – our knowledge of the world – owes as much to the resisting reality as to our self-produced ideas. (Popper, 1979: 68n.)

Science progresses by finding out what is 'not false'. The rigorous elimination of falsehoods can progress our understanding of nature, society, and in our case children and young people by permitting a progressively stronger relationship to ultimate truth, which Popper called ***verisimilitude***. Objective knowledge is that which has been definitely *disproved*. It then follows that all scientific statements have to be formulated in a way that makes it possible to determine if a statement is false. Typically these statements are posed as testable predictions or **hypotheses.** We *deduce* whether our theory ('self-begotten ideas') expressed via an hypothesis is resisted by empirical reality. For this reason Popper's method is known as the *hypothetico-deductive method*. For example, there might be a theory that the day of the week is a causal factor in violent behaviour by children; thus 'all children become violent to their parents on each and every Monday'; the statement is 'scientific' because it implies that if any child is not violent on any Monday then we can demonstrate that the statement is false. In other words (thankfully) it would be an error to think that Mondays are invariably associated with violence by children towards their parents.

Some statements are 'unfalsifiable' and must be avoided by scientists. Such statements will be *logically true* or concern a belief which is untestable. For example,

Daily Horoscope – 5 December 2002 First name: **Sandy.** Sun Sign: **Virgo.** Gender: **M.**

Today will be the perfect day to let go of the pressures around you, Sandy. Indeed, people around you might seem a little bit disorganised and out of it, and *your day planning could fall down the drain*. Nothing will seem to be in order. Don't be too alarmed as it is only temporary. Try to use this situation to your advantage by putting your own goals and ideas into clearer order.

My 'day planning could fall down the drain' – the 'could' implies that it might not. My 'day planning' might be all right, but it might not. This kind of statement is unfalsifiable. Logically, it can never be false. Popper also argued that moral statements, belief in God, Marxism and Freudian psychoanalysis were also unfalsifiable. There were no inherent tests within these canons of work that could ultimately disprove their tenets. Their propositions, like those of religious statements, might even be true but there was nothing in such theories that could be tested to determine if they were false. Therefore they were unscientific and intending scientists should leave them well alone.

Thomas Kuhn's paradigms

Empiricist, inductivist, falsificationist, hypothetico-deductivist philosophies of science have been both a description of what science is and does and of what science ought to be. For example, Popper suggested that the inductivist model was wrong and that during the historical phase of its domination the best scientists were essentially hypothetico-deductivists in practice – whether they knew that or not! The crucial issue about successful and significant scientific empirical inquiry was that it was founded on the right method – whether inductive or hypothetico-deductive. The right method cuts across our opinions and viewpoints and links us to the underlying 'objective' reality that is sometimes masked by our opinions. Yet what if this line of argument was just another opinion? It would mean that the so- called 'right method' was something that was socially produced between the people undertaking the study or experiment in question. It would also mean that the so-called right method could not guarantee any link to objective knowledge. Perhaps then, in social and psychological research – including research with children and young people – we should place less emphasis on scientific method because other methods are as valid and reliable as anything that science can provide. This was one possible reaction to the ideas of Thomas Kuhn.

Thomas Kuhn (1922–96) originally trained as a theoretical physicist before turning to the history of science and latterly to philosophy. In *The Structure of Scientific Revolutions* (1996), first published in 1962, Kuhn set out his view that science in general was not characterised by a single method. Rather, scientists share similar sets of *beliefs* about the way in which particular problems exist and a set of implicit and explicit agreements on how such problems can be understood (Burton, 2000: 15). A mature branch of science has a 'paradigm', a basic set of assumptions or ways of problem solving. To be accepted as a paradigm, a theory must seem better than its competitors, but it need not, and in fact never does, explain all the facts with which it can be confronted. A paradigm guides the research efforts of scientific communities but paradigms are not persistently stable. According to Kuhn paradigms develop historically and are subject to sudden transformations when previously held beliefs are shattered by intellectual revolutions. These 'paradigm shifts' offer groundbreaking novelties of fact or theory.

Kuhn implied that whether empirical research is oriented to verification or falsification, scientists/empirical researchers essentially attempt to bolster their pre-existing ideas of the way in which the world operates. Facts are not 'objectively' collected (inductivist/empiricist), neither do scientists really select tests which would disprove their theories (falsificationist); rather they select activities which would tend to *support* existing theory. During periods of 'normal science', scientists attempt to bring professional preconceptions, accepted theory and accepted fact into closer and closer agreement. Scientists are typically intellectually conservative. Generally speaking they ignore 'bad results' or facts which significantly contradict their theories. Yet anomalies build up over time to provoke intellectual dissatisfaction. The conservatism of scientists does not apply to all scientists, all of the time. When particular paradigms have been exhaustively explored (often by young scientists whose indoctrination is incomplete) an alternative paradigm is considered which explains existing facts as well as if not better than the existing theory or paradigm. Kuhn offered in argument the historical example of the emergence of Copernican theory that the Earth revolves around the Sun in preference to the Ptolemaic theory that the Sun revolves around the Earth. This is but one example. There are many more.

The move between paradigms happens when an existing scientific paradigm cannot resolve an intellectual crisis either by effectively explaining the issue at hand or by deciding to 'put aside' the problem until more adequate observational or experimental tools are available. 'Paradigm wars' ensue in which two incommensurable views of the same problem compete with one another until the new paradigm supplants the old one. Kuhn suggested that the view that all science is underwritten by a common underlying practice is mythic. Objective knowledge is formed by the particular paradigm and cannot either be verified or falsified as if there were a 'resisting reality' in the way that Popper suggested. Our understanding of the world may become increasingly sophisticated and refined as we pass through different paradigms but it is doubtful, in Kuhn's view, if there has been any real progression towards understanding an ultimate truth. Rather, the result will be a plethora of different ways of understanding truth in the natural and social world. Just as Darwin exposed the reality that although a species will develop from one to another and diversify, so too will our intellectual sophistication. Plants, animals or ideas do not evolve towards anything. Kuhn's view of the science of natural phenomena has striking similarities to the development of post-structuralism in the social sciences (see below).

Empiricism, inductivism and hypothetico-deductivism have been widely used in the social sciences. Applied to empirical research with children and young people this implies that there are social or psychological facts that can be separated from values concerning children and young people. Hence we find that psychology as a social science has often relied upon experimental methods. B.F. Skinner (1904–90), the main proponent of behavourism, and Piaget (1896–1980) differed in the focus and content of their work but both used experiment to suggest that certain psychological 'facts' existed about how individuals learn or develop. Within the 'scientific paradigm' these 'facts' did not imply any particular moral outlook. Early sociologists, like Emile Durkheim, asserted that there were 'social facts'. By the study of 'social facts' sociologists could gain an understanding of the way in which society operated and 'controlled' human behaviour. He argued that individuals in society were constrained in their behaviour by collective ways of thinking, expressed in law, religion, the division of labour and social institutions. He used the phenomenon of suicide to demonstrate 'social facts', arguing that different social conditions produced different rates of suicide independently of the individual motivations of the people concerned. For example, suicide rates fell in times of war because society experienced a greater degree of integration, i.e. despite the problems citizens were more likely to feel they belonged and that there were shared goals to be achieved.

The structuralist paradigm(s)

The structuralist paradigm overlaps with the scientific paradigm. Certainly many structuralists would want to be considered as scientists. Some scientists would see some structuralists as holding hopelessly value-laden or unfalsifiable views, arguing that their 'facts' were determined by their values and theoretical conceptions rather than by objective reality. Since structuralism and science are to some extent interwoven, this section sets out the structuralist position (in so far as this can be coherently put) in order that the reader can contrast this with the scientific position. Arguably Marx and Durkheim selected 'facts', then empirically collected them to 'prove' or illustrate the conceptions with which they started. Some have argued that other structuralists (see below) like Chomsky, Piaget and Lévi-Strauss do exactly the same thing and thus they in their turn are not 'scientific'. Yet this 'fault', according to Thomas Kuhn (see above) is 'normal science' and is to be expected; values 'choose' which problems are to be addressed by scientists, values 'choose' which methods of investigation are to be chosen, values 'choose' which theories should be highlighted or used. Hence, the firm distinction between 'fact' and 'value' outlined earlier in this chapter which seemed to allow 'value-free' 'objective knowledge' seems less clear cut. What we shall do now is to illustrate four different structuralist accounts across different disciplines of empirical study: Sociology, Anthropology, Psychology and Linguistics. Despite the emergence of post-structuralism these illustrations retain viability as starting points for empirical research.

Sociology

Durkheim, a sociologist, theorised that all societies have a social structure made up of social institutions that perform functions analogous to those of the body. Each society had to have a manufacturing heart, a blood supply of trade, and a brain-like state. Societies had evolved by a social form of natural selection. The normal pattern within any society was social stability unless its social institutions were faulty in some way. Sociologists helped by informing relevant social institutions on how best to perform their functions; the goal of social science was to help maintain social order. Hence, empirical research might inform teachers about the social structures and 'social facts' influencing the education of children and young people.

Karl Marx was also a 'structuralist', arguing that society has a social structure based on social class. This led to conflict rather than the social harmony that Durkheim envisaged. Social classes created civil organisations for themselves through which they sought to win influence and control; their success led to the creation of the state, which held other class interests in check, permitting the ruling class to maintain wealth, status and continuing power. The institutions and structures thus created were not free from conflict. The dominant social class always had to coerce or persuade other social classes to live in accordance with its wishes and interests. The education system's role might be to provide skilled and passive labourers for a labour market favouring the best interests of employers (capitalists). Yet children and young people growing up to become members of the subordinate (working) class might not accept this passively. Like the class struggle in industry there will be a class struggle within the classroom and between teachers and their employers. Empirical research with children and young people might then demonstrate the existence and subtleties of class conflict in the classroom (Willis, 1977).

Anthropology, psychology and linguistics

The term 'structuralism' is used in anthropology, psychology and linguistics to assert the objective existence of universal *structures of mind*, as is apparent in the works of the anthropologist Claude Lévi-Strauss, the psychologist Jean Piaget and the linguist Noam Chomsky. However, these theorists differ as to what constitutes structures of mind. Nevertheless, the common link is through the early work of Saussure (1857–1913) who was interested in the structural properties of language. The structures were the relationships between *units*, i.e. the sound-units within a particular language, known as *phonemes* (there are 31 in English that build words) – and *rules* i.e. grammatical rules which link words. Such rules exist in all languages so are *universal* in human societies. Societies could be characterised in terms of similarities and differences between these rules. The rules themselves might emanate from the structure of the mind or brain.

Noam Chomsky argued that language was an innate human ability. He asserted that young children could construct an infinite number and variety of sentences as a result of listening to adults talking. He proposed that this implied a comprehension of the grammatical rules underlying ordinary sentences. Chomsky differentiated between the words and sounds we hear which he termed 'surface structures', and the mechanisms by which the underlying meaning of speech is understood, which he called 'deep structures'. All humans, including children and young people, form sentences by producing surface-structure words from deep-structure rules via sets of 'grammatical transformations'. According to Chomsky, these 'deep structural' rules are fundamentally similar in all languages. They correspond to innate, genetically transmitted universal mental structures in human beings.

The anthropologist Claude Lévi-Strauss applied this idea to the study of myth and ritual of various cultures throughout the world. Lévi-Strauss replaced Saussure's sound unit, the *phoneme*, with the *mytheme*, the unit within a myth or ritual. He argued that such units can be found in all cultural artefacts, myth, kinship and marriage patterns, literature, dance, any performing art or method of communication between humans. Communication involves a layering and comparing of classifications of what we perceive. The classifications are bound together with rules analogous to grammatical rules. Fundamental to this is the rule of binary opposition. Binary oppositions are embedded within language and reflect basic universal structures of mind; for example, good and evil, night and day, yin and yang, black and white, joy and sadness, conscious and unconscious, on and off, positive and negative, raw and cooked, male and female, mind and body, public and private, live and dead, nature and culture. We construct meanings from layering binary oppositions both in speech and cultural artefacts. Lévi-Strauss argued that we are *bricoleurs*; we are like 'odd job' men or women who put together makeshift constructions using binary oppositions to build the walls of the cultural 'house' that we live in. People might seem to differ according to culture but cultures are expressed through universally similar structures of mind.

> Verbal categories provide the mechanism through which *universal* structural characteristics of human brains are transformed into *universal* structural characteristics of human culture. (Leach, 1970: 38, quoted in Bottomore and Nisbet, 1979: 584)

The significance of this is that any human behaviour can be 'deconstructed' and its elements broken down into its constituent units and rules. This can be applied to children and young people, to their myths and rituals of 'growing up'; to their narratives of how they describe themselves and to the cultural products they form an audience for, e.g. the deconstruction of youth culture. Cultural phenomena that might seem bewilderingly complex can be deconstructed into their elements and better understood.

Jean Piaget identified himself as a 'structuralist'. His 'structure' was the *schema*. Immanuel Kant originally used the concept of the schema to break the stalemate between the empiricists, who argued that knowledge has its origins in the external world, and the rationalists, who argued that knowledge is a product of the mind. Piaget argued that schemas are interposed between *a priori* properties of the mind and *a posteriori* raw sensory data. According to Piaget, the early schemas of the child consist of biologically based reflexes that organise the child's interactions with the environment. Over time biological schemas allow adaptation to the environment. Further aspects of Piaget's account of child development are described in Chapter 11 of this book. Piaget argued that

> a structure is a system of transformations. In as much as it is a system and not a mere collection of elements and their properties, *these transformations involve laws* [i.e. rules]: the structure is preserved or enriched by the interplay of its transformation laws, which never yield results external to the system nor employ elements that are external to it. In short, the notion of structure is comprised by three key ideas: the idea of wholeness, the idea of transformation, and the idea of self-regulation. (Piaget, 1970: 5)

Durkheim, Marx, Chomsky, Lévi-Strauss and Piaget identified structures in quite different ways. Moreover, there are other significant theorists whom we have not mentioned who can be classified under the term 'structuralist'; e.g. Max Weber and Sigmund Freud. Yet there are general similarities: there is a unit, call it a phoneme, mytheme, social fact, social class. And there is a rule, call it grammar, binary opposition, organic harmony or class conflict. Empirical research is then used to demonstrate the reality of such structures and rules, and to describe the ways in which they have an impact on social and psychological life. In practice there are many different 'structures' that can be identified as having explanatory potential. There may be disagreement between structuralists about which structure should take explanatory precedence; cross-cutting that, there will be debates about whether certain structures have any material or actual existence. But the common theme is that a 'structure', whether social or mental, is important to explanation; these structures can be variously applied to empirical research with children and young people.

The interactionist paradigm

The structuralism of Durkheim and Marx related well to relatively settled if dynamic polities in Europe. The situation in the USA was entirely different. By the late nineteenth century the USA had a vast frontier and faced mass immigration from various nationalities, e.g. the Irish, Russian, Polish and Italian, as well as internal migration from the South northwards. Any existing notion of an American nation-state was under threat. Society seemed both geographically unbounded and in its urban centres bewilderingly diverse. How could these diverse cultures be reconciled with each other, never mind with the WASPish (White, Anglo-Saxon, Protestant) assumptions of the elite? Such were the primary concerns of academic sociology in the USA at the end of the nineteenth century, centred in the city of Chicago.

Out of these concerns a paradigm emerged which focused on *meanings* that individuals and groups attributed to their social circumstances as opposed to 'facts'. Influenced by evolutionary thought, sociologists like W.I. Thomas (1863–1947) and Robert E. Park (1864–1944) stressed that cultures were in conflict because they were in competition for space. Migrations had occurred throughout history and had resulted in new and repeated cultural conflict. Nevertheless the wealth created by industrial society and democratic states fashioned a capacity to contain and possibly eliminate conflicts based on cultural artefacts like race, religion or other traditional cultural forms. Rational communication – *interaction* – was to provide the bridge between cultures. But how can traditional cultures be moved towards 'rationality'?

Following William James (1842–1910), Park argued that we all share 'a certain blindness' about each other produced by our cultural 'masks'. When we present ourselves to each other we 'wear' the histories and meanings of the cultural groups to which we belong rather than our individual, private 'selves'. We are often unaware of our own or other cultural masks; we assume that the person, culture and cultural group to which a person belongs is identical. This process occurs out of evolutionary necessity in hazardous contexts; historically we have relied on our cultural group for individual survival. Park suggested that by the second half of the nineteenth century in the USA at least this requirement had been made potentially redundant. Modern social circumstances afforded opportunities for members of different cultural groups to meet and exchange views as individual strangers. Processes of migration, urbanisation and occupational specialisation isolated persons from their natal cultures and created opportunities for individuals to associate and rationally communicate without their 'masks'.

Yet, might not these new opportunities lead to 'throwing the baby out with the bathwater'? If people were deprived somehow of their original culture they would lose their social, intellectual and moral compass. The answer therefore was the empirical investigation of each other's 'masks' and their meanings to inform communication between 'individual strangers'. Research had to go beyond the assertion of cultural conflict in order to illustrate the meaning of particular conflicts. This could only be done empirically, e.g. W.I. Thomas's *Polish Peasant in Europe and America* (Thomas, 1995, originally published between 1918 and 1920).

These considerations were echoed in the social psychology of George Herbert Mead (1863–1931). He argued that 'mind' and 'self' emerged out of social processes of communication between people. He resisted ideas of causality which suggested that the environment or biology determined behaviour, for example, any structuralism. Rather we had to comprehend individual *perspectives* within social situations.

> Even when we consider only sense data, the object is clearly a function of the whole situation whose perspective is determined by the individual. There are peculiarities in the objects which depend upon the individual as an organism and the spatio-temporal position of the individual. It is one of the important results of the modern doctrine of relativity that we are forced to recognize that we cannot account for these peculiarities by stating the individual in terms of his environment. (Mead, 1938: 224)

During the twentieth century relative affluence changed the nature of sociological inquiry in the USA. If it was important to discover the perspectives and meanings behind the mask of national and ethnic culture how much more so between different *generations* of Americans? The concept of the 'generation gap' emerged. Hence studies of youth subcultures materialised, perhaps led by the 'social problems' like rock and roll, innovative sectarian religions or anti-Vietnam-War protest which had captured the imagination of the young to the consternation of the old. Central to this interpretation of meaning in social interaction, or *symbolic interactionism*, was the concern for the freedom of action of the individual within his/her cultural context. The extent to which a culture can control and coerce individuals by defining what it means to be 'normal' became very important. For example, Erving Goffman in a series of papers and books alerted us to the notion of a 'total institution'. Total institutions create rules of behaviour that are difficult to escape. He posed as an example the mental asylum.

Goffman denied any psychiatric or psychological explanation of non-normal behaviour which featured psychoses, personality disorders, or similar. Rather he suggested that 'madness', i.e. 'non-normal behaviour', existed because some people simply did not want to abide by traditional cultural rules. Goffman viewed mental illness as a 'social stigma' or 'stereotype' rather than as a material disease. Even in total institutions – asylums, concentration camps, private boarding schools, etc. which attempt to define and control the meaning of normal behaviour in leisure, work and private spaces – there is always room for individual expression of meaning. Goffman chose the extreme example of mental asylums to argue that individuals can still escape the (oppressive) constraints of their culture and 'reinvent' themselves. But the very existence of rules or norms of behaviour means that we can stray from the norm or be accused of straying and become outcast. Empirical research into, for example, 'teen culture' can illustrate particular norms and meanings within such cultures, and demonstrate means of promoting, policing and punishing in accordance with such norms.

This view was enhanced by the work of Howard Becker (1928—) who contended that

> Social groups create deviance by making the rules whose infraction constitutes deviance and by applying those rules to particular people and labelling them as outsiders. From this point of view, deviance is *not* a quality of the act the person commits but rather a consequence of the application by others of rules or sanctions to an 'offender'. The deviant is one to whom that label has successfully been applied; deviant behaviour is behaviour that people so label. (Becker, 1963: 9)

Becker's viewpoint has been influential in criminology but also in education, where he argued that teachers 'labelled' children. The labels given to children tended to be 'self-fulfilling prophecies' (Hargreaves, 1967; Rosenthal and Jacobson, 1968): that is, the idea that by predicting that something will happen we unconsciously take steps to ensure that it will happen. A pupil may somehow become stereotyped as 'stupid' irrespective of his/her cognitive ability; teachers will be less motivated towards such a pupil and consequently the pupil will tend to fail and feel a failure. 'Intelligence' can be attributed in much the same way with the opposite results. Empirical research becomes a process of collecting 'qualitative data' that highlights implicit values and ethical judgements which create stereotypes.

Symbolic interactionism may be credited with laying the seedbed of ideas concerning the emergence of the 'new sociology of childhood' in the 1990s. In the late 1970s, Norman Denzin, a symbolic interactionist opened up the sociological study of childhood as a new venture in sociology. He argued:

> Children must be viewed as historical, cultural, political, economic, and social productions. There is nothing intrinsic to the object called 'child' that makes that object more or less 'childlike'. Accordingly, children as they are known in current

social and psychological theory may in fact be historical and cultural products of the nineteenth and twentieth centuries. (Denzin, 1977: 2)

In effect, this follows on from Becker. With Becker there was nothing 'intrinsic' to being a criminal. With Goffman there was nothing 'intrinsic' to being mentally ill. If deviance is a label, simply being a child is also a label – though not a pejorative one. While recognising the contribution of Piaget, Denzin sought to reverse the normal polarity of the study of children, i.e. how do children become adults?

> My intentions are to reverse the usual scheme of sociological analysis, which typi-
> cally asks how young children become adult like. Rather, I shall ask how it is that
> children do not act adult like. (Denzin, 1977: 58)

Such thoughts tend to presage concerns expressed by a variety of authors in the 1990s. The concern of symbolic interactionists to deny 'intrinsic' qualities is echoed in the ideas which emerged in the late twentieth century, variously known as post-structuralism, post-modernism and social constructionism. Whether these terms actually constitute a paradigm is open to debate; they tend to celebrate different levels of truth rather than attempt to clarify a particular method to arrive at a definite truth.

The post-structuralist and social constructionist paradigm(s)

> Traditional psychology looks for explanations of social phenomena inside the
> person, for example by hypothesising the existence of attitudes, motivations, cogni-
> tions and so on. These entities are held to be responsible for what individual
> people do and say, as well as for wider social phenomena such as prejudice and
> delinquency. Sociology has traditionally countered this with the view that it is
> social structures (such as the economy, or the major institutions such as marriage
> and the family) that give rise to the social phenomena that we see. Social con-
> structionism rejects both of these positions, and regards as the proper focus of our
> enquiry the social practices engaged in by people, and their interactions with each
> other. Explanations are to be found neither in the individual psyche nor in social
> structures, but in the interactive processes that take place routinely between
> people. (Burr, 1995: 7–8)

There are affinities between the interactionist and post-structural para-
digms. Both focus on meaning and the use of language. Post-structuralism tends to assert that all knowledge is contingent, that is, located within the communication shared by people. We construct knowledge together, i.e. socially in groups. Hence what we know is *socially constructed*. This is also referred to as 'discourse'. No knowledge exists outside of socially constructed discourses. Discourses define what can be described as a 'fact', what is worth knowing about and how it can be known. Science is as much

a discourse as any other communication between people and thus cannot be 'value-free' – so there are affinities between this view and Kuhn's scientific paradigms.

Post-structuralism is linked with post-modernism. It has been argued that 'modernism' is a trend in thought and practice emergent since the Enlightenment which suggested that progress was possible through the powers of (1) *reason* over ignorance; (2) *order* over disorder; (3) *science* over superstition. Modernity was revolutionary in relation to what had gone before. However, at the end of the twentieth century modernist and structuralist accounts were questioned. The modern world had brought the era of industrial capitalism and scientific thinking but it had also brought in the world of Auschwitz, of the possibility of nuclear war, the horrors of Nazism and Stalinism, of neo-colonialism, Eurocentrism, racism, pollution, global climate change and Third World hunger. Progress was doubted and the salience and robustness of the modernist 'powers' doubted too. There is the sneaking suspicion that the horrors of modern times were associated with its underpinning ideas. The rule of reason, order and science created a *powerful illusion* of freedom and progress that obscured their devastating effects. Our illusions have therefore to be 'deconstructed' (Lyotard, 1984; Foucault and Rabinow, 1984; Deleuze, 1988).

Cultural workers, artists in general and social analysts have to go beyond modernism into post-modernism/post-structuralism. Whereas social constructs like 'sexuality', 'gender', 'nation', 'race', 'ethnicity', 'poverty', 'child development', 'childhood', 'youth', 'child abuse', 'schizophrenia' and 'depression' at one time seemed quite stable, scientific or objective they are now to be perceived as fluid. In post-modernism, 'identity is not unitary or essential, it is fluid or shifting, fed by multiple sources and taking multiple forms' (Kumar, 1997: 98; see also Bell, 1973; Hall, 1996).

Post-structuralism and social constructionism suggest that empirical research aimed at discovering the essential 'X-factor' 'behind' an event, e.g. criminal behaviour, as caused either by genes or by poverty, is misguided. Instead empirical research ought to be concerned with collecting and analysing discourse in terms of its content, authorship, authority, audience and goals (Worral, 1990: 8). This could be at the level of small actual or virtual networks or large scale discourses that carry across the whole of society. Any analysis of such data is capable of multiple readings, multiple truths. Jacques Derrida (1930—) suggested that all discourse is ambiguous, so a final and complete interpretation is impossible.

The point of all this is to reveal which discourses are more powerful in their context, even if the context is capable of bearing more than one meaning. 'The concept of power is vital to discourse analysis by way of the theoretical connection between the production of discourses and the exercise of power' (Punch, 1998: 227). This has relevance to empirical research with children and young people in so far as social constructs such as 'children', 'childhood', 'child development' and 'young people' are part of discourses which need to be unpicked to reveal the nature of how power is exercised.

At the large scale level this is important in terms of describing if and how children are subordinated to adults. Beyond this, empirical research with children and young people can reveal how they in turn create and use discourses in relation to adults or in relation to other children and young people. The focus of empirical research is then about how children and young people achieve 'agency'; that is, agency refers to the ability of a social actor to engage in the process of construction of meaning or identity in such a way as to influence the form that that meaning or identity takes.

Concluding remarks

This chapter has outlined a number of current paradigms of empirical research. The version of empiricism presented here may be regarded as naïve; certainly empiricists responded to the challenge posed by falsificationism, and falsificationism has responded to Kuhn's ideas. Structuralism in its various forms still has its adherents despite post-structuralism and post-modernism. We have not tried to argue a case for preferring one paradigm over another. Instead this chapter serves to introduce intending researchers to some of the issues involved. This should assist in framing research questions. The most vital of these is to consider what kind of question your question is. Do you want to engage in discovery and exploration by counting or collecting facts in order to make generalisations? Do you want to assess or test what 'causes' a social or psychological event? Do you want to illustrate how class, race or gender impacts upon individuals or groups? Do you want intellectual empathy with different individual or cultural perspectives? Do you want to understand how the interests of individuals and groups can be made powerfully manifest by the use of language through discourse? The data required to answer each of these kinds of questions will differ. Maybe your 'view of the world' impacts on the type of question you want to ask as does the nature of what you wish to study. Being aware of the different paradigms and philosophies of research helps us to be clear about what kind of data we want, and the strength of that data in relation to the paradigm it is part of.

References

Becker, H.S. (1963) *Outsiders*, New York, Free Press.
Bell, D. (1973) *The Coming of Post-Industrial Society*, London, Heinemann.
Bottomore, T. and Nisbet, R. (1979) 'Structuralism', in Tom Bottomore and Robert Nisbet (eds), *A History of Sociological Analysis*, London, Heinemann.
Burr, V. (1995) *An Introduction to Social Constructionism*. London, Routledge.
Burton, D. (ed.) (2000) *Research Training for Social Scientists*, London, Sage.
Chalmers, A.F. (1978) *What Is This Thing Called Science?* Open University Press.

Chalmers, A.F. (1999) *What Is This Thing Called Science?* 3rd edn, Buckingham, Open University.

Dawkins, R. (1994) 'The Moon is not a calabash', *Times Education Supplement*, 30/09/94, pp. 17–18.

Deleuze, G. (1988) *Foucault*, London, Athlone.

Denzin, N. (1977) *Childhood Socialization: Studies in the Development of Language, Social Behaviour, and Identity*, San Francisco, Jossey-Bass.

Derrida, J. (1974) *Of Grammatology*, Baltimore, Johns Hopkins University Press.

Derrida, J. (1978) *Writing and Difference*, Chicago, University of Chicago Press.

Derrida, J. (1981) *Dissemination*, Chicago, University of Chicago Press.

Foucault, M. and Rabinow, P. (1984) *The Foucault Reader*, New York, Pantheon Books.

Fraser, A.C. (1959) *John Locke: An Essay Concerning Human Understanding*, New York, Dover.

Goffman, E. (1988) *Asylums: Essays on the Social Situation of Mental Patients and Other Inmates*, Harmondsworth Penguin Social Sciences. First published 1961.

Hall, S. (1996) 'The meaning of new times', in D. Morley and K-H. Chen (eds), *Stuart Hall: Critical Dialogues in Cultural Studies*, London, Routledge.

Hargreaves, D.H. (1967) *Social Relations in a Secondary School*, London, Routledge and Kegan Paul.

Hughes, J. (1990) *The Philosophy of Social Research*, 2nd edn, London, Longman.

Kuhn, T.S. (1996) *The Structure of Scientific Revolutions*, Chicago, University of Chicago Press. First published 1962.

Kumar, K. (1997) 'The post-modern condition', in A.H. Halsey, H. Lauder, P. Brown and A.S. Wells (eds), *Education: Culture, Economy, and Society*, Oxford, Oxford University Press.

Leach, E. (1970) *Claude Lévi-Strauss*, New York, Viking Press; London, Fontana.

Lyotard, J.-F. (1984) *The Postmodern Condition: A Report on Knowledge*, Manchester, Manchester University Press.

May, T. (2001) *Social Research: Issues, Methods and Process*, Buckingham, Open University Press.

Mead, G.H. (1934) *Mind, Self and Society*, Chicago, University of Chicago Press.

Mead, G.H. (1938) *Philosophy of the Act*, Chicago, University of Chicago Press.

Piaget, J. (1965) *Etudes Sociologiques*, Geneva, Librairie Droz.

Piaget, J. (1970) *Structuralism*, New York, Basic Books.

Popper, K.R. (1979) *Objective Knowledge: An Evolutionary Approach*, Oxford, Oxford University Press.

Punch, K.F. (1998) *Introduction to Social Research*, London, Sage.

Robson, C. (2002) *Real World Research*, Oxford, Blackwell.

Rosenthal, R. and Jacobson, L. (1968) *Pygmalion in the Classroom*, New York, Rinehart and Winston.

Thomas, W.I. (1995) *The Polish Peasant in Europe and America: A Classic Work in Immigration*, (ed.) Eli Zaretsky, Urbana, University of Illinois Press (November). First published 1918–20.

von Wright, G.H. (1971) *Explanation and Understanding*, London, Routledge.

Willis, P. (1977) *Learning to Labour: How Working Class Kids Get Working Class Jobs*, Farnborough, Saxon House.

Worral, A. (1990) *Offending Women*, London, Routledge.

SECTION 2 RESEARCH RELATIONS

6 Power
CHRIS ROBINSON AND MARY KELLETT

In 2002 the Scottish Parliament was considering legislation to prohibit the smacking of children. Research into the views of children on smacking found that over 90 per cent of those who took part were opposed to smacking (Scottish Executive, 2002). However the adults of Scotland, in the main, did not support a ban on smacking and the proposal was dropped from the legislation in 2003. The power of adult views took precedence.

As Taylor (2000: 21) noted, it is adults who write about and debate the issues of rights for children and this might be seen as indicative of the power relations which confine children to subordinate roles in their societies. Power is a complex subject and is referred to in many contexts in other chapters in this book. Here, however, the main focus is on power relations in *research* with children and young people. We cannot begin to examine this dimension unless we have an understanding of power relationships between adults and children in society generally. Therefore an important part of this chapter discusses theoretical frameworks of power and how these relate to research with children and young people. The contribution of feminisms, in all their different forms, points us to the power differentials around gender in wider society and reflected within the family. The rethinking of power by Foucault and others, as having multiple forms and micro levels, is important in thinking about researching children's lives. We also explore how researchers' views about child status affect notions of power relations and how this impacts on the research process. Specific issues of age, competence, knowledge and experience are examined and generational factors discussed. Research examples are drawn upon to illustrate the contextual power conflicts that are at work. Chapter 14 of this book concentrates on power relations and research in the majority world and therefore in this chapter we will be looking in particular at the minority world. We begin by looking at a definition of power.

What is power? 'The ability of individuals or groups to make their own concerns count, even when others resist. Power sometimes involves the direct use of force, but is almost always accompanied by the development of ideas (ideologies) which justify the actions of the powerful' (Giddens, 1995: 54). Power then is not just about force but the creation of knowledge. As the opening sentences of this chapter show, children's knowledge can be disregarded and they can still be controlled by force, however benevolently that may be constructed by adults. Through communication we are able to perceive and exercise power.

> The freedom to communicate will depend not only on the availability of appropriate communication mechanisms and sensitive interpretation, but also on the power relations in the exchange and attitudes established over time. (Detheridge, 2000: 114)

Detheridge was writing about research with children with severe learning difficulties, but the principles she addresses apply to all research.

Theories of power

We begin this section by recognising, briefly, the contribution of sociological thinking to understanding power in research with children and young people. The term 'sociology' has no single orthodoxy, paradigm or style of research but the aim remains to try to explain the role of power in people's lives, how society works and order is achieved. Until quite recently, however, such explanations were focused on the world of men, with little regard for the worlds of women and even less the worlds of children (Anderson, 1983; Abbott and Wallace, 1990; Abbott, 2000). Feminists were critical of the portrayal of the family as 'natural' and unchanging (e.g. Barrett and McIntosh, 1982; Grant, 1993; Oakley 1980; Oakley and Williams, 1994). There were widespread debates within and between feminists about the role and expectations of the family. Black feminists were very critical of white feminists of all persuasions, arguing that the paradox of the black experience had been ignored. 'On certain dimensions Black women may more closely resemble Black men; on others white women; and on still others Black women may stand apart from both groups. Black women's both/and conceptual orientation, the act of being simultaneously a member of a group and yet standing apart from it, forms an integral part of Black women's consciousness' (Hill Collins, 1997: 200).

Feminist approaches have criticised sociology both for theorising in male terms and for developing methods that reinforced power relations within society (e.g. Abbott and Wallace, 1990; Reinharz, 1992; Farganis, 1994). There are many variants of feminism, which cannot even be glimpsed within this one chapter, but a key theme in all is that gender is central in the construction and framing of knowledge.

> Feminist approaches are bound together by the recognition of the central role that gender plays in the lives of people. Its contribution is a set of writings that start from the world as women see it and its objective is to bring to the fore a perspective that has been missing. (Farganis, 1994: 8)

Feminism has increasingly, since the 1980s, developed from 'working on women' to 'theorising gender' (Kemp and Squires, 1997: 10), recognising that any change in the status of women will affect men, and the concept of 'masculinities' enables the exploration of different and oppressed forms of masculinity. The 1980s witnessed growing concern about and research into the lives of men, the complexity of power and oppression and that there has been a departure from polarised assumptions that 'all men' oppress 'all women'. These developments are important to us when we consider research with boys and girls and young men and women, for example the influence of the concept of 'masculinities' in research with young men. Wright et al. (1998: 243) researched 'masculinised discourses of African Caribbean youth within education' and acknowledged the importance of feminist researchers' recognition of the reproduction of gender divisions within education; this work highlighted and helped to address the educational performances of young women in school. It also led to the development of work that shows how schools contribute to the formation of varied male identities. As we will be discussing later in this chapter, much research with children and young people takes place in the 'public' sphere of school.

Important to us in thinking about power in the lives of children and young people is the concept of public and private aspects of life and the family. A number of feminist writers have discussed these topics and we draw upon the work of Bell and Ribbens (1995) and Ribbens and Edwards (1998). They suggest that the concepts are relevant for understanding the divisions within the lives of people in Western society, not just within the labour market, but in terms of the meanings which men and women accord the notion of public and private. Collins (1990) has recognised the significance not only of gender to these concepts, but also of race and class. Again these are complex terms, which are difficult to deal with briefly, but core elements can contribute to our thinking about the position of children, who have limited power within the private area of family life. Studies of children in the home are often reliant on reports by their parents or carers: for example Dosanjh and Gurman (1998) looked at Punjabi childrearing practices through the eyes of parents. Increasingly however research is conducted with children and young people and their views are sought directly, for example in the work of Atkin, Ahmad and Jones (2001) into how young South Asian deaf people negotiate relationships and identities and work by Barker (1997) on British Asian girls' multiple identities.

The concepts of public and private are not easy to define. It is too simplistic to suggest that the public sphere is only male and the private is only female, but this distinction has some purchase nonetheless. For example feminist geographers (e.g. Katz and Monk, 1993) have deployed the terms in contributing to understanding women and girls' oppression. Fear by women and girls of being in public places is constructed in such a way that their freedom is restricted and violence within the home is ignored. These concepts are relevant in understanding the different experiences of boys and girls and in ensuring that research with children and young people takes into account the impact of gender, race and disability in offering different world views of the participants in research.

Generational issues

Power relations in child research are reinforced by more general cultural notions that exist between children and adults in society at large. Generational issues feature prominently in this respect. Alanen (1992) maintains that there is a form of 'generational ordering' at work in the way children are contained in the 'private' world of the home and the family and excluded from the 'public' world of politics and economics. Mayall (2000: 120) argues that the asymmetrical power relationship of childhood versus adulthood is a principle of social organisation:

> Adults have divided up the social order into two major groups – adults and children, with specific conditions surrounding the lives of each group: provisions, constraints and requirements, laws, rights, responsibilities and privileges. Thus, just as the concept of gender has been key to understanding women's relationships to the social order, so the concept of generation is key to understanding childhood. This means that the adult researcher who wishes to research with children must confront generational issues.

Mayall was faced with these kinds of generational issues in her study on child health care (1996). When trying to elicit information about children's views, even at the most informal level, Mayall was aware of the power dynamics at work, particularly in the authoritarian context of a school classroom. She attempted to dilute this by interviewing children with a friend of their choosing, 'At ease with each other, and thereby, perhaps, more confident with the third, adult participant' (Mayall, 2000: 123) and by allowing children to take control of the conversation agendas. But no measure could entirely bridge the pupils' innate sense of power differential across the generation gap.

One of the obstacles in the path of participatory research with children is the use of age as a delineating factor in competence. This legacy from the dominant period of developmental psychology is being robustly challenged (Woodhead and Faulkner, 2000) and opening up the debate about social experience being a more reliable marker of maturity and competence (Solberg, 1996; Alderson, 2000; Christensen and Prout, 2002). Nor is age necessarily a barrier to participation in terms of methodology, as has been demonstrated by Clark's (2004) imaginative 'Mosaic' approach where very young children actively participate in data collection.

A factor that sustains unequal adult–child power relations is a belief that adults have superior knowledge. Undoubtedly this is the case in some areas of life but with regard to childhood – in the sense of what it is like to be a child – then it is children who have the superior knowledge, as Mayall (2000: 122) states,

> I want to acquire from them (children) their own unique knowledge and assessment of what it means to be a child; for though I can remember some things

about being a child, I may have forgotten much, and childhoods may vary and have probably changed over the years since I was a child.

Anthropological participant observation such as that undertaken by Mandell (1991) where the researcher tries to blend into children's worlds in the 'least-adult' role can be hard to sustain (see Thorne, 1993). Even though the researcher attempts to minimise power relations by trying to be 'one of them', she cannot easily dispel the central adult characteristic of having power over children (Mayall, 2000). Cross (2002) in her research with school children in Jamaica and Scotland writes about the value of relating to the children in different contexts which in themselves altered the power relations between herself as a researcher and the children. Working in Jamaica, Cross discussed in depth how she approached her research:

> my analysis was one of negotiating and defining differences through play and work. Children's relative power within these activities was often highlighted by conflicts that arose during these activities. We did not discuss socio-economic theory; we did discuss its more relevant situated manifestation as experienced in bullying and school punishment. The terms of engagement were through popular icons, Bounty Killer not Giddens. (2002: 99)

Cross recognises the importance of the community of children and the power relations between them.

Researchers' perspectives on children

The ways in which researchers view children are pivotal to the power relations that ensue between researcher and participant. Christensen and Prout (2002: 480) outline four ways that children and childhood have been identified in research: the child as object, the child as subject, the child as social actor and the child as participant/co-researcher.

The first of these research approaches views children and young people as objects acted upon by others rather than social actors in their own right. From this perspective, children and young people are seen as dependent, incompetent and not able to deal appropriately with information. They have to be 'protected' by caring adults who take on the role of 'interpreters' of their lives. This orientation of research relies heavily on adult accounts and adult perspectives. The research process all but circumvents the children themselves, denying them the competence to understand, give consent or contribute to the research. In her work on child abuse Kitzinger (2000) has noted that this image of children as needing protection denies children access to knowledge and power and can actually increase their vulnerability to abuse.

The second viewpoint positions children as subjects, putting them more into the foreground of the research process and orienting this towards a child-centred perspective. However, although the appropriateness of involving children and young people is acknowledged it is tempered by judgements about their social maturity and cognitive ability. Adult researchers exert power in determining whom to include and exclude (e.g. they may include only children older than a certain age, and exclude those with learning difficulties) and choose whether to adopt methodologies to accommodate varying levels of maturity and competence. Begley (2000) notes that researchers rarely talk directly with children with Down's Syndrome, and that a failure to ask people with learning difficulties for their views continues to be common practice.

In the third perspective of children as social actors they 'act, take part in, change and become changed by the social and cultural world they live in' (Christensen and Prout, 2002: 481). The concept of this research perspective is of children having an autonomous status (Thorne, 1993; Cosaro, 1997) in the sense of them being viewed as social actors in their own right rather than 'parts' of an 'other' such as part of a family, part of a school, etc. This research approach does not necessarily make a distinction between adults and children and there is no automatic assumption that methodologies will need to be adapted according to age or that different ethical standards will apply.

The fourth researcher perspective is concerned with children having an active participant role in the process of the research (Thomas and O'Kane, 1998; Clark, 2004) building on the UN *Convention on the Rights of the Child* (General Assembly, 1989) recommendation that children should be informed, involved and consulted about all activities that affect their lives – including research. Increasingly, this mode of active participation is developing into a quasi-partnership of children as co-researchers. Here, the balance of power between adults and children can be volatile and changeable. A crucial aspect is the degree to which adults share (or hold back) knowledge and control. Hart (1992) uses the metaphor of rungs on a ladder to illustrate different levels of children's involvement. On the bottom rung is the 'pretence of shared work' (Alderson, 2000) characterised by manipulation and tokenism.

Some research examples are genuinely empowering for the participant children. One such example is the Participation and Education Group Project (1998) where young people – some as young as eight years old – were involved in investigating how unhealthy schools can be. They drew up the agenda and also chaired the planning meeting (in which they politely reminded adults not to talk down to children nor interrupt them when they were speaking!) Howarth's report (1997) about Bangladeshi teenagers researching the play and leisure needs of Bangladeshi children in Camden carries a similar message of active participation and genuine power sharing. Here, the young researchers did an audit of play provision and interviewed 83 children, their parents, community workers and head teachers. They were able to analyse why so few children used the play facilities and to recommend how to make them safer and more attractive.

The transition from viewing children as objects to viewing them as social actors is not simply a matter of ideological reflection, it has a real impact on the conduct of research practice – on the initial choice of topic, the nature of design and type of methodology. There is an imperative to engage with children at an active rather than a passive level, what Christensen (1999) refers to as 'cultures of communication'. Otherwise child and childhood researchers are vulnerable to criticisms similarly levelled by other margin-alised groups – e.g. minority ethnic communities and disabled people – about not adequately engaging with the social culture of those groups.

The regulation of childhood

Children and young people, as discussed in Chapter 3, are frequently thought to require surveillance. The nature of surveillance and control was important in different ways to Donzelot and Foucault. Both identified families and children as being subject to state 'guidance'. Foucault (1980) argued that childhood became the nursery of the population to come and was therefore identified as requiring regulation and surveillance.

Foucault has written extensively about power and developed a meaning of the term which does not translate easily from French. The term in English includes a range of meanings, including conspiracy. In keeping with the post-modern tradition Foucault rejected the notion that one single theory could explain the distribution of power. His work was complex, developing and changing throughout his career and in this section we are only glimps-ing aspects of it. He never claimed that his work constituted a conceptual whole; rather he referred to it as offering a set of propositions. Foucault sought to answer a series of questions about how power is exercised. He proposed to identify a threefold process by which people become subjects: firstly, through the objectifying sciences, such as biology and economics, secondly, by binary divisions into good and bad, and thirdly by considering how people become created or create themselves as subjects. He opened up the possibility of thinking about power at different levels and argued that it was most effective when it was undetected. His argument that power must be studied from the 'bottom up' is relevant to considering research into the experiences of children and young people. At a macro level he argued that from the sixteenth century a new concept of governmentality was developed which led to techniques of individualisation. At this level power is deployed to control those who pose a risk to society. Kendall and Wickham (1996) suggested that 'therapy' constitutes government at an interpersonal level. At the micro level, Foucault (1982) referred to 'agonism', the state of permanent provocation between those with power and those they are seeking to influence and control.

An ascending analysis, Foucault argued, showed how the mechanisms of power at the micro level of society have become part of the dominant methods of power relations. Foucault believed that by paying close atten-tion to the detail of practices, the sources of power and the discourses through which they were expressed could tell us about the way power could be exercised. For example a study of 1960s child welfare practices in the west of Scotland (Robinson, 2002) which looked at the records of intervention into the lives of children from poor working class families and children from travelling families found different discourses of the acceptability of parental standards of care. Working class children who were missing from home for long periods were deemed to have 'run away from home', indicating concern about what was happening at home or suggesting that the child was becoming unruly and therefore a potential reason for intervention by those in authority. Travelling children who were away from home for long periods were described as 'wandering from home' and this was seen as a 'normal' part of their childhood experience and rarely a cause by itself for professional intervention.

Foucault did not develop an extensive analysis of gender in his work on power and oppressed groups. He recognised the uneven distribution of power and his analysis encompassed different ways in which power could be exercised. Foucault's work was never explicitly feminist. For some feminists, he has offered new ways of thinking about how women are controlled within a patriarchal system.

Child abuse

We cannot discuss issues of power relations in research with children and young people without examining the important subject of child abuse and the exercise of adult power in this area. The failure of the recognition of gender as central to understanding why abuse occurs was evident in early approaches to child abuse. Early studies tended to look for factors in the family or in the personality of the child, 'The child can himself trigger off or provoke some of the responses that subsequently lead to what can be severe physical abuse' (Bentovim and Boston, 1987: 60). The critique of patriarchal approaches to child sexual abuse arose in considerable part from feminist redefinitions of the 'family'. Later studies recognised the powerlessness of children within the family situation and researchers began to talk to children directly about their experiences of the helping systems (Butler and Williamson, 1994; Farmer and Owen, 1995; Farmer and Boushel, 1999). Westcott (1998) recognised that nowhere are the ethical and practical dilemmas of research so clearly highlighted as in this area. She contrasted her approach to children 'opting in' rather than 'opting out', noting that the power imbalance between the researcher and the child limits the child's capacity to give or withhold informed consent.

Morris (1998) in her research with young disabled people who are cared for away from home describes how the research was undertaken by researchers who were themselves disabled and shared a disability rights perspective. The project was advised by a reference group of young people who had experienced living away from home. The study is presented in a way that enables the young people's voices to be heard. For example Maeve's account of being taken into care because of physical abuse.

I was a bit frightened you know, a bit

I was a bit sad. And a little bit unhappy and a bit upset. Because I

Was away from home, because of my dad.

Can't remember what they said to me.

I was frightened a bit upset.

I ran away once when I was 15. I had to go to the police station.

I went to my mum's house. And got told off a bit.

Morris's study highlights the lack of attention given to the views of young people, often about major decisions in their lives, such as moving to another unit or going home to live.

Hendrick (1998) concluded that the 'contemporary child' had been recognised increasingly as a person with needs and wishes, but that since the murder of James Bulger in 1993 public and legal attitudes towards children have hardened. Child abuse inquiries from Maria Colwell in 1975 and Jasmine Beckford in 1985 to that of Victoria Climbie in 2003 comment critically on the unwillingness of adults to actually talk to children. 'To begin with a cruel paradox: in spite of all the care and concern, the easiest thing to do in child abuse work is to lose the child's perspective' (Moore 1985: 1). Talking to children about their views and feelings is often still not part of adult discourses. Access to children's views has been addressed in some studies of child protection summarised by Gough (1995) with the conclusion that children's views are rarely taken seriously. There is little evidence to suggest that this has changed since Gough's study. Recent studies of children's experience of child sexual abuse (e.g. Parton and Wattam, 1999) found that abused children were very concerned for their families and were anxious not to be the cause of the family breaking up.

The contribution of Roland Summit's (1984) work to understanding this reluctance has concentrated on what he called 'the reluctant discovery' of child sexual abuse and why it is so difficult for abused children to be heard.

If adult society can learn to believe in the reality of child sexual abuse, there is opportunity for unprecedented advances in the prevention and treatment of emotional pain and dysfunction. If adults cannot face the reality of incestuous abuse, then women and children will continue to be stigmatised by the terrors of their own helpless silence. (Summit, 1984: 167)

It has to be said that some aspects of Summit's work have been criticised (see for instance Hill at http://users.cybercity.dk/~ccc44406/smwane/

Antipodes.html last accessed 26/08/2003), although his work on 'adocentrism' has been influential in thinking about the powerlessness of children.

> The victim of child sexual abuse faces disbelief, retaliation, and revictimisation at each level of disclosure within the world of adults. It is not only the court and the community of men that are so incredulous of sexually exploited children. The basic reason for disbelief is 'adocentrism', the unswerving and unquestioned allegiance to adult values. All adults, male and female, tend to align themselves in an impenetrable bastion against any threat that adult priorities and self-comfort must yield to the needs of children. (Summit, 1984: 179)

'Adocentrism' has at its root the power of adult society, male and female. Summit recognises the differential power structure and acknowledges the lack of power of many women. However, the term remains at a general level. 'Adult values' are not defined precisely, and how 'allegiance' to them is sustained was not developed. Summit's concept is limited by its inclusiveness. Nevertheless, Summit's work can alert us to the power relations which exist between adults and children and how these impact not just on what is researched but on how it is conducted and how the findings are disseminated.

The ' rediscovery' of child sexual abuse was and is still in some respects resisted and the 1980s saw wide-ranging literature in North America and Western Europe on the causes of abuse and methods of treatment.

> The increasing awareness of child sexual abuse among professionals has its origin in two related but very different sources. The first is the growing children's rights movement which in the historic context of the human rights movement is following the women's rights movements. The second source is the increasing knowledge and concern about child health and child mental health. (Furniss, 1995: 4)

The increasing recognition of abuse of boys and that some abusers are women (Elliott, 1997) undermines a concept of abuse as endured only by females. Children are structurally dependent and it is important to sustain an intergenerational perspective. The fate of children who are not believed when they seek to communicate their abuse is frequently discussed within the literature. As Furniss (1995) noted, not only do their families disbelieve them, but also entire legal codes are built on unsubstantiated opinion that children are less reliable witnesses than adults. Kitzinger (2000) recognises the tensions and contradictions in the study of abused children and stresses the importance of recognising and questioning the social construction of childhood.

Studies of working with abused children have increasingly examined and discussed the role of the power of the researcher and sought to ensure that children are not further disempowered by the research experience.

Devine (2002: 307) maintains that children's social positioning is an active process that is continually evolving in the light of expectations and evaluations:

With regard to children's citizenship, where adult – child, teacher – pupil relations are framed in terms of voice, belonging and active participation, children will be empowered to define and understand themselves as individuals with the capacity to act and exercise their voice in a meaningful manner on matters of concern to them.

Research relations in context

In this final section we examine the effect of location and context on power relations in child research. We focus on the context of school for three reasons. Firstly, children in the minority world spend a large proportion of their childhood at school. Secondly, a great deal of child research is undertaken in school locations and thirdly, school is a context where the adult–child power imbalance is particularly acute. Citizenship is a compulsory curriculum subject for some ages of pupils in England and Wales. Current discourse about citizenship emphasises the recognition of difference and giving voice to those currently excluded. Where do children feature in this debate? Can children be equal in terms of citizenship? The concept of participation is central to any definition of citizenship (Devine, 2002). Writers such as Cockburn (1998) and Roche (1999) challenge the traditional stance of excluding children. For children to have a voice and identify themselves as citizens, there has to be acknowledgement of their status as social actors in their own right. Yet, ironically, the school environment lends little credence to the actuality of child citizenship status. For example children were not able to voice their protest against the 2003 Gulf War without fear of truant labelling and threats of prosecution. While women in the workplace are successfully challenging oppressive dress codes on a platform of human rights, girls are still struggling, in some schools, to overturn prejudice about the wearing of trousers. At a time when European directives are advising on maximum weekly employment hours for the working population, children have little power to challenge the exhaustive hours the government expects them to work in order to achieve 'minimum standards and targets'.

Some writers (e.g. Morrow and Richards, 1996) have questioned the ethics of research where children are 'captive subjects'. In schools the balance of power is heavily skewed towards adults, and children are least able to exercise participation rights. Adults control children's use of time, occupation of space, choice of clothing, times of eating – even their mode of social interaction. So how does this impact on the nature and outcomes of school-based research?

One of the first considerations is the degree to which children can exercise freedom of choice with regard to participation in research. Much has been written about informed consent (Morrow and Richards, 1996) and the ethics of including competent children in that process (Alderson, 1995) but less attention is given to children and young people's right to *dissent*. How often does a child turn up for school and find an adult lurking in the back of the classroom scribbling notes? It could be an OFSTED inspector, it could be someone doing an assessment or appraisal on the class teacher, it could be a student teacher – or it could be a researcher. The reality is that at best a note will have been sent to parents informing them of the visitor and giving them an opportunity to raise objections; at worst, nothing will have been done at all. In either scenario it is unlikely that *children themselves* will have been consulted. Some would argue the impracticality of consulting 36 children every time a researcher comes to observe in their classroom and that chaos would ensue if an individual child exercised a right to object. How could that child be educated on that day? To exclude the child from the classroom would be an infringement of his/her human rights. The proper course of action would be for the researcher to be refused access to the classroom, but this rarely happens on the basis of a child's dissent. Real power in such instances lies with adults – with the parents and teachers.

A second consideration is the power exerted in terms of influence with regard to hierarchies of what it is important to study at school. Subjects that are valued as core learning such as maths, language and science dominate the timetable in comparison to marginalised subjects like art, music and PE, conveying implicit messages about their relative merits. Children are not consulted about the weighting of subjects in the timetable despite evidence (see Pollard and Triggs, 2000) that they find these subjects more appealing. Neither are they consulted about the distribution of work/play time. The absence of children's voice in decisions about the organisation of their time and space in school goes against the concept of children as social actors with the right to a voice. UN's *Convention on the Rights of the Child* article 31 relates to the right of the child to rest and leisure and to engage in play and yet there appears to be an expectation that these entitlements do not relate to anything that happens in school hours.

> School and schooling is experienced as something 'done to' the children, legitimized by a discourse which prioritizes adult/future-oriented needs and expectations over present lived experience. The emphasis lies with the preparation of children as future citizens, equipped with the skills (productivity, competitiveness, comportment and control) to contribute as adults to the needs of modern industrial/postindustrial society. (Devine, 2002: 312)

This emphasis on equipping children to lead productive, 'fulfilled' adult lives ignores their right to a productive, 'fulfilled' childhood, especially if the two ideals are antithetical. It accords with Prout's (2000: 304) reference to a tension between increased recognition of children as persons in their own right with a capacity for self-realisation, and the intensification of control and regulation that characterises British late modernity. A way forward is through more active participation of children in initiatives like school councils where children have a voice, and peer support groups (Alderson, 2000; Osler, 2000). However, these initiatives are sometimes tokenistic with a lone child voice not given parity amid a dominant adult culture.

Print et al. (2002) suggest that a way forward is to facilitate the development of children's 'political literacy' through active decision making and participation in all aspects of school life.

In this chapter we have only been able to glimpse the complexities of power relations in respect of children and young people within societies and the research processes. One of the key theoretical tools offered by feminist and post-structuralist approaches is that of deconstructing dichotomies such as rural/urban, and the contributions of feminisms in all their different forms have alerted us to the power differentials around gender within wider society and reflected within the family. The rethinking of power by Foucault and others, as having multiple forms and micro levels, is important in thinking about researching children's lives. The ways in which adults contemplate children affect all areas of their lives. We reviewed four key ways in which children and childhood are addressed by researchers and discussed the issues of generation, age, competence and citizenship. Finally we examined the effect of power in the adult-dominated context of school. This chapter has shown how researchers can take seriously power differentials between themselves and children and seek to address these in the design, implementation and dissemination of their work. Some of these are ethical questions and will be addressed by Priscilla Alderson in the next chapter.

References

Abbott, P. (2000) 'Gender', in G. Payne, (ed.), *Social Problems*, Basingstoke, Macmillan.

Abbott, P. and Wallace, C. (1990) *An Introduction to Sociology: Feminist Perspectives*, London, Routledge.

Alanen, L. (1992) *Modern Childhood? Exploring the Child Question in Sociology*, Research Report 50, Jyvaskyla, Finland, University of Jyvaskyla.

Alderson, P. (1995) *Listening to Children: Children, Ethics and Social Research*, Barkingside, Barnado's.

Alderson, P. (2000) *Young Children's Rights*, London, Jessica Kingsley.

Anderson, M.L. (1983) *Thinking about Women: Sociological and Feminist Perspectives*, New York, Macmillan.

Atkin, K., Ahmad, W. and Jones, L. (2001) 'Young South Asian deaf people and their families: negotiating relationships and identities', *Sociology of Health and Illness*, 24(1): 21–45.

Barker, C. (1997) 'Television and the reflexive project of the self: soaps, teenage talk and hybrid identities', *British Journal of Sociology*, 48(4): 611–628.

Barrett, M. and McIntosh, M. (1982) *The Anti-social Family*, London, Virago.

Begley, A. (2000) 'The educational self-perception of children with Down's syndrome', in A. Lewis and G. Lindsay (eds), *Researching Children's Perspectives*, Buckingham, Open University Press.

Bell, L. and Ribbens, J. (1995) 'Isolated housewives and complex maternal worlds: the significance of social contacts between women with young children in industrial societies', *Sociological Review*, 42(2): 227–262.

Bentovim, A. and Boston, P. (1987) 'Sexual abuse – basic issues – characteristics of children and families', in A. Bentovim, A. Elton, J. Hildebrand, M. Tranter and E. Vizard (eds), *Child Sexual Abuse within the Family: Assessment and Treatment*, London, Wright.

Butler, I. and Williamson, H. (1994) *Children Speak: Children, Trauma and Social Work*, London, NSPCC/Longman.

Christensen, P. (1999) 'Towards an anthropology of childhood sickness: an ethnographic study of Danish school children', PhD thesis, University of Hull.

Christensen, P. and Prout, A. (2002) 'Working with ethical symmetry in social research with children', *Childhood*, 9(4): 477–497.

Clark, A. (2004) 'The mosaic approach and research with young children', in V. Lewis, M. Kellett, C. Robinson, S. Fraser and S. Ding (eds), *The Reality of Research with Children and Young People*, London, Sage.

Cockburn, T. (1998) 'Children and citizenship in Britain', *Childhood*, 5(1): 99–117.

Collins, P. H. (1990) *Black Feminist Thought: Knowledge, Consciousness and the Politics of Empowerment*, Boston, Unwin Hyman.

Cosaro, W. (1997) *The Sociology of Childhood*, Thousand Oaks, CA, Pine Forge Press.

Cross, B. (2002) 'Children's stories negotiated identities: Bakhtim and complexity in upper primary classrooms in Jamaica and Scotland', PhD Thesis, Edinburgh University.

Detheridge, T. (2000) 'Research involving children with severe learning difficulties', in A. Lewis and G. Lindsay (eds), *Researching Children's Perspectives*, Buckingham, Open University Press

Devine, D. (2002) 'Children's citizenship and the structuring of adult–child relations in the primary school', *Childhood*, 9(3): 303–320.

DHSS (1974) *Report of the Committee of Inquiry into the Care and Supervision Provided in Relation to Maria Colwell*, London, HMSO.

Dosanjh, J.S. and Gurman, P.A.S. (1998) 'Child-rearing practices of two generations of Punjabis: development of personality and independence', *Children and Society*, 12: 25–37.

Elliott, M. (1997) *Female Sexual Abuse of Children*, Chichester, John Wiley and Sons.

Farganis, S. (1994) *Situating Feminism – From Thought to Action*, London, Sage.

Farmer, E. and Boushel, M. (1999) *Child Protection and Family Support*, London, HMSO.

Farmer, E. and Owen, M. (1995) *Child Protection Practice: Practice Risks and Public Remedies*, London, HMSO.

Foucault, M. (1980) *Power/Knowledge: Selected Interviews and Other Writings 1972–1977*, (ed). Colin Gordon, New York, Pantheon.

Foucault, M. (1982) 'The subject and power'. An Afterword to H. Dreyfus and P. Rabinow, *Michel Foucault: Beyond Structuralism and Hermeneutics*, Chicago, University of Chicago Press.

Furniss, T. (1995) *The Multi-professional Handbook of Child Sexual Abuse*, London, Routledge.

General Assembly of the United Nations (1989) *The Convention on the Rights of the Child*, New York, United Nations.

Giddens, A. (1995) *Sociology*, 2nd edn, Cambridge, Polity Press.

Gough, D.A. (1995) *Child Abuse Interventions – A Review of the Research Literature*, London, HMSO.

Grant, J. (1993) *Fundamental Feminism: Contesting the Core Concepts of Feminist Theory*, London, Routledge.

Hart, R. (1992) *Children's Participation: From Tokenism to Citizenship*, London, Earthscan/Unicef.

Hendrick, H. (1998) *Children, Childhood and Society*, Cambridge, Cambridge University Press.

Hill Collins, P. (1997) 'Towards an Afrocentric epistemology', in S. Kemp and J. Squires (eds), *Feminisms* , Oxford, Oxford University Press.

Howarth, R. (1997) *If We Don't Play Now, When Can We?* London, Hopscotch Asian Women's Centre.

Katz, C. and Monk, J. (1993) *Full Circles: Geographies of Women over the Life Course*, London, Routledge.

Kemp, S. and Squires, J. (eds) (1997) *Feminisms*, Oxford, Oxford University Press.

Kendall, G. and Wickham, G. (1996) 'Governing the culture of cities: a Foucauldian framework', *Southern Review*, 29(2): 202–219.

Kitzinger, J. (2000) 'Who are you kidding? Children, power and the struggle against sexual abuse', in A. James and A. Prout (eds), *Constructing and Reconstructing Childhood: Contemporary Issues in the Sociological Study of Childhood*, London, Falmer Press.

Kritzman, L. D. (1988) *Michel Foucault. Politics, Philosophy, Culture. Interviews and Other Writings, 1977–1984*, New York, Routledge.

Mandell, N. (1991) 'The least-adult role in studying children', in F. Waksler (ed.), *Studying the Social Worlds of Children*, London, Falmer Press.

Mayall, B. (1996) *Children, Health and the Social Order*, Buckingham, Open University Press.

Mayall, B. (2000) 'Conversations with children: working with generational issues', in P. Christensen and A. James (eds), *Research with Children: Perspectives and Practices*, London, Routledge Falmer, pp. 120–135.

Moore, J. (1985) *The ABC of Child Abuse Work*, Aldershot, Gower.

Morris, J. (1998) *Still Missing Volume 1: The Experience of Disabled Children and Young People Living Away from their Families*, York, Joseph Rowntree Foundation.

Morrow, V. and Richards, M. (1996) 'The ethics of social research with children: an overview', *Children and Society*, 10(2): 90–105.

National Commission of Inquiry into the Prevention of Child Abuse (1996) *Childhood Matters, Vol. 1.*, London, The Stationery Office.

Oakley, A. (1980) *Women Confined: Towards a Sociology of Childbirth*, Oxford, Martin Robertson.

Oakley, A. and Williams, S.A. (1994) *The Politics of the Welfare State*, London, University College London Press.

Osler, A. (2000) 'Children's rights, responsibilities and understandings of school discipline', *Research Papers in Education*, 37(2): 143–159.

Participation and Education Group (1998) *Schools Can Seriously Damage Your Health: How Children Think School Affects and Deals with Their Health*, Gateshead, PEG.

Parton, N. and Wattam, C. (eds) (1999) *Child Sexual Abuse: Responding to the experiences of children*, Chichester, John Wiley.

Pollard, A. and Triggs, P. (2000) *What Pupils Say: Policy and Practice in Primary Education*, London, Continuum.

Print, M., Ornstrom, S. and Skovgaard Neilsen, H. (2002) 'Education for democratic processes in schools and classrooms', *European Journal of Education*, 37(2): 193–210.

Prout, A. (2000) 'Control and self-realisation in late modern childhoods'. Special Millennium Edition of *Children and Society*, 14: 304–315.

Reinharz, S. (1992) *Feminist Methods in Social Research*, Oxford, Oxford University Press.

Ribbens, J. and Edwards, R. (eds) (1998) *Feminist Dilemmas in Qualitative Research – Public Knowledge and Private Lives*, London, Sage.

Robinson, A. C. (2002) 'Children in good order. A study of constructions of child protection in the West of Scotland', PhD, University of Stirling.

Roche, J. (1999) 'Children's rights, participation and citizenship', *Childhood*, 6(4): 475–493.

Sawicki, J. (1991) *Disciplining Foucault. Feminism, Power and the Body*, New York, Routledge.

Scottish Executive (2002) www. childrenareunbeatable.org.uk.

Solberg, A. (1996) 'The challenge in child research from "being" to "doing"', in J. Brannen and M. O'Brien (eds), *Children in Families: Research and Policy*, London, Falmer Press, pp. 53–65.

Summit, R. C. (1984) 'Beyond belief – the reluctant discovery of incest', *American Journal of Orthopsychiatry*, 56: 167–181.

Taylor, S.A. (2000) 'The UN Convention on the Rights of the Child', *in* A. Lewis and G. Lindsay (eds), *Researching Children's Perspectives*, Buckingham, Open University Press.

Thomas, N. and O'Kane, C. (1998) *Children and Decision-Making: A Summary Report*, University of Wales, Swansea: International Centre for Childhood Studies.

Thorne, B. (1993) *Gender Play: Girls and Boys in School*, Buckingham, Open University Press.

Westcott, H.L. (1998) 'Perceptions of child protection casework: interviews with children, parents and practitioners', in C. Cloke and M. Davies (eds), *Models of Participation and Empowerment in Child Protection*, London, Pitman.

Woodhead, M. and Faulkner, D. (2000) 'Subjects, objects or participants? Dilemmas of psychological research with children', in P. Christensen and A. James (eds), *Research with Children: Perspectives and Practices*, London, Routledge Falmer.

Wright, C., Weekes, D., McLaughlin, A. and Webb, D. (1998) 'Masculine discourses within education and the construction of black male identities amongst African Caribbean youth', *British Journal of Sociology*, 49(2): 241–260.

7 Ethics
PRISCILLA ALDERSON

This chapter reviews different aims and approaches used when examining ethical questions in research with children. It considers why ethics matters, and whether ethics is simply an optional extra or a vital theme running through every aspect of research. The chapter discusses how ethical insights can be useful to researchers, and who carries ethical responsibilities. The next sections consider some of the ethical questions that arise throughout research projects with children and suggest how you could think about these, both when you do your own research and also when you read other people's research reports. The conclusion discusses how ethics is often a matter of trying to find a balance between opposite extremes. Ethical standards in research with children have changed greatly in the past 30 years. Modern standards of research ethics may depend on modern transparent research methods and more recent respectful relations between researchers and children.

Introduction

What is research ethics?

The notion of research ethics is fairly new. It grew out of ancient professional codes such as the medical Hippocratic oath from the fifth century BC. During the 1940s, publicity about Nazi research made people aware that research could no longer be seen simply as part of care, such as routine medical care. The Nuremberg Code (1947), written by lawyers, stressed the dangers of research and insisted that willing unpressured consent should be asked for. Children were assumed to be too immature to be able to consent, and were therefore banned from taking part in research projects that would not benefit them.

However, in 1963 concern about the children born with deformed limbs after their mothers took thalidomide during pregnancy led doctors to insist, on the value of research and the dangers of using under-researched treatments. The *Declaration of Helsinki* (WMA, 1964/2000), written by doctors, set out more detailed ethical research standards. Yet examples of researchers using children as 'guinea pigs' in dangerous experiments continued to be reported (Pappworth, 1967).

Slowly, doctors accepted that they have extra duties to patients who take part in research. During the 1970s, US lawyers and philosophers began to set up the new discipline of medical ethics staffed by ethicists (Beauchamp and Childress, 2001). Their ideas have spread around the world into networks of research ethics committees, which vet medical, psychological and, increasingly, welfare and educational research. There have also been great changes since around 1990 in social scientists' willingness to listen to children seriously.

Ethical frameworks

Ethicists teach that the rules for ethical research are based on three main ways of thinking about what is 'good' research:

- *The principles* of respect and justice concern doing 'good' research because it is the right, correct thing to do, such as always respecting children as sensitive dignified human beings, trying to be fair, and using resources efficiently.
- *Rights based research* also involves respect, and children's rights have been listed under '3 Ps': *providing* for basic needs (the best available health care, education); *protection* (from harm, abuse, neglect, discrimination); and *participation* (United Nations, 1989; Franklin, 2002). Participation rights that are vital during ethical research include children being well informed, and having their own views listened to and respected by adults. Rights based research ethics tends to listen to children and their views on what is 'good' research rather than relying wholly on adults' principles and values.
- *Best outcomes based ethics* means working out how to avoid or reduce harms and costs, and to promote benefits. For example, research might evaluate the benefits and problems for children and teachers who use a new reading scheme, compared with groups using an older scheme or the hoped for benefits to future classes that can use the research findings.

These three, and other ethical approaches, all have strengths and gaps, which are widely debated (Beauchamp and Childress, 2001). The main approaches have been listed here to help you to identify which approach you tend to prefer, and which ones are used in research reports that you read, whether or not the chosen approaches are clearly stated.

Why do ethics and the status of children in research matter?

Safeguards

As already mentioned, medical research can be very dangerous and even lethal. Fortunately, social research (including sociological, psychological, educational, welfare and market research) does not kill or maim children. Yet researchers may upset and worry children and parents, embarrass them, or betray them, for example by making false promises. Researchers may produce misleading findings that result in policies that can damage children's lives.

Moral questions about power, honesty, and respecting or abusing people arise throughout the research process. One serious ethical problem, though seldom mentioned by ethicists, is the risk of published research reports increasing shame, stigma and disadvantage for whole groups of children and young people, such as teenage parents. Ethical review can help researchers to be more aware of such risks and problems and of how to deal with these.

Some people see a conflict between science (sound rigorous research methods) and ethics. For example, a researcher who is too careful not to upset anyone might exclude the more anxious-seeming children from a project, which then ends up with limited and misleading findings. I hope this chapter will convince you that high standards in science and in ethics can work well together. Ethics is about helping researchers to be more aware of hidden problems and questions in research, and ways of dealing with these, though it does not provide simple answers.

Researchers rely on the public to take part in research, to fund much research, and to respect and use research findings. If this co-operation is to continue, then researchers have to keep, and be seen to keep, high ethical standards. Public anxiety about the removal of children's organs without consent, partly for research, at Alder Hey Hospital in Liverpool, shows how views about research ethics, consent and rights may suddenly change, especially when children are involved. Doctors assumed that it was kinder not to ask parents. Parents tended to say they would have consented to research if they had been asked, but they were very angry that they were not informed. Similar changes might happen in social research, so that it could be useful to gain foresight about social research from the hindsight of the history of medical research.

Researchers need to be aware that some medical journals refuse to publish reports of projects that have not had research ethics committee approval. This standard might spread to other journals. Ethical standards keep rising and researchers need to keep abreast of them.

The safeguards of research ethics, such as applying to an ethics committee for approval, take time, but they can protect the people who take part in research, and also the researchers, for example from criticism or litigation.

Ethical status of children in research

There are three main levels of involving children in research. The three terms used here are often confused – children treated as objects are mis-called participants. Yet these three terms can show crucial power differences in children's status.

Unknowing objects of research are not asked for their consent and may be unaware that they are being researched. This includes covert research such as through one-way mirrors, and deceptive research such as when researchers ask one question but are really looking for answers to another, perhaps unspoken question. Then there is research when, even if children are asked for their views, no one explains why, or what will be done with the replies. In the past, parents and teachers were asked to report on (what they assumed were) children's views and feelings, because children were seen as unreliable – an example of how research can simply reinforce inaccurate prejudices instead of questioning them. Imagine a Victorian husband being assumed to be able to report completely his wife's views, and you have some idea of the present power differences between many adults and children.

Aware subjects are asked for their informed, willing consent to being observed or questioned, but within fairly rigid adult-designed projects such as questionnaire surveys.

Active participants willingly take part in research that has flexible methods: semi-structured interviews with scope for detailed personal accounts, exploring topics through focus groups or drama, diaries, photos or videos, paintings or maps created by the children. Increasingly, children are involved in planning, directing, conducting and/or reporting research projects (Alderson, 2000a, 2000b).

The advantages of children having greater control over producing and analysing data are that they may enjoy the research process far more (they know that they can drop out if they wish), and that the findings may more accurately report children's own views and experiences. The ethical risks of greater participation are that, if children contribute and reveal far more about themselves than they intended, they might later feel greater regret, shame or anger if researchers produce disrespectful reports. Adult researchers still hold the power to interpret and write reports.

Models of childhood

When planning research or reading research reports, picturing the model of the child in the researchers' minds helps to identify their ethical relationship with children in the project. It can also reveal how this relationship influences the research. Examples include: the innocent child needing protection; the child at specific Piagetian stages; the deprived disadvantaged child needing resources and services; the criminal child requiring control; the ignorant child who needs education; the excluded child who may need special shelter or opportunities; the disabled child who is the victim of personal tragedy or of a rejecting society; and far less often, the strong resourceful child who shares in solving problems and creating new opportunities. It is as if we put children into a small glass cage called childhood, and then examine how they perform within the cage's restrictions, instead of looking critically at the cage itself, its causes and effects.

The book *Games People Play* (Berne, 1964) shows how people tend to be drawn into an unhappy destructive triangle of playing the victim, the rescuer or the persecutor. Much research about children re-enacts this game. Berne proposes the solution of everyone moving beyond the game and working together towards ethical, honest and mutually respectful relationships. In research, this involves moving beyond simple stereotypes of children as victims or villains to see that everyone, children and adults, has needs and strengths, failings and skills. Researchers can then work respectfully with and for children to explore their complex and wide ranging views and experiences. They may, for example, combine reports of children's social, political and economic state with children's own views about these broad issues, as illustrated in Box 7.1 (on p. 104).

Combining children's own views with political and economic research

A new report analysed national and local data on children to produce the first regional report on *The State of London's Children* (Hood, 2001). The report showed unexpectedly high levels of poverty and numerous problems for London's children. It sets standards for regular reviews, to check how London's children fare in future. The respectful report is based on the UN *Convention on the Rights of the Child* (UN, 1989). The report's methods reflect the ethics in quoting many children's views. These bring the report to life, showing the real impact on children's lives of the political and economic data. The quotes are drawn from a survey of 3,000 children that was designed and conducted with the help of young people (Office of Children's Rights Commissioner for London, 2001). Children are shown to be actively concerned, part of the solution and not simply the problem.

Planning the research

The cherry or the cake? Ethics as an afterthought or a vital theme throughout the research

Some researchers see ethics as an afterthought and an annoying extra hurdle. They have planned their detailed project, raised the funds and then they even have to get research ethics committee approval. A paragraph or two about ethics is quickly written and added rather as decoration, like a cherry on a cake. Ethics is, however, far more useful when it is seen as a vital part of the whole recipe. It provides questions and standards that inform and are mixed into every aspect of the project, as considered in the next sections. Many ethical questions arise at each stage of a project, especially in research with fairly powerless groups such as children.

In later sections, some issues that might not at first seem to have ethical aspects will be reviewed. This is partly to help you to ask your own questions, either during your own research or when you are reading between the lines of other researchers' reports. What is missing? What are the hidden values and standards? Sometimes solutions are suggested. Sometimes questions are raised simply so that you can think about your own answers. All the questions link to ethics in terms of potential harm or benefit, and honesty, fairness and respect.

Using ethical guidelines and committees – ticking a box or soul searching?

Formal ethical guidelines (see list at end of chapter) can provide useful checklists. Yet some have gaps. Whereas some respect children (NCB, n.d.; CCS, n.d.; RCPCH, 2000; BSA, 2002, section 30), others say little about them (BERA, 1992; JUCSWEC, 2002; SRA, 2003). Surprisingly the SRA revised guidelines (2003) discuss the pros and cons of obtaining consent mainly by citing literature from the 1970s and early 1980s, although there have been great changes in ethics since then. Some are rather casual about covert (secret) research – not asking for consent or even telling people that you are observing or recording them or reading their records (BPS, 2000). This is often seen as unethical, or as allowed only if there are very good, unavoidable reasons for doing so. Yet researchers sometimes use guidelines with their let-out clauses, such as permitting covert research, as simple tick-a-box lists. If researchers end up with low standards, but also believe they are doing 'ethical research', this can be worse than if they had not heard about ethics. Guidelines are more valuable if they are used to ask hard searching questions about all aspects of research. The government insists that all research conducted with people through the health and social services meets high ethical standards (DH, 2002).

Like the guidelines, ethics committees can help to raise awareness and standards. Yet there is a risk that, once they have committee approval, researchers may feel they can be more casual than they otherwise would be. They might say, 'This family seems to be very worried and upset by the research, but the committee has said the project is OK, so it must be ethical to go on involving them'. In research teams with strict hierarchies, if junior researchers who interview children find that the children are unhappy about the research, they may find it hard to convince the project director that changes should be made. The director may blame the juniors for being inefficient, or say that the design cannot be changed because it has been approved, and it is too complicated to reapply to the ethics committee. These kinds of transfer and denial of responsibility undermine ethical standards, which depend on everyone concerned (the whole research team, ethics committee, funder and institution) sharing responsibility to ensure methods of respecting the groups with least power – children and young people.

Funders

Research, including consultancies, evaluations and audits, often begins with raising funds. Are there any funders whose 'dirty money' you would not accept, such as baby milk or arms firms? Have you thought about funders' possible motives, with the 'story' that they would like the research to tell about children, and how that story might serve funders' interests? A sportswear firm, for instance, might be very keen on surveys that show how children 'need' their goods to avoid stigma, bullying and social exclusion. Researchers should check at the start that they have a 'freedom to publish' contract, in case funders want to suppress or alter the findings.

Aims

Research usually has an underlying, often unspoken, moral agenda. The implicit aim may be to show children's weakness, failings, faults and deficits. The motive here may be to rescue, protect or provide for children by 'proving' that they need more educational, social or psychological support, in a bid to gain increased resources for such support – and more clients for the practitioner-researchers and their colleagues.

While some children might indeed need such help, there is a risk that this research overstates children's problems and their reliance on adults' solutions. Research reports can thereby, perhaps unintentionally, increase public prejudices and pity for children's supposed weaknesses. The history of the women's movement shows how men were fond of doing 'scientific' research that 'proved' women's deficits, their inferior dependence on men's protection. Women's status changed only when they were able to show that they could be men's equals and were therefore entitled to equal rights.

The 3 Ps help to clarify hidden aims and motives in research designs: to protect or provide for children or to participate with them in joint projects. Children's vital participation rights are respected when adults see that children are willing and able to exercise these rights. Although children are not fully equal to adults, their status only rises when the strength and good sense of many children is respected. In contrast to research about children's assumed deficits and failings, participatory research in its topics, methods and practical involvement with children and young people aims to show their competencies. Even with the youngest children, research concerned with their agency can show how they contribute to their family life and communities, based on respect for children's creativity, their own reasonable views and values and how they make sense of the world. Box 7.1 provides an example illustrating some of these points.

Box 7.1 Practical and valuable research by the youngest children

A run-down housing estate was being upgraded. Almost by chance, an adult asked children about the plans. Eventually, ten children aged 3–8 years did a survey of the other children's views. They wrote a report about their results, adding their photos, maps and drawings. They met senior council officers to discuss the report, and advised that the play area should not be put on the edge of the estate as planned, beyond a busy road. Instead, the play area was set in the centre of the estate, where children could safely play without needing adults to be with them (Newson, 1995).

Children's own meanings

Researchers showed children photographs of each main area of their family centre. They asked the children which areas they liked best and least. The book area was the least popular place. The research might seem to show that the children were immature, or they needed adults to ensure that the book corner was used more. Perhaps better books should be chosen.

Yet through asking and observing the children, the researchers found that the children disliked the way that the book corner was used – to keep them quiet and constrained, such as when the staff tidied up, and to read stories to large groups. The staff and children began to use the book corner and other areas more freely, and to have smaller story groups (Miller, 1998).

Children have views and motives that researchers cannot take for granted. Ethical research includes sensitive methods for discovering children's own views and meanings.

You might like to think about how open or hidden aims and motives serve various interest groups, and also influence research methods and findings, when you plan or read about the following kinds of research:

- Programmes to test, evaluate or audit an intervention or service (such as when OFSTED inspects a school and consults the children).
- Projects for training new practitioners. Should student teachers and nurses ask children's permission before writing practice case studies about them? And, if they do not, does this train students to do unethical research?
- Surveys of young people's views in high crime areas, on how they would help to prevent crime.

- Campaigns that collect children's and adults' views, such as to protest against threatened closure of a local playground.

Access

Access is one of the hardest stages of research with children. Their many gatekeepers (parents/guardians, teachers, doctors, social workers, who work and care for them) can both protect children but also silence and exclude them (see also later section on consent).

Ideally, research is opt-in rather than opt-out. This means that researchers do not see lists of children's names and addresses. A nurse or teacher may invite the parents/guardians and children to opt-in to the research project, and to post back their consent or refusal – or they can refuse by not replying at all. The ethical opt-in approach takes time and tends to obtain lower response rates, but it does respect people's privacy and free choice.

While many children can quickly be accessed through schools or hospitals, will such formal settings constrain their responses? They might talk more freely at clubs or playgrounds. Unfortunately, fears about stranger-danger in Britain further limit researchers' informal access to all kinds of children. Increasingly, researchers will need police clearance before contacting children.

Sampling

How can researchers ensure that samples of children are selected fairly, to include minority groups and children of both sexes and with a range of ages, abilities, ethnicities, social backgrounds or languages? This list raises many practical questions, such as how to include children with speech and language and learning difficulties (Morris, 1998). Care should be taken with a few groups with many health and social problems, that risk being involved in too many research studies.

Information, consent and competence

Information

Researchers can write simple clear leaflets that adults can read and explain to very young children or those with learning difficulties. It is important to use simple language and diagrams, and pictures can help. The leaflets should be in the first language of those to whom they are addressed. Large print, a pale background and non-glossy paper help children with poor sight. A coloured A4 sheet folded into an A5 leaflet looks more reader friendly. It is worth trying out draft leaflets with children and seeking their critical views. Before research sessions such as interviews, you could go through the leaflet with the child, who may not have read or remembered the leaflet. If you then invite questions, you may pick up common worries or queries that can be resolved.

Ethics committees require that leaflets should explain the nature and purpose of the research: Why is it being done? What are the main questions? Who might benefit from the findings? What might participants gain – if anything? Any risks or problems should be explained, with a brief summary of the methods and timetable, and any activities participants will be asked to do. The leaflet should explain how and where to contact the researchers (address, telephone and email) and should give the research ethics committee number if there is one. Several points can be headed 'Your rights', as illustrated below.

Example from a research information leaflet for children

Research and your rights

- It is for you to decide if you want to talk to me.
- You do not have to say 'yes'.
- If you do say 'yes', you do not have to do the whole interview.
- We could stop when you want to, or have a break.
- If you do not want to answer some of the questions, you can just say, 'pass'.
- Before you decide whether to help me, you might like to talk about this project with your parents or with a friend.
- I will keep tapes and notes of the interviews in a safe, lockable place.
- When I talk about the research and write reports, I always change people's names, to keep their views anonymous.
- I would not talk to anyone you know about what you have said, unless you talk about the risk of someone being harmed. If so, I would talk with you first about what could be done to help.

Even if you do not have to write an information leaflet for children, it is well worth doing so. Besides helping the children to know and decide about your research, writing a leaflet will help you to think very clearly about the nature and purpose of your work. This is likely to improve the standard of your research, and also make it easier to explain to children and adults. See the ethical guidelines (at end of chapter) and Alderson and Morrow (2004) for full details of the necessary information to give, to enable children and parents to give informed consent.

Consent

Consent is a key issue in research with children and raises hard, often unresolved, questions. Do we always have to obtain parents' as well as children's consent, even for young people aged 12, 15 or 17 years, as some guidance advises? Parents can give vital support to children who wish to refuse, but should we be barred by parents' refusal when the children or young people want to join the research? (There is clear agreement that the young child's reluctance and refusal must be respected in medical research.) Is a head teacher's permission sufficient or ought we to ask every child in the school who might be observed? How do we do research with whole classes, if one or two children object? How can we reduce the risks of children being either coerced into joining a project, or else unwillingly excluded and silenced? All these questions are still being debated. One way forward is to discuss the questions with relevant groups of children and adults and to work towards some answers with their help.

Continuing consent during longer projects involves checking that children are still willing to carry on. Sometimes people are afraid to refuse. Researchers need to watch out for cues and gently check how they feel. Sometimes I have ended interviews early, or not gone back to people who gave consent, because I felt that they were uncomfortable about the research but did not want to say so. I interviewed parents in intensive care baby units, and many times I kept away from parents who looked extra anxious and tired. This can make the project longer and harder, to complete, it may exclude very important groups, and maybe some of the parents would have liked to talk to me if I asked them.

Competence

When are children old enough to be competent to consent? There is no simple answer to this question. Much depends on each child's own experience and confidence, the type of research, and the skill with which researchers talk with children and help them to make unpressured informed decisions. Children aged three years upwards have willingly taken part as researchers, as illustrated previously.

Some people propose standardised tests to assess competence, but these tests may result in unduly high thresholds of competence that many children and some adults fail to reach. Instead, their competence to consent to research can be assessed by asking the children how much they understand about the project and their rights. This turns the session into a two-way test, not only of the children but also of the researchers. How well have they informed and listened to the children? The session can then change from being a test into being a time for sharing more ideas, so that the children can give a more informed and unpressured consent or refusal. Adults must be wary of underestimating children's understanding, and of misinterpreting their responses negatively when the children might have valid reasons of their own for refusing.

Methods of collecting, storing, analysing, reporting and disseminating data

Disrespectful methods

Disrespectful and even abusive methods should not be used with children. These include:

- not respecting their privacy and confidentiality rights;
- making covert observations, such as through one-way mirrors, secretly doing case studies, video and audio tapes;
- discussing the children openly without altering their names or hiding their identity;
- assuming that children are not yet able to speak for themselves;
- asking adults (parents, teachers) for their views about a child's beliefs and behaviours but not also asking the child;
- asking only negative and standard questions about children instead of also asking about each child's strengths, achievements and unique individuality;
- using questionnaires with adult-centred questions such as 'what is your housing status?' that might make children look foolish;
- labelling children without asking about their own reasons, which might make sense of their actions and views;
- testing them in labs, without seeing that being in a strange place can unsettle and distract them and thereby lower their competencies;
- routinely using upsetting methods, such as the tolerance of strangers test to see how babies react if their mother suddenly leaves them with a stranger;
- using deception, such as telling a child not to touch something, without giving any reason, then secretly watching to see how long the child obeys;
- talking down to children;
- publishing results that reinforce negative stereotypes about children and young people.

There is a double standard when researchers assume that children will not know or mind about these methods, which adults would refuse to accept for themselves. Besides involving direct harm and disrespect, such methods bring further harms. When people of any age are used and deceived without their informed consent, they are less likely to perform well. Failures are misleadingly recorded as if they are the true record and children of that age cannot achieve any better. The self-perpetuating myths then stop many adults from even trying to help children to achieve more. Children then continue to be underestimated and disrespected. Thus negative attitudes to children feed into negative research methods that produce negative findings and reports, and the whole cycle continues, as can still happen with women and members of ethnic minorities.

Respectful methods

Researchers who, with children's consent, observe and talk with them find that children are far more competent in their real everyday lives than they are in labs. One example is how young children with long-term problems who have surgery can have great understanding and courage (Alderson, 1993). So too can young children in Africa and Asia who take part in the 'adult world' of work and street life (Johnson et al., 1998). Research methods and findings from the 83 per cent majority poorer world are forcing researchers into new respect for British children's competence. The research methods include people making time and space maps, photos and videos, dramas and exhibitions about their daily lives, so that the methods reinforce the ethical findings about children's competence.

Children and young people now share in planning, conducting and reporting research, and then meeting policy makers to see how it can be used (for example, Cockburn et al., 1997). 'Dissemination' means sowing seeds. If the seeds of change produced by practical research are to grow, then researchers may have to do more than simply write academic papers. They may need to use the mass media, conferences and policy committees, to see that a wider public knows about their research and applies it. Does this go against older ideas about detached objective research? Objectivity itself raises ethical questions, if it means refusing to question injustice and dishonest traditions. Researchers can be fair, honest, open-minded and self-critical, and yet also respect children and contribute practical and emancipatory findings, as much feminist research shows (Hood et al., 1999).

Conclusions: finding a balance

This brief review has raised only a few of the many ethical questions that arise in research with children. The aim has been to alert you to such questions and suggest ways to start addressing them. As mentioned earlier, ethics helps researchers to be more aware of hidden problems although it does not provide easy answers.

Often, the problems at first seem to be about conflicting opposites: science or ethics, encouraging children's participation or protecting children by excluding them from research. And yet ways to balance these seemingly opposite values can often be found, as discussed through this chapter, and as this closing section summarises.

While working to complete projects on time and to budget, sometimes researchers also have to be ready to slow down and wait until children are ready to take part. This need not be a simple clash between scientific efficiency and ethical respect. Adjusting the pace to suit the children may help them to make a far more worthwhile contribution to the project. Ethics can strengthen scientific method.

Ethical guidelines and advice are most useful when they are taken seriously in order to ensure high standards. Children benefit when everyone concerned carries ethical responsibility, instead of denying or transferring it to others. The three frameworks of doing good, rights, and balancing harms and benefits offer such broad guidance that researchers have to work out how best to apply them in the context of each project.

Informing and involving children may block certain research methods, such as covert or deceptive research. However, if researchers rethink their questions and methods in more transparent and honest ways, they may gain more interesting and worthwhile findings. One example is not to do secret case studies of truanting children, but instead to discuss their research with informed and consenting children and parents. The researchers may then learn far more about children's motives, reasoning and ideas on how their truanting might be resolved.

This second approach means moving away from traditions that treated children as static unthinking objects. Instead, it respects children as dynamic reasoning agents – a more realistic, productive, and also ethical approach. Modern ethics fits and encourages modern research methods with children as real participants.

Ethics questions can also alert you, when you conduct research or read other researchers' reports, to underlying issues. What are the hidden values and interests? Who benefits? How is power used, abused or shared? Are children seen as problems, villains or contributors? Do the researchers aim to rescue, or criticise, or respect children?

Being aware of their moral relationship with the children can guide researchers towards solving the many ethical and practical problems arising through the research process: from access and informed consent to managing the data and dissemination. Ethical standards, high or low, weave into all parts of the research fabric and shape the methods and findings. Modern medical ethics has forced medical researchers to change their methods. They now do less risky research with children, and they inform, respect and protect children to a greater extent. It is important that social researchers also take ethics very seriously. This will ensure the adoption of methods which are respectful of children, as well as attention to ethics at every stage of the research that they conduct or read about.

Codes and guidelines

British Educational Research Association (1992) *Ethical Guidelines,* Slough, BERA.
British Psychological Society (2000) *A Code of Conduct for Psychologists,* Leicester, BPS.
British Sociological Association (2002) *Statement of Ethical Practice,* Durham, BSA.
Centre for the Child and Society (n.d.) *Code of Practice for Research Involving Children,* Glasgow, CCS.
Department of Health (2003) *Research Governance Framework for Health and Social Care,* London, DH.
Joint University Council Social Work Education Committee (2002) *A Code of Ethics for Social Work and Social Care Research,* London, JUCSWEC.
Medical Research Council, *Personal Information in Medical Research,* www.mrc.ac.uk/ethics
National Children's Bureau (n.d.) *Guidelines for Research,* London, NCB www.ncb.org.uk/research/guidelines.htm, last accessed on 23/05/03.
Nuremberg Code (1947) www.med.umich.edu/irbmed/ethics/Nuremberg/Nuremberg Code.html, last accessed on 23/05/03.
Royal College of Paediatrics and Child Health (2000) 'Guidelines on the Ethical Conduct of Medical Research Involving Children', *Archives of Disease in Childhood,* 82: 177–182.
Social Research Association (2003) *Ethical Guidelines,* London, SRA.
World Medical Association (2000). *Declaration of Helsinki,* Fernay-Voltaire, World Medical Association (1964).

References

Alderson, P. (1993) *Children's Consent to Surgery,* Buckingham, Open University Press.
Alderson, P. (2000a) *Young Children's Rights,* London, Jessica Kingsley.
Alderson, P. (2000b) 'Children as researchers', in P. Christensen and A. James (eds), *Research with Children,* London, Routledge/Falmer.
Alderson, P. and Morrow, G. (2004) *Ethics, Social Research and Consulting with Children and Young People,* Barkingside, Barnardo's.
Beauchamp, T. and Childress, J. (2001) *Principles of Biomedical Ethics,* New York, Oxford University Press.
Berne, E. (1964) *Games People Play,* Harmondsworth, Penguin.
Cockburn, T., Kenny, S. and Webb, M. (1997) *Moss Side Youth Audit Phase 2,* Manchester, Manchester City Council and Manchester Metropolitan University.
Edwards, C., Dandini, L. and Forman, G. (eds) (1998) *The Hundred Languages of Children,* 2nd edn, London, Ablex/JAI Press.
Franklin, B. (ed.) (2002) *Revised Handbook of Children's Rights,* London, Routledge/Falmer.
Hood, S. (2001) *The State of London's Children,* London, Office of Children's Rights Commissioner for London.
Hood, S., Mayall, B. and Oliver, S. (eds) (1999) *Critical Issues in Social Research,* Buckingham, Open University Press.

Johnson, V., Ivan-Smith, E., Gordon, G., Pridmore, P. and Scott, P. (eds) (1998) *Stepping Forward,* London, Intermediate Technology.

Mayall, B. (2002) *Towards a Sociology for Childhood,* Buckingham, Open University Press.

Miller, J. (1998) 'But we didn't mean to do that!' *Co-ordinate,* 67: 5–6.

Morris, J. (1998) *Don't Leave Us Out! Involving Disabled Children and Young People with Communication Impairments,* York, Joseph Rowntree Foundation.

Newson, C. (1995) 'The patio projects', *Co-ordinate,* 45: 10-11.

Office of Children's Rights Commissioner for London (2001) *Sort It Out!* London, OCRCL.

Pappworth, M. (1967) *Human Guinea Pigs,* London, Routledge and Kegan Paul.

United Nations (1989) *Convention on the Rights of the Child,* New York, United Nations.

8 Involving Children and Young People as Researchers
ADELE JONES

This chapter explores issues and practice implications for involving children and young people as researchers. Inquiry and exploration are central to the ways that children learn and develop, however while the role of researcher makes use of children's inquisitive capacities, children cannot be held to be responsible for research. This responsibility lies with the organisation or academic institution and the practitioners or academics who initiate children's involvement. At the very least there will be responsibility for ensuring that objectives and outputs are achieved and there are also responsibilities to children who participate and those who are the subjects of research. These responsibilities involve the exercise of professional (adult) authority. This 'authoritative adult' is referred to within this chapter as the adult researcher. By emphasising adult or professional authority, relative to this, the position of the child-researcher – as subordinate, is also established. This is a power inequality that cannot be levelled out through superficial attempts at egalitarianism. Wilkins, writing in *Research in Social Care & Social Welfare: Issues and Debates for Practice* defines egalitarianism in research as giving equal value to the perspectives of all participants (Wilkins, 2000). This is not a simple matter in relation to children, since *their* rights are mediated through adult perspectives. This raises questions as to whether democratisation in research involving children is possible, and what gains there may be for young people who are researchers. This chapter seeks to explore these questions and to examine what they mean for practice.

The first part of the chapter, 'Issues for reflection' describes the context within which the shift from the child being regarded as an object of study to becoming subject or 'actor' in creating knowledge is taking place. Issues of power, constructions of childhood and notions of children's rights are also discussed. In the second part, a framework for research is developed and its implications for practice explored and in part III research examples are drawn upon to illustrate children's involvement in specific stages of the research process. In conclusion, the chapter identifies some important principles for involving children as researchers.

Part I: Issues for reflection

Power and representation

The involvement of children in research, as researchers as well as informants, is a practice that has emerged out of social action research although its application is not limited to these forms of research. The term 'social action research' refers to the collective range of emancipatory, participatory and developmental research approaches that have emerged out of critical opposition to traditional positivist approaches (see for example, Humphries, 1994; Mohanty et al., 1991). The political struggle for recognition, representation and equality is the common thread that runs through these forms of research which are linked to issues of oppression and marginalisation in that they:

- seek social change;
- question divisions created between the personal and the political, the personal and the professional, theory and method;
- make claims for inclusion and 'voice';
- challenge the privileged status given to the notion of scientific validity and highlight the ways in which this major locus of debate and posturing serves both to mask and perpetuate power and status within established research communities;
- assert that the position of research informant or subject is one of 'knowing' as well as a source of what might be 'know-able';
- reveal the limitations of traditional positivist approaches to research;
- have led to participative methods of inquiry.

These advancements in social science research together with the increasing recognition of children's rights of expression (article 12, UN *Convention on the Rights of the Child*, 1989) summarise the context within which children's involvement in research has evolved from them being regarded simply as objects of study to sharing their own insights and undertaking research themselves. An increasing groundswell of opinion supports the view that children are important in generating knowledge. Indeed, it can be argued that knowledge about children is incomplete unless it takes into account the knowledge that children have of themselves.

There is a growing body of literature on the role of children and young people as researchers (Hill, 1997; Alderson, 2000; Boyden and Ennew, 1997). The value of these methodologies, which lies not least in the opening up of dialogue about the power dynamics of research, is undermined when they are applied uncritically or when they make use of methods that would be rejected in any other setting. There are good and there are bad ways for children to be engaged in research. 'Good' research requires careful attention to epistemological and methodological issues and the adoption of a critical reflective approach to research practice. Although established here as an essential bedrock for working with child-researchers, critical reflection, which arises out of a critical theory paradigm (Rubin and Babbie, 2001), is important in the forms of research referred to above, although it tends to be applied primarily in the interpretation of findings. Critical reflective practice in studies that involve children as researchers includes analysis of 'adult'-self as researcher, scrutiny of theory and assumptions and the capacity to be within, part of and at the same time reflect on the dynamics of interactions within which one engages children. Reflection must be both *precursor* to children's involvement (examination of own behaviour, values and role) and also *concurrent* with children's involvement (examination of the research process as it unfolds). Critical reflective practice provides opportunities for learning and growth and helps to avoid the inadvertent exploitation or coercion of children.

In scrutinising taken-for-granted assumptions about children and in exploring ideas about *how* to negotiate their role in research, questions about rights, constructions of childhood and the ways in children's involvement in research may result in their politicisation are brought to the fore.

Politicisation and rights

It is argued that research is never apolitical (Fonow and Cook, 1991); indeed, some forms of social action research make explicit the political implications of their aims. Politics, it is said, belongs to any situation. It is often contended, however, that children should be protected against political activity, and that private life and public life should be separated so that children are free to develop their capacities untainted and unburdened by adult activities (Arendt, cited in Elshtain, 1997). What Arendt railed against first and foremost was the exploitation of children for political ends. She argued that children were unnecessarily burdened by such activities and that left in their own private spaces they would thrive and claim (or reject) political positions later on. Children *are* vulnerable to political exploitation, however; Arendt's position was based on a view of childhood that is available only to *some* children and which minimises the struggles of others. In a study of immigration proceedings, Jones argued that children were politicised by their experiences of asylum or deportation. She suggested, for example, that young people's claim to self-defined identities and their rejection of representations that demean them (such as media images of asylum-seekers) is a political act (Jones, 2000a; 2000b). There are many examples throughout the world of children and young people operating as political actors in order to improve their conditions. The role of children in ending apartheid in South Africa, for instance, is a powerful illustration that they may need to engage in political action in order to be freed from burdens that constrain their development. As Elshtain suggests, politicisation is sometimes necessary in order that children 'may return to the playgrounds to which they belong' (Elshtain, 1997). Other social commentators have reflected on the ways in which social life *itself* inducts children into politics: '... that children are never spared politics. Every child must take his or her bearings in a particular time and place' (Coles, 1986, in Elshtain, 1997: 120).

Views about children's involvement in politics are heavily influenced by constructions of childhood. In Arendt's vision they are presented as innocent, vulnerable and in need of protection and special treatment. While these are needs that children have, an overemphasis on protection can result in a denial of the child as political or self-determining subject and is difficult to reconcile with a conceptualisation of rights that accords status to children's knowledge. Dominant (Western) discourses on children's rights often sustain the separation of the personal and the political and consequently perpetuate the powerlessness of children and young people (Jones, 2000a; 2000b). This happens as a consequence of regarding the child as having a special and separate status, disconnected – disembodied, as it were – from the families, communities and the context in which they live their lives. It is also linked to the emotional and social investments often placed in sentimentalising childhood as the kind of place from which adults have emerged or wished they had emerged.

> We – we adults in late modernity – have such a stake in locating innocence somewhere, in some site or condition of being, we often assign children the task of creating or embodying such for us...Stories of political children draw us away from innocence into something far more complicated and morally ambiguous. (Elshtain, 1997: 123)

Much has been achieved through the universal language and standards on children's rights. However, in actuality it is the material conditions of children's lives and macro-level decisions (societal and global) that determine what rights children have. And, it is cultural and social values, disability, sexuality, gender inequality together with micro-level decision making within families that determine how these rights are expressed or realised. Children's rights are both general *and* specific and are always sited in the historical, economic and political environment in which claims for rights are made.

The child as researcher runs *counter* to prevailing ideas, and involving children in research requires a commitment to seeing that children are not separate from the worlds they inhabit. Political processes at both macro and micro levels govern these worlds and children have long demonstrated their readiness to participate in political struggles. For these young people, the separation of the personal and political does not exist: '[C]hildren as workers, patriots, and protestors are powerful evidence of the ways in which these categories, and the realities towards which they gesture, bleed into one another' (Elshtain, 1997: 125).

Part II: Implications for practice

It is beyond the scope of this text to explore children's role as researchers in relation to the many different epistemological and methodological approaches that exist. The focus here is on social action research. This is because of its relationship to critical theory. Critical theory is the theoretical framework through which concepts of empowerment and advocacy, applied usually to research procedures and research subjects but utilised in this instance in relation to the child-researcher, can be embedded within the process. This does not mean that children's contributions cannot be utilised in other forms of inquiry, indeed the issues and principles raised are widely applicable. This section of the chapter provides the reader with a framework for involving children as researchers and discusses its practical application. The framework does not promote the uncritical use of the concept of empowerment and suggests that a precursor to this must be the identification of structures that prevent children's participation and the creation of environments that facilitate it.

A framework for involving children as researchers

All stages of a research project potentially present opportunities for the involvement of the child-researcher; however, most studies utilise children's skills at particular points or for particular tasks. It is helpful to clarify these from the outset, although they should not be regarded as fixed since flexibility and the capacity to respond to changes are essential aspects of ongoing reflection. It may be, for instance, that children are unable to participate as planned; they may develop different areas of interest or skills, or a particular focus may become a dead-end that has to be abandoned. Involving children as researchers requires attention to six key processes:

- Identification of barriers and boundaries
- Negotiation
- Planning and design
- Access
- Creating the work environment
- Reflection

Identification: identifying barriers and establishing boundaries

As with children and young people's participation in other spheres of social life, research is not isolated from the structures and processes that affect their involvement. In determining the role children are to play it is likely that there will be some barriers to participation. These barriers may exist as material reality or they may have been constructed at the conceptual level and while some can be dismantled, others will remain. Barriers may even need to be erected to set the boundaries for young people's participation, as in this example. In a study of child protection services for black children and families (Butt and Jones, 1995), a young person who had been in local authority care was recruited to carry out interviews with other young people in care. In the course of the study, one respondent revealed that she was soon to become homeless. The young researcher identified so closely with this other young person's experiences that she invited her to stay temporarily at her home. The situation gave rise to some difficulties for both young people and external help was needed to move the homeless young person to a more appropriate placement. Establishing boundaries for the young researcher's *own* role and also for the participation of the young people whose experiences she was investigating might have prevented this situation from arising.

It is useful to distinguish those barriers that obstruct children's involvement and might need to be dismantled or challenged, from those that should remain. The adult researcher must also identify (in consultation with others, including children) the boundaries that will need to be in place to protect the rights of the child who is 'researched' as well as the child who is researcher. These boundaries must be clearly understood by all parties. Barriers to children's participation include:

- Funding criteria which restrict the role of children
- Aspects of the research considered inappropriate for children
- Lack of knowledge, skills or abilities for particular tasks
- Limited time or interest of the child
- Project time scale allowing insufficient time for children's inclusion
- Access or communication barriers, for example a child-researcher with mobility impairments may be unable to interview other children in their homes
- Adult perceptions and the social status of children resulting in their restricted access to certain processes
- Children's perceptions that influence the role they play
- Factors such as gender, race, religion and culture that create social pressures or expectations that impact on children's participation

In some instances, barriers might be reframed to establish boundaries. In the list above, there are several examples that could be used in setting boundaries. For instance, while it may be considered acceptable for a child to interview another child about socio-economic circumstances, adult views about children would make it unacceptable in many social contexts for a child to interview an adult on the same topic. If this is identified as a barrier, the adult researcher can address it by discussing and establishing boundaries about the topics, informants and settings that would be appropriate.

Negotiation: negotiating engagement and clarifying roles

The stages and tasks of the research should be described and the aspects of work available to child-researchers clearly identified. Children and young people and where appropriate their parents or caregivers should be asked what interest there is (or might be generated) in participating. It is important to engage children with the 'idea' of the research: this involves preparatory work, talking through the research problem and the types of activities children might undertake. It is almost always beneficial to involve the parents and caregivers of children and young people. Usually parental consent is required, but the role of parents and other family members may extend beyond this. First and foremost, family members are concerned to ensure that their children will not be manipulated or harmed; secondly, family members must satisfy themselves as to the worthiness of the project; and thirdly where support is offered this will often extend beyond the formal hours of a research project. This support can be invaluable.

In negotiating with children and their families, the adult researcher must be clear about how 'open' the agenda is, whether children have access to all parts of the research process and whether there can be equality in the decision making. Choice rarely exists as an absolute freedom: what is important is that the limitations as well as the possibilities are made explicit. Children should have the opportunity to explore what research means (there are various methods for doing this, for example getting children to devise and carry out surveys about things of interest to them such as food, pop stars, etc., developing interview skills through role playing, discussing the experience of being interviewed, hearing and recording each other's views and analysing the results). Children also need to understand how their participation fits into the bigger picture and what the benefits or drawbacks might be for them. The respective roles that children are to play must be clearly understood and the specific skills children have or may need to develop should be identified.

Planning and design: devising appropriate methods

Unlike other approaches, studies that involve children as researchers require not only that methods fit the research aims, but also that methods 'fit' the child-researcher. It is also important that the links between method and theory are made explicit and what is taken as 'read' be fully explored:

> the art of producing theory is important because it signifies who and what is held to be important…When researchers and funders present theory as the least important aspect of the process, they must realise that this indicates not that theory is absent – it never is – but that the theoretical positions that underpin the research have been presented as taken-for-granted. In this lies the danger of perpetuating ethnocentric or universalist assumptions. (Jones et al., 2002: 4)

Feminist scholars have argued that theory and method should not be treated as disconnected. This standpoint is useful both for sustaining critical reflective practice and also in practical application. By teasing apart, constructing and articulating theoretical positions, the research project becomes 'anchored' to a set of principles which can guide the process.

In a study of black children with caring responsibilities by the Bibini Centre for Young People (Jones, Jeyasingham and Rajasooriya, 2002), there were extensive discussions among and between the different participants. The discussions were contentious as people grappled to scrutinise meanings behind terms such as 'carer', 'children's rights' and 'black perspective'. Hallowed positions were challenged, tensions between children's and parents' rights were explored and, slowly and painfully, theoretical positions were elucidated and a set of principles established. Children's views were an essential part of this process. The principles are important in themselves, as they set the study in a specific social and political context; however, the process of arriving at agreement on what they should contain was invaluable. The voice of the child influenced the principles in several ways, for example in the attention given to children's strengths; their problems, such as school exclusion, and in making visible the work young carers do.

It is useful to involve children who are to be researchers in 'let's talk' sessions, informal yet focused discussions using creative communication methods. Sessions such as these can be part of the preparation for engagement; they allow the participants to explore meanings (including each other's) and concepts, to challenge stereotypes, and to check out assumptions. They provide early opportunities for the adult researcher to assess the child-researcher and vice versa. For children they allow them to flex and develop the faculty for explanation, interchanging ideas, communication and seeing self as a subject of knowledge. They also enable the adult researcher to gain an insight into children's broader perspectives on human experience as well as their opinions on the research project. There are many useful texts on approaches for exploring children's meanings (see for example, *A Journey of Discovery: Children's Creative Participation in Planning*, Save the Children, 1999). In devising research methods to fit the child-researcher, the adult researcher must take into account the age and abilities of the child and any relevant social factors.

Access: accessing resources for communication and participation

In the assessment of children's abilities and interests, attention must be paid to issues of language, communication styles and support needs. It may be necessary, for example, to arrange sign language interpreters to support deaf children or to have other interpreters available to facilitate children's involvement in cross-cultural research. Physical access is also an important consideration. Depending upon the nature of the child's work, specific arrangements may be needed to remove barriers for children who have mobility impairments. Other disabled young people may need assistance with personal care in order for them to participate fully. The resource and time implications of facilitating children's participation are often considerable but should not be circumvented. The process usually results in unexpected learning and gains for all involved and it is neither complicated nor arduous to deal with these matters. Children and their families are often their own experts on support needs and are likely to suggest creative ways of meeting them. Providing transport, food and refreshments can be important in sustaining children's involvement. These are things that adults take for granted, but children may find it difficult to organise their own transport or to plan in advance for meals. It is also the responsibility of the adult researcher to ensure the health and safety of children and to create a working environment that is safe and supportive. This means evaluating the places, conditions and times that particular research activities happen. If children are to be involved in carrying out interviews in people's homes for example, measures may need to be put in place to ensure their safety. Some points to consider here include: joint interviews with adult researchers, organising transportation, appraising the interview setting beforehand, alternative interview venues and so on.

Creating the work environment

The child who is a researcher is involved in real work and attention must be paid to the creation of a positive work environment. While child-researchers may not be formally employed, it is helpful to think of them as child-workers and to ensure that the conditions they will be working within comply with standards. In addition to ensuring that activities are non-hazardous, non-exploitative and do not interfere with schooling, arrangements must be made for any necessary training, for support, supervision and compensation.

The adult researcher must identify whether training is needed, how this can be provided and what form it should take. The training should equip young people with skills for carrying out their work and also for addressing broader issues, such as ethics in research. Training should be age/ability appropriate. In addition to training, it is important to set up systems for support and supervision. In the Bibini Centre Project referred to earlier, the support system set up for the duration of the project included access to 24 hour telephone contact with one of the adult researchers, regular formal supervision, an interview feedback form, de-briefing after each interview and a support group. Support and supervision are necessary to ensure that:

- research objectives are met;
- research principles are followed;
- problems or concerns are addressed at an early stage;
- any emotional effects of the research are identified and appropriate support provided;
- the young person's ongoing development as a researcher is facilitated;

- gaps in skills, training or resources are identified;
- young people have opportunities to input their views.

One issue that is often neglected is what material benefits there are for child-researchers and how children should be compensated for their time. The benefits for adults of doing research are rarely made explicit; this is partly because such discussions may be regarded as 'tainting' the ethics of research, or because the benefits, though unstated, are well established. For instance, adult researchers may also be salaried staff, or they may be paid for their work on a particular project. They may also benefit in other ways, for example from published work and career advancement. Children and young people do not gain in these ways and while they may derive benefits in terms of increased confidence and satisfaction, their work must count for more than this; they should receive material benefits. Some examples of benefits include: acquisition of research skills; certificates for training courses attended; references to supplement school or college achievements; job references; financial compensation; non-monetary compensation. It can be difficult to pay children and young people for their work. Parents may not wish money to be given to their children. Furthermore receiving cash may affect welfare benefits or may be added to the household income and children may prefer to benefit directly from their work. In these circumstances providing vouchers that can be exchanged for goods from stores is one option. For other young people, involvement in the research provides a viable and safe form of earning valuable income for themselves and their families.

Reflection: reflection, monitoring and review

Reflection, monitoring and review should take place periodically during the project. It is advisable to schedule opportunities for reflection in the research timetable otherwise this can get overlooked or sacrificed to work that is considered more pressing. The research team should meet together to talk about progress, process, issues and feelings. This provides a formal opportunity to deal with conflicts and concerns that have arisen and is a useful mechanism for keeping all partners informed. The structure and method for conducting these sessions should facilitate and promote the expression, exchange and hearing of views. This may mean confronting behaviours within the team (mainly those of adult researchers) that dominate or inhibit interaction and using purposively designed strategies for inclusion.

Part III: Examples from practice

In this section, three examples of social action research are drawn upon to illustrate the way in which children can be involved in research design and data collection and the interpretation and dissemination of findings. It is important to note that in the research examples that are described, children were not involved simply because of their child status, but were invited to participate on the basis of other qualifying factors. In the first example, the study of black young carers, by the Bibini Centre for Young People, children with first-hand experience of providing support to someone who is ill or disabled were considered the real 'experts' on their situation. While this did not mean that they were seen as experts for other young people, it was felt that research about young carers needed to acknowledge and make use of this expertise. The second example, research carried out by the International Labour Organisation on the worst forms of child labour, sought the views of child labourers and utilised child labourers in obtaining those views. The approach was based on the recognition that 'although adults' perceptions are not devalued, the adults themselves are no longer considered to be the sole authorities on children's lives' (Boyden and Ennew, 1997, cited in ILO, 2002: 63). The third example, a study on children and migration, carried out by the University of the West Indies together with a child guidance clinic, involved children affected by separation from parents in the dissemination of findings. The meanings young people attributed to the findings were, in this instance, considered to be more important than other interpretations and the dissemination process therefore sought to address their voicelessness.

While adult researchers are not usually selected on the basis of their identification with the research problem, with children this may be the case. There can be both benefits and drawbacks to this approach. Benefits are that the child may have increased interest, sensitisation and motivation as well as important insights. Furthermore, it can be helpful for children who are research informants to feel that the person they share the information with has some understanding of their situation and can understand their particular way of seeing the world. However, as with adults, children can become over-involved or be put in touch with experiences that so closely resemble their own that they may have difficulty separating out the issues. While the research examples described made use of children's experiential knowledge of the research problem, clearly this is not always necessary and may not even be desirable in some instances.

What is important here is the acknowledgement that children can play a significant role in carrying out research because they are children and not only because they are a particular kind of child who has a particular kind of experience that links to a specific research problem. It is not that being a child carries an essential property that of itself brings value to research; however, unimplicated in creating hegemonic discourses, children and young people can provide valuable insights regardless of their individual backgrounds.

Involving children in research design and data collection

Invisible Families: The Strengths and Needs of Black Families in which Young People have Caring Responsibilities (Policy Press with the Joseph Rowntree Foundation, Jones, Jeyasingham & Rajasooriya, 2002).

This study investigated the circumstances and views of children who were caring for parents or relatives who were disabled or ill. Children of different ages were involved in different activities. For instance 13 children aged from 5 to 16 years were involved as child-to-child researchers and worked on the formulation of the research design while three young people over 16 were recruited as peer researchers to gather data through interviews.

Research design

An initial three-day consultation event familiarised children with the research process and enabled them to influence the areas of investigation necessary to reflect their experiences. The forum also dealt with the dynamics of young carers from different racial and cultural backgrounds, searching out differences and commonalities. Time was given to play and social interaction as children made it clear that 'playtime' and 'socialising' were spaces and experiences that were scarce and precious, since so much of their time was taken up with caring responsibilities. Gradually, a focus on the research project was established. Ground rules set out the responsibility the adult researchers had for listening to and learning from children (as opposed to setting rules for children's behaviour). Exercises were devised to help children both to reflect on their individual circumstances and to work collectively on the kinds of questions that would enable them to find out more about what being a carer means. The young people recognised that some of the information was sensitive and that they might feel vulnerable and exposed if they were sharing details about their home lives. They interviewed each other to identify the questions that it would feel 'safe' to answer. In these exercises and explorations young people were both informants and researchers. Some very rich information was produced and these early findings were fed back into the research process and used to develop the research design. Two interview schedules were devised, one for parents and other family members and one for children and young people. This process gave rise to questions about identity, religion and ethnicity, experience of family life, work children do to support disabled family members, the impact of tasks, the division and allocation of work, other factors affecting children and family life, experiences of services, wishes and aspirations.

Involving young people in collecting data

Three young people were recruited as peer researchers. The peer researchers interviewed other young people while the adult researchers carried out interviews with parents, other family members and agencies. The role of peer researcher was considered appropriate for young people over the age of 16 because of the level of responsibility, maturity and skills needed for carrying out interviews. A four-day training course was developed in which the young people learned about research methods and developed interviewing skills. Interactive methods such as role play and video recording sessions were used. The training also included:

- Protecting the rights of the researched (e.g. confidentiality)
- Ensuring own health & safety
- Dealing with any child protection issues that might arise
- Interviewing techniques
- How to go where children are
- Planning for things that go wrong
- Recording interviews
- Preliminary data analysis.

Peer researchers were matched to research informants on the basis of gender, language and culture, young people's wishes and levels of confidence. Professional boundaries were established and the peer researchers were equipped with skills and strategies for terminating interviews that they might find uncomfortable or distressing.

Involving children in interpreting findings

Involving children in the interpretation of data provides particular challenges depending upon whether the focus is on transforming quantitative data into generalisable findings or whether interpretation seeks to achieve depth in understanding meanings. In both instances children's contributions are easily marginalised. A critical issue in the involvement of children in interpreting findings is the authority given to the child's voice. It is not that the child's voice has ontological status simply because children have been excluded from the production of knowledge, but in including children and young people's understandings of the phenomena they observe, measure or are part of, new possibilities are opened up. Although not writing about children, relevant here is Foucault's argument that 'in refusing to privilege discourses of the powerful, [we] create a space for the release of "an insurrection of subjugated knowledge"' (Morgan 2000: 121, citing Foucault, 1980).

Reflection on interpretation within many studies would lead to questions such as, Why is *this* particular aspect being emphasised? What linguistic devices are used to portray a particular version of the interpretation? Why this version? What discursive practices do the choices of language belong to, create or undermine? How are status and credibility achieved in the theory formulations arising out of interpretation? In involving children in interpretation, we might also ask what other versions children might offer.

Since 1998, with the establishment of the Statistical Information and Monitoring Programme on Child Labour (SIMPOC), the International Labour Organisation has undertaken research in several countries to understand the complex social and economic features of child labour. The approach to research developed by the ILO is summarised in this statement:

> Qualitative and quantitative data are indivisible. It is not possible to count something until there is first a definition of what is to be counted – therefore the issue must be understood qualitatively. Questions cannot be framed for surveys without knowing what words and concepts will be understood by community members, including children. Statistics can only be correctly interpreted through an understanding of the context in which they have been generated. Collection of qualitative data is particularly important for the worst forms of child labour, which will not yield up their secrets to customary forms of survey…or similar conventional instruments. (ILO, 2002: 14)

The experiences of the ILO demonstrate the need for children's contributions both to what is known about child labour and also in action to eliminate harmful forms of child labour. In a consultation event held in the United Republic of Tanzania, children stressed the importance of being *informed* (about the effects of some types of labour), of *participating* (in activities and forums) and being *involved* (in designing programmes to eliminate child labour within their communities) (ILO, 2002: 65). Children have had an increasingly significant role in research on child labour, particularly in interpreting findings. Research findings increase knowledge about the scale and complexity of the problem; however, children can identify what the findings mean to *them* and their perceptions are important in planning corrective measures. In a conference to discuss the findings of international studies on child labour, delegates were disturbed by the scale of dangerous work being undertaken by children and sought to establish consensus on the abolition of all forms of child labour. While children present at the conference did not disagree with the information presented, their views about what these findings meant were influenced by their perspectives as child labourers and differed in fundamental ways from the adults. Children did not accept that work was necessarily negative or exploitative. For many of them their contributions were important for the survival of the family, furthermore, many children thought it was actually important for them to be able to work.

> 'Nearly all child labour is intolerable and nearly all is criminal,' contended Neil Kearney, General Secretary of the International Textile, Garment and Leather Workers' Federation, reinforcing his case with a sampling of dire examples of child exploitation. 'If the agenda of those pushing for action on intolerable forms results in other child labour being ignored I think future generations of working children will never forgive us.'
>
> It was in this context that the children's delegates gave their countervailing message loud and clear, urging not abolition but regulation. Action should be taken, they said, to eradicate the most pernicious forms of child labour. But, in the absence of a real assault on the root causes of poverty, children had to have the right to work. It was not work but exploitation in the workplace that had to be targeted, and not only that of children. Was it any better to be exploited after the age of 15?

'We say "yes" to work, "no" to exploitation; "yes" to work, "no" to ill-treatment; "yes" to work, "no" to abuses; "yes" to work, "no" to social exclusion,' intoned Ana Maria Catin Torrentes (17), of the Movement of Working Children and Adolescents in Nicaragua ... 'Through my work I felt I was part of society,' said Vidal. 'I felt responsible and proud that I was contributing by paying for my education and that of my brothers and sisters.' Work should not be the possession of any group, he argued, but a universal right, available to both children and adults. (*New Internationalist*, July 1997 at http://www. newint.org/ last accessed 17/09/03)

The ILO believes that unless children are involved in interpreting findings then action arising out of research may result in more harm than good. An example of this was the Harkin Bill (United States 1993) which called for a boycott of all goods manufactured using child labour. This led to thousands of child workers being dismissed, many of whom then faced destitution (ILO, 2002: 89).

Children's role in dissemination

Children of Migration: A Study of the Care Arrangements and Psychosocial status of Children of Parents who have Migrated (The University of The West Indies with the Department of Child Psychiatry, Eric Williams Medical Sciences Complex, Jones, Sharpe and Sogren, 2003).

This research example explores the role of children in disseminating findings. The study examined indicators of depression among 146 children (aged 13–16) in a secondary school in Trinidad, half of whom were living with substitute caregivers because their parent or parents had migrated. The study raised important questions about the limitations of attachment theory (Bowlby, 1973) in understanding adolescents' emotional needs and challenged the strategies that adults use to justify the decisions they make when they sever children's attachments. This, of course, is a *particular* interpretation of one of the study's findings; there are others. It is emphasised here because it relates directly to the method selected for dissemination. The study found that children separated from parents through migration were more than twice as likely to demonstrate indicators of depression (low self-esteem, difficulties with interpersonal relationships, negative mood, anhedonia and ineffectiveness) than other children and there were differences in the manifestation of problems depending upon age and gender. Moreover some of the problems were of such a serious nature as to warrant professional intervention. Importantly, the study revealed that families used a range of 'devices' to promote to the external world that all was well within the child's world, even when it was not, making it extremely difficult for the child's pain to be recognised. During the study children went to considerable lengths to ensure that their involvement in the research would signal to others the extent of their distress. In some instances, children assumed the identity of other children or forged caregivers' consent in order that they could take part. When explored further, these children made it clear that they saw participation in the study as a means of ensuring they were listened to.

The findings of all studies raise implications for a range of audiences and methods for dissemination should be tailored accordingly. For example an academic audience might best be reached through an article in a professional journal; policy makers and practitioners through training and research reports; families through seminars or written information; and young people themselves, through advice on rights and key findings. Each of these audiences may require a specific approach in terms of the language and methods used. While there is no reason why children should not be involved in disseminating findings to all of these audiences, there will be limitations in terms of time, skills and interest that may impact upon the decision making. At the dissemination stage careful consideration should be given to the wishes of children as well as to how children's perspectives and skills might best be used. This is likely to result in identifying specific aspects of the dissemination process for children's involvement. For example, it might be considered particularly important to have children read over a report to identify language or terms that are ambiguous, or to eliminate unnecessary jargon.

In the research example described above, children's perceptions and skills were utilised both in sharing findings and in challenging three observations: families' denial about the effects on children of separation; a perception that children should be seen and not heard (upheld by powerful social traditions); and the assumption parents held that increased economic benefits of migration were worth other social costs. A 'Theatre in Education' drama company was hired to portray the main themes of the study to an audience made up of parents, surrogate caregivers, family members and teachers. The company designed and staged an interactive play performed by professional actors. Periodically the drama was 'freeze-framed' – the actor would switch places with one of the children from the study who would then act out in his or her own way their interpretation of the particular issue being explored. This mix of professional actor-adult/child-research informant provided a status and credibility to the children's performances that would have been difficult to achieve had they staged a play by themselves. The professional actors gave authority to the child's voice, the drama served as a foil to preserve confidentiality and the 'act' provided a mask for children to express their emotions and yet preserve the external presentation of self.

Conclusion

This chapter has set out the political and social context for the involvement of children and young people as researchers. It has discussed some key issues and examined what these mean for practice. The insights generated by approaches that are inclusive of children and young people's perspectives increase our understanding of the world. However, in order to refine and improve the research methods that make use of these approaches it is necessary to reflect on the ways in which the structures created by adults limit children's contributions:

> to chisel through the authority from which adults/professionals speak and to create the space in which the meaning children and young people ascribe to their experiences challenge hegemonic approaches. (Jones, 2000b: 44)

Furthermore, the structures that limit children's involvement mean that the environments through which their participation is made possible and meaningful do not exist; they must be created. An important stage in this process is to clearly articulate and apply the principles that must underpin children's involvement. Research methods that involve children and young people as researchers should seek to ensure:

- clarity about the role and purpose of children's involvement;
- transparency and agreement about which children (and why) will be the partners in the research;
- consent from the child and, where appropriate, parents or other caregivers;
- that children's work is counted. This includes ensuring that there are material benefits for the child-researcher;
- that research tasks that are identified are appropriate and 'do-able' and take into account children's views, age and abilities as well as relevant social and cultural factors;
- that the language, methods and processes of research are made accessible to children;
- adequate support to facilitate children's participation with attention at the practical level, i.e. skills, knowledge and resources needed; and the discursive level – reflection on issues of power, rights, ideas and perspectives;
- that children are not subject to harm, exploitation, coercion or adult manipulation;
- there are adequate support systems in place;
- understanding and agreement about how far the study (and the child-researcher) should go in prying into the lives of other children.

References

Alderson, P. (2000) 'Children as researchers', in P. Christensen and A. James (eds), *Research with Children*, London, Falmer Press.

Bowlby, J. (1973) *Attachment and Loss*, Volume II: *Separation, Anxiety and Anger*, London, Hogarth.

Boyden, J. and Ennew, J. (eds) (1997) *Children in Focus: a Manual for Participatory Research with Children*, Stockholm, Rädda Barnen.

Butt, J. and Jones, A. (1995) *Taking the Initiative: A Study of Child Protection Services to Black Children and Families*, London, NISW, REU and NSPCC.

Elshtain, J.B. (1997) 'Political children: reflections on Hannah Arendt's distinction between public and private life', in M.L. Shanley and U. Narayan (eds), *Reconstructing Political Theory: Feminist Perspectives*, Cambridge, Polity Press, pp. 109–127.

Fonow, M.M. and Cook, J.A. (1991) *Beyond Methodology: Feminist Scholarship as Lived Research*, Bloomington and Indianapolis, Indiana University Press.

Foucault, M. (1980) 'Prison talk', in C. Gordon (ed.), *Power/Knowledge*, New York: Pantheon, pp. 37–54.

Hill, M. (1997) 'Participatory Research with Children', in *Child and Family Social Work*, London, Blackwell, pp. 171–183.

Humphries, B. (1994) 'Empowerment and social research: elements for an analytic framework', in B. Humphries and C. Truman, *Re-thinking Social Research*, Aldershot, Avebury and Ashgate, pp. 185–203.

Humphries, B. (ed.) (2000) *Research in Social Care & Social Welfare: Issues and Debates for Practice*, London and Philadelphia, Jessica Kingsley.

International Labour Organisation (2002) *A future without Child Labour: Global Report under the Follow-up to the ILO Declaration on Fundamental Principles and Rights at Work*, Geneva, ILO.

Jones, A. (2000a) '*UK immigration policy and practice: a study of the experiences of children and young people*', PhD thesis, Manchester Metropolitan University.

Jones, A. (2000b) 'Exploring young people's experience of immigration controls: the search for an appropriate methodology', in B. Humphries (ed.), *Research in Social Care & Social Welfare: Issues and Debates for Practice*, London and Philadelphia, Jessica Kingsley, pp. 31–47.

Jones, A., Jeyasingham, D. and Rajasooriya, S. (2002) *Invisible Families: The Strengths and Needs of Black Families in which Young People have Caring Responsibilities*, Bristol, Policy Press and Joseph Rowntree Foundation.

Jones, A., Sharpe, J. and Sogren, M. (2003) *Children of Migration: A Study of the Care Arrangements and Psychosocial status of Children of Parents who have Migrated*, St. Augustine, Trinidad, The University of the West Indies, (unpublished research report).

Mohanty, C.T. (1991) 'Cartographies of struggle: Third World women and the politics of feminism', in C.T. Mohanty, A. Russo and L. Torres (eds) (1991) *Third World Women and the Politics of Feminism*, Bloomington and Indianapolis, Indiana University Press, pp. 1–47.

Mohanty, C.T., Russo, A. and Torres, L. (eds) (1991) *Third World Women and the Politics of Feminism*, Bloomington and Indianapolis, India University Press.

Morgan, S. (2000) 'Documentary and text analysis: uncovered meaning in a worked example', in B. Humphries (ed.), *Research in Social Care & Social Welfare: Issues and Debates for Practice*, London and Philadelphia, Jessica Kingsley, pp. 119–131.

Rubin, A. and Babbie, E. (2001) *Research Methods for Social Work*, Belmont, CA, Wadsworth.

Save the Children (1999) *A Journey of Discovery: Children's Creative Participation in Planning*, London, Save the Children.

Shanley, M.L. and Narayan, U. (eds) (1997) *Reconstructing Political Theory: Feminist Perspectives*, Cambridge, Polity Press.

United Nations (1989) *Convention on the Rights of the Child*, New York, United Nations.

Wilkins, P. (2000) 'Collaborative approaches to research', in B. Humphries (ed.), *Research in Social Care & Social Welfare: Issues and Debates for Practice*, London and Philadelphia, Jessica Kingsley, pp. 16–30.

9 Gender
ROB PATTMAN AND MARY JANE KEHILY

In this chapter we will explore some of the issues that arise in the process of doing qualitative research on gender in the lives of children and young people. Our discussion will focus upon examples of research that can be described as self-reflexive and young-person-centred. In using the term 'self-reflexive' we refer to a style whereby the interviewer reflects upon the ways in which identities are produced and negotiated within the context of the research process. This approach to research with children and young people commonly uses methodological approaches that can be described as ethnographic – drawing upon a range of research methods such as participant observation, semi-structured and open-ended interviews with groups and individuals. Overall, such studies aim to contribute to our understanding of social relationships and social categories from the perspective of the respondents themselves. In this context the relationship between the researcher and researched becomes a central dynamic in the study, shaping the research encounter in particular ways that impact upon the contours of the project and the findings (see Frosh et al., 2002). Rather than asking what kind of information is being elicited from boys and girls concerning their attitudes to gender, our aim in this chapter is to provide a critical commentary upon doing research of this kind. Throughout the chapter we reflect upon the many ways in which gender is in play throughout the research process. We will also consider how, in the very process of research, gender identities are being negotiated and constructed.

The chapter will consider the following research issues:

- Gaining access to the social worlds of children and young people
- The influence of the gender of the researcher
- The difficulties associated with researching boys and girls in single sex groups
- Men researching girls
- Interviewing boys and girls together

The following section introduces the concept of gender and discusses some contemporary perspectives that have emerged from research in this field.

Perspectives on gender

Contemporary perspectives on gender often point to a dichotomy between essentialist and social constructionist ways of looking. Essentialism is commonly understood to rest upon biological arguments which posit that gender differences are genetically determined and that each gender carries with it a set of physical, emotional and psychological characteristics. Social constructionist perspectives, on the other hand, suggest that gender is shaped by and through the society in which we live. There are many different social constructionist perspectives on gender. However, they all share the idea that becoming male or female is a social process that is learned through culture: in the family, in school and in social interactions more generally. Viewing gender as culturally specific also suggests that notions of gender are not fixed but may in fact change over time and place. Social constructionist perspectives frequently point to the ways in which gender can be understood as relational. In other words, what it is to be male is often defined in relation to what it is to be female and vice versa. Correspondingly, the gendered identities of masculinity and femininity can be seen as a mutually defining and mutually exclusive relationship. In this respect the relational aspect of gender produces categories sustained by binary opposites which may be invoked in stereotypical ways:

masculinity	femininity
strong	weak
active	passive
hard	soft
rational	emotional

Dualisms such as these may be seen as part of a tradition of Western thought which has many consequences for us as gendered human beings. One often unacknowledged consequence has a direct bearing on sexuality and sexual identity. Sexual desire invoked through gender arrangements is premised upon the widely held assumption that if you are a man you will inevitably be attracted to a woman and if you are a woman you will inevitably be attracted to a man. Rich (1980) refers to this as 'compulsory heterosexuality'; the largely unspoken policing of sexual desire in culture which makes same sex relationships marginal and even taboo. The assumed dominance of a heterosexual order in societies places heterosexual relationships at the centre as 'normal' and normalising and thereby indicates that all other forms of sexual relationship remain 'deviant' and 'abnormal'.

How do these ideas about gender relate to doing research with children and young people? Researchers interested in gender issues within this age group have traditionally focused upon the school as a key site for study. The concept of the 'hidden curriculum' has been used by school-based researchers to acknowledge that much of what young people do at school remains outside the scope of normal pedagogic practices. Moreover, what is learned by students may not fit with the intended aims of teachers and educational policy makers (for a discussion of these themes see Hammersley and Woods, 1976; Whitty, 1985). Qualitative school-based research from the 1970s suggested that through participation in school routines, students learn to conform or resist the official culture of the school (see for example Rosser and Harré, 1976; Willis, 1977). We would like to suggest that the 'hidden curriculum' can also be seen in terms of learning gender. Within the context of the school much informal learning takes place concerning gender roles and relationships. Gender-appropriate behaviour for example is both learned and practised in friendship groups and play activities. A rich vein of research on gender has exposed the gender inequalities that exist between young men and women and the implications of this for those working with young people (e.g. Connell, 1987; Lees, 1986, 1993; Griffin, 1985; Kenway et al., 1998; Weiner and Arnot, 1987; Arnot and Weiler, 1993; Arnot et al., 1999; Gordon et al., 2000). This body of work has the effect of 'making visible' the experience of girls and points to the need to address gender inequalities in school. Gordon, Holland and Lahelma (2000) explored issues of inequality as a spatial dynamic as well as an effect of power relations. Their innovative approach to themes of marginalisation and participation demonstrates the complexity of gender arrangements and the need for a reformulated notion of 'citizenship' to take account of gender relations.

Further research has explored the intersubjectivity of gender and class and particularly girls' troubled relationship with femininity and academic achievement (Walkerdine et al., 2000). Walkerdine et al. illustrate the many ways in which 'growing up girl' involves modes of embracing or eschewing educational success that incur psychic costs. Recent work on masculinities has contributed to the literature on gender by exploring the recognition that boys too are gendered subjects, engaged in the struggle for masculine identities (e.g. Epstein et al., 1998; Mac an Ghaill, 1994; Gilbert and Gilbert, 1998; Pattman et al., 1998; Lingard and Douglas, 1999). Many of the studies we have referred to illustrate the ways in which diverse sexualities can be spoken through the various masculinities young men come to inhabit. Being a lad may involve the cultivation of a hyper-heterosexual identity, while being a 'wimp' implies occupying a feminised or asexual identity that may easily translate into being called 'gay'. In this sense, sexuality underpins the location of young men's masculinities and can be seen to structure gender arrangements more generally.

Further research has drawn attention to the links between gender and sexuality and particularly the heterosexist structure of school relations by acknowledging gay and lesbian identities in school (e.g. Epstein and Johnson, 1998; Mac an Ghaill, 1994; Trenchard and Warren, 1984; Sears, 1992; Britzman, 1995; Nayak and Kehily, 1996). This literature provides us with valuable insights and ways of understanding the power relations involved in the deployment of gender and sexuality as social categories.

Such studies indicate that gender and its relationship with sexuality is not biologically given but is created through institutional and lived practices. Moreover, schools can be seen as sites for the *production* of gendered and sexualised identities rather than as agencies that passively reflect dominant power relations (Kehily, 2002). The homophobia of young men, the sexual reputations of young women; and the pervasive presence of heterosexuality as an 'ideal' and a practice further mark out the terrain for the production of gendered and sexualised identities. Furthermore, such social learning is overt and explicit rather than hidden. These considerations have implications for the process of social learning in childhood and adolescence, particularly in relation to gender. Some of these issues are discussed below. The following sections of this chapter take a look behind the literature to discuss some of the issues that arise during the process of carrying out qualitative research on gender in the lives of children and young people.

Gaining access to the social worlds of children and young people

Understanding the world from the perspective of children and young people involves researchers recognising that it is their respondents who are the 'experts'. The girls and boys who participate in the study can be seen as keepers of the knowledge and insights that researchers hope to glean. This shift in epistemological status from the adult to the child or young person disrupts the usual social relations that take place in schools and families. However, the research relationship is not an unproblematic inversion of normative social relationships. Researching gender with children and young people involves moments of negotiation, identification and reflection. The point we want to emphasise is that a young-person-centred approach to research is dependent upon forging positive personal relationships. Becoming accepted by children and young people to the point where they are willing to share their experiences with you involves time, active listening and mutual respect. Corsaro's (1985) ethnographic study of children in a nursery school in the US describes the process whereby he became accepted by the children as 'Big Bill', the adult who hung out in the home corner. In a UK-based study of primary school girls in Year 5 (Kehily et al., 2002), Kehily was invited to become an 'honorary member' of the 'diary group', a girls' friendship group that met in the playground to discuss friends, boyfriends and puberty. In both cases it could be argued that the gender of the researcher and their approach to children and young people played a significant part in the research.

Frosh et al.'s (2002) interview-based study of 11–14-year-old boys in London, UK addressed how gender can be produced rather than simply elicited in research, and focused on how the boys responded to being positioned as social actors and experts about themselves and their relations with others by a male interviewer. Interviews with individuals and groups were conducted by Rob Pattman. They were semi-structured and encouraged the boys to express themselves in 'narrative' terms – as freely as possible, elaborating on issues of importance to them, with the interviewer adopting a non-judgmental and self-affirming approach. One of the findings of this research was how the experience of being interviewed conflicted with the expectations of most of the boys, and the surprise and pleasure many of the boys expressed at being able to talk at length about their feelings and relationships. This was in part because they imagined the interviewer would be more like a didactic teacher figure, firing questions, putting them on the spot and sitting at the top of the table, rather than in a circle. This caricature of the interviewer, informed by media representations and a societal context in which children rarely discuss their lives with adults, is one that school-based researchers frequently have to overcome. Other researchers conducting school-based ethnographies and interviews have reflected on how they came to be seen by pupils *not* as figures of authority in the way they positioned teachers (see e.g. Kehily and Nayak, 1996; Thorne, 1993; Davies, 1989). In the following section we will discuss some of the research issues that arise as a consequence of the researcher gaining access to the social worlds of children and young people. In particular we will focus upon the gender of the researcher and differences that emerge between one-to-one interviews and group interviews.

The gender of the researcher

In the group interviews in Frosh et al.'s study, 'the boys were much more invested in asserting themselves against girls' (p. 37), for example ridiculing girls for imagining they were more mature than boys, for wanting to play football with boys, for being favoured by teachers and for liking 'girl power' (see also Prendergast and Forrest, 1997; Gilbert and Gilbert, 1998; Kenway et al., 1998). It may be that Pattman, as a male interviewing young men, may have unwittingly contributed to this polarisation of gender in the all-male peer group. As Frosh et al. (2002) found, some boys interviewed in groups accounted for the rapport they established with the interviewer in terms of their shared gender and their assumed shared distancing from females.

> *Maurice:* It's not like talking to a woman (.) if you was like a woman we couldn't talk about the things we've talked about, we couldn't talk to a teacher about porn mags and things like that [*laugh*].
> *Benny:* Yeah we couldn't say things about the girls cos she might disagree. (p. 37)

Frosh et al. found that the same boys when interviewed individually praised girls for their maturity and sensitivity in contrast to boys. It was mainly in individual interviews that boys criticised other boys for being 'uncommunicative, thick-skinned, aggressive and uncaring' – characteristics that were often key motifs of masculinity created in group interviews. These boys were producing 'softer' versions of masculinity, in the sense of being less loud and funny and speaking about emotions and relations in ways which would be derided as 'soft' and 'wimpish' with a group of boys or even with adult males.

The interviewer reported on the irony of some boys interviewed individually confiding in him – a man – about their problems, yet idealising women and girls as sympathetic and supportive listeners. Rather than letting this pass, he challenged these boys to reflect upon how they were polarising gender. For example John was asked what would happen 'if a boy rather than a girl was "quite tender and comforting towards you."' (p. 192). John defined himself as 'hard' and talked graphically about his commitment to fighting, yet spoke in a serious, reflective and critical way about this, and expressed sadness about not seeing his estranged father. He idealised girls and women as people with 'fairer voices' who would sympathise with him about his relationship with his father. Responding to the interviewer he said:

John: He'd be pushed aside.
RP: By you? Would you push him aside?
John: Well, depends if, depends if the boys would push him away first or if I don't get to hear him he might just be bugging me or something so I just push him to the side and then I feel sorry for them because they're trying to help me and then I don't, then I get angry and I'll lose my temper.

While responding to John's idealisation of girls in relation to boys, the interviewer seems to be challenging him to consider how invested *he* is in sustaining tough and hard relations with other boys. What is striking is the reluctance of John to say *he* would 'push him aside', presumably because he had been 'critical of boys for being so unsympathetic and emotionally disengaged' and because he had developed a close relationship with the interviewer that enabled him to be so. When John generalises that 'he'd be pushed aside' the interviewer asks if he would do this. John 'admits' he might push him aside, though qualifies this with 'just' as if diminishing the effect of his action. But he also speaks of getting angry, 'as if he knows he has missed an opportunity' (p. 192). This view of John's was co-constructed in the sense that it emerged as a result of the sort of relations being forged between interviewer and interviewee. Here the interviewer appears to be picking up on John's attachment to him as a caring and interested man who challenged him to reflect upon his longing for these kinds of relations and his investment in a particular male identity collectively constructed and performed in opposition to versions of 'softness'. Such moments of engagement between the researcher and respondent point to the fluidity of gender as a social category and the way it may be shaped by the research space.

The insularity of girls' groups and the problems this poses researchers

In the previous section we focused upon the responses that emerged in research contexts where the interviewer and the interviewee were both male. The discussion pointed to some of the ways in which masculinities may be produced in the process of doing qualitative research. We have drawn your attention to the ways in which masculinity is constructed in relation to femininity. Many of the studies point to the difficulties and tensions that can be associated with the concept of masculinity. In this section we turn our attention to girls and some of the difficulties associated with doing qualitative research with girls.

In an ethnographic study of working class girls in a youth club in Birmingham, UK, McRobbie (1978) suggested that 'it seems that it is more difficult for a woman to be "one of the girls" in this situation, than for a similarly aged male to be "one of the boys."' She suggested that this was because of their reluctance to participate in the 'team spirit of the club' and also the girls' construction of her as a figure of authority. Rather than addressing girls as marginal and peripheral figures in relation to the organised activities in the club and in relation to adult figures like herself, McRobbie centres her research upon the girls and addresses the difficulties posed by this. The girls, she found, tended to construct women 'in terms of their place in the family', or if not, 'as middle class figures of authority – teachers, careers advisors, social workers and so on' (p. 40), which was how, McRobbie claimed, they saw her. Her difficulty in 'gaining entry as a researcher' also stemmed from the 'cliquishness, insularity and exclusiveness' of the small groups the girls developed. In these the girls 'elevate out of all proportion a distinctly feminine ideology', preferring 'fashion, beauty and female interests to the team spirit of the club'. These girls, McRobbie suggests, were constructing their femininity and creating spaces for themselves through this kind of opposition. McRobbie took her difficulties of relating to these girls as a starting point for investigating the kinds of feminine identities they are forging rather than as confirmation of their essential cliquishness and passivity.

Hey (1997) in her ethnographic study of girls' friendships contested the 'fantasy of imagining that our feminism secures for us [as feminist researchers] the privilege of "becoming one of the girls" through wishing away the differences between us and them' (p. 49). Echoing McRobbie, she claimed that 'in electing to study girls and their cultures I was already committed to accessing precisely those spaces designed to keep intruders out' (p. 45). Hey provided a graphic account of how early on in the research she arranged to follow a particular working class girl only to be publicly rebuked by her when she went to collect her. '"It's that woman!" she yelled, running to the back of the classroom'. This incident, according to Hey, illustrated not only 'the salience of class antagonism' at the school, and how she was being constructed as a middle class outsider, but also girls' commitment to small and exclusive friendship groups. Their 'social and psychological investments' (p. 47) in these, she suggested, are reinforced by the school's failure to address their lived experiences of gender power relations.

Both McRobbie and Hey attempted to develop closer relations with girls to enable them to be more girl-centred and to investigate how they saw themselves and others. McRobbie, for example, served the girls coffee at the youth club and was careful not to look too closely at them or to question them at disco nights. Trying to build a good relationship with them by dancing with them at the disco, was, however, counterproductive, as one woman youth leader found to her cost. 'The girls…saw this as an infringement to their private territory and made this hostility clear.' These tensions reveal just how united the girls' groups were by their opposition to 'outsiders'. Significantly, 'male leaders expressed no such difficulty in participating in the boys' activities' (p. 40). Through a sustained attempt to build up relationships, Hey managed to engage in sports activities with the girls, go to cafés and even bunk off school with some of them. While some of these activities may present a challenge to teachers and parents, it should be noted that the tradition of participant observation in ethnographic research prioritises 'hanging out' with respondents in order to understand actions from their perspective.

Resistance to Hey's research came not just (initially at least) from some of the girls, but also from male teachers and boys. The teachers constructed the research as 'feminist' and subversive and tried defusing the threat it was seen to pose through mocking humour, and the boys 'had taken upon themselves the role of conveying collective male disapproval'. One boy 'challenged' her 'right to study girls' in the class in which she was present and others stared at her and gave 'mild verbal abuse'. Hey viewed this as 'male resistance to being ignored' and saw it as expressing 'both boys' jealousy as well as power' (p. 44). This, as we have already pointed out, is supported by recent school-based research in Britain and Australia which has noted a tendency for boys to construct themselves as victims of feminism and teachers' sexism, and to respond to this by asserting themselves in macho ways.

Men researching girls

Historically male researchers have been criticised by feminist writers for unconsciously marginalising girls in qualitative research. McRobbie and Garber (1976), for instance, critiqued Willis's (1972) treatment of girls as peripheral figures in his study of motorbike subcultures. They argued that this reflected his failure to focus on how he as a man may have influenced the ways girls positioned themselves in relation to him.

> Willis does comment on some of the girls' responses to questions – giggling, reluctance to talk and their retreat into cliquishness. Are they typical responses to a male researcher, influenced by the fact that he is a man, by his personal appearance,

attractiveness, etc? Or are the responses influenced by the fact that he is identified by the girls as "with the boys"? Or are these responses characteristic of the ways girls customarily negotiate the space provided for them in a male dominated and defined culture? (McRobbie and Garber, 1976: 210)

In his study of racism and gender identities in a primary school, Connolly (1998) reflected on how being an adult man limited his interactions with girls so that he was unable to address what we have seen was a key dimension of girls' lives – their small friendship groupings.

The very nature of the girls' friendship networks, located in more private and intimate groupings meant that I, as both an adult and a male, found them almost impossible to access.

This, he suggested, was compounded by his own tendency to 'identify with the essentially public nature of the boys' field' (p. 138). Similarly, Willis's (1977) study of working class boys in a West Midlands comprehensive school in the UK has been critiqued for his over-identification with 'the lads'. The non-conformist 'lads' became the main protagonists in Willis's study and overshadowed the presence of other groups within the school such as girls, teachers and the low-status boys known as 'ear'oles'. Such selective focusing could indicate the dominance of certain groups over others. However, the interpretive lens could also point to Willis's status as 'wannabe lad', identifying with one group at the expense of others on the basis of shared affiliations. Many of the difficulties involved in carrying out cross-gender research of this kind may be attributed to issues of gender identification. In the course of field relationships, researchers identify with respondents they recognise as like themselves in some way, where exchanges and events may be familiar and may, in some cases, be reminiscent of earlier childhood experiences. We return to this theme below.

Mixed gender interviews

Though we have focused on research which addresses gender as relational, we have not addressed issues raised by interviewing boys and girls in mixed groups. Many boys who had been interviewed in all-male peer groups, in Frosh et al.'s study, expressed 'horror' at the prospect of being interviewed with girls. This was the response, for example, from one group of boys:

James: They'd be hogging the tape not giving us a chance to speak.
Benny: They'd be saying, 'Oh that's not true, you lot do this, you lot do that'
...
Joey: They'll be a big argument in that.
Benny: Oh my God.
Marvin: Ohh.

Frosh et al. (2002) interpreted this as 'part of the collective gender performance in which boys were engaged, constructing themselves with much humour in opposition to easily offended, serious, obsessively talkative and bossy girls' (p. 38). Yet in most of the mixed gender interviews they conducted the boys expressed surprise that they were able to engage with girls without hostility. For though the girls seemed quite elitist, acting like teachers and addressing boys as rather slow and stupid pupils, they also related to them as potential friends. It appeared that boys in these interviews were not (as in many single sex group interviews) patronising, nor did they attack girls for being 'soft' but, to some extent, they identified with the girls' concerns with the boys' monopolisation of football and playground space and disruptive behaviour in class. Most of the girls welcomed the opportunity to speak about themselves and boys, and interpreted the male interviewer's interest in the problems they spoke about concerning their relations with boys as evidence of his 'siding' with them. This may encourage girls to respond positively to the interviewer and express themselves fluently. Many researchers have, however, observed how boys try to assert themselves in relation to girls in the classroom often by being 'naughty' or through the threat of this (see for example, Spender, 1982; Francis, 1998; Connolly, 1998; Gilbert and Gilbert, 1998). These 'performances', as some researchers have found, characterise mixed gender interviews.

Our focus in this chapter has been with people's investments in what they say and how they construct gender through talking about themselves and others in specific kinds of qualitative research (see Hollway and Jefferson, 2000 for a discussion of these themes). Respondents, however, are not free, unfettered authors creating themselves out of nothing. They are constrained by the positions made available to them in longstanding popular cultural discourses (Foucault, 1979) and, as in many of the examples cited, the positions available to young men and women remain very different. Sometimes differences may exist at the level of language use. In an interview-based study of young people in the UK, Holland et al. (1998) found differences between the ways in which young men and women spoke about sexual matters. In contrast to young men who were 'comfortable' with 'embodied sex talk', young women 'drew on euphemisms or faced difficulties in expressing their experiences'. While mixed gender interviews may serve to reproduce longstanding gender inequalities and polarities, mixed gender interviews may encourage girls to respond to the boys in ways that challenge the 'oppressive' construction of boys as subjects and girls as objects of a sex drive (Hollway, 1989).

Gender as a feature of Western childhood: remembering the 'inner child'

One of the characteristics of the research we have discussed in this chapter is that it addresses young people as social actors. This raises questions about the research relationship; the positioning of the (adult) male/female researchers and the young male/female researched. Thorne (1993) argued that in order to be young person centred we must resist our tendency to identify as fully developed and free thinking adults by constructing children, in contrast, as 'developing' and as 'passive recipients of socialisation' (p. 13). This, she suggested, entails remembering (rather than splitting and forgetting) the kinds of masculine or feminine identities one inhabited as a child and the sorts of relations one established with other boys and girls. In her ethnographic study of gender relations at an elementary school in the US, she found that the sorts of feelings she developed for particular girls evoked feelings similar to those she had as a child. These were tied to the ways she positioned herself in the past in hierarchical relations with other girls. Significantly, she identified with girls, not boys, through memories, which suggested, perhaps, how gender segregated many childhood experiences tend to be. Since these feelings influenced how she reacted to the girls in her research and the amount of time and attention she devoted to them, recollecting 'the child within' was central to understanding the research. She wrote, for example, of how she realised how 'obsessed' she was with 'documenting' one girl's 'popularity'.

> 'The rich get richer,' I thought to myself as I sorted out yet another occasion when Kathryn got extra attention and resources. Then I realised the envy behind my note-taking and analysis and recalled that…when I was a fourth and fifth grader of middling social status, I had also carefully watched the popular girl, using a kind of applied sociology to figure out my place in a charged social network. (Thorne, 1993: 24)

With another girl, Beth, Thorne felt 'aversion rather than envy'. For Beth had few friends, and sitting next to her at lunch, which Beth invited Thorne to do, 'brought minimal social yield'. Thorne responded 'vaguely' to her invitation ('maybe, we'll see') much as she had done when she was at school and another unpopular girl 'was trying to cling to me and I didn't want her social encumbrance' (p. 25). Reflecting upon herself in this way, Thorne provided powerful insights not only into how girls construct hierarchical relations between themselves, but also into her own investments in focusing on particular girls. Becoming conscious of this enabled her to reflect upon these relations: 'Instead of obsessing over Kathryn and avoiding Beth…I tried to understand their different social positions and experiences, and those of other girls and boys' (Thorne, 1993: 27).

Conclusion

The issues we have discussed in this chapter have important implications for gender identities and in particular for conducting research on gender with children and young people. These can be seen in terms of the need to focus upon young people's cultures, to recognise children and young people themselves as *expert* commentators on their social world. This approach involves developing appropriate and self-reflexive ways of relating to boys and girls. Frosh et al. (2002) argued that the sorts of young-person-centred interviews they conducted and the supportive and non-judgmental relations established between interviewer and interviewees could and should be replicated in other research settings. Their study demonstrated that boys were extremely engaged when being interviewed at length by an adult who *listened* to them and *showed interest* in them. Furthermore, we also saw how these kinds of young-person-centred discussions could be highly creative in challenging negative behaviour and promoting more equitable gender relations. As Mac an Ghaill (1994) and Frosh et al. (2002) have shown, male researchers can relate to boys in 'softer' ways. Through the research encounter boys may form attachments and identifications with the interviewer that enable and encourage them to become critical of popular versions of masculinity based around bullying, misogyny and homophobia. By encouraging boys to be critical of popular forms of masculinity, Frosh et al. stressed that it is important not to blame boys but rather to highlight the contradictory ways boys act in groups in contrast to when they are 'on their own'.

The studies of McRobbie and Hey challenge researchers to reflect upon their relations with girls and whether they contribute to the marginalisation of girls by taking boys' monopolisation of spaces for granted and constructing girls as peripheral figures. How, as female (and male) adults, they can relate to girls in young-person-centred ways which are not perceived as intrusive, should be of key concern not only to researchers, but to youth workers and teachers. Mixed gender interviews, as we saw, offered possibilities for breaking down and renegotiating gender polarities. It may be that boys and girls need to be split into relatively small groups if they are to engage in supportive and self-reflexive dialogue with each other and to become less invested in emphasising gender difference. Finally, Thorne's commitment to young-person-centred relations with children invites adults researching and working with children to reflect upon their own investments in distancing themselves from children and to 'remember the child within'. In such moments of reflection researchers may consider the ways in which they identify with some children while distancing themselves from others. By reflecting upon our own girlhood/boyhood we may learn some important lessons about the social connectedness of research – ourselves in relation to the young people we study.

References

Arnot, M. and Weiler, K. (1993) *Feminism and Social Justice in Education, International Perspectives*, London, Falmer.

Arnot, M., David, M. and Weiner, G. (1999) *Closing the Gender Gap*, Cambridge, Polity Press.

Britzman, D. (1995) 'What is this thing called love?', *Taboo: Journal of Culture and Education*, 1: 65–93.

Butler, J. (1990) *Gender Trouble*, Cambridge, Polity Press.

Connell, R.W. (1987) *Gender and Power: Society, the Person and Sexual Politics*, Sydney, Allen and Unwin.

Connell, R.W. (1995) *Masculinities*, Cambridge, Polity Press.

Connolly, P. (1998) *Racism, Gender Identities and Young Children*, London and New York, Routledge.

Corsaro, W. (1985) *Friendship and Peer Culture in the Early Years*, Norwood, NJ, Ablex.

Davies, B. (1989) *Frogs and Snails and Feminist Tails*, London, Allen and Unwin.

Epstein, D. (ed.) (1994) *Challenging Gay and Lesbian Inequalities in Education*, Buckingham, Open University Press.

Epstein, D. and Johnson, R. (1994) 'On the straight and the narrow: the heterosexual presumption, homophobias and schools', in D. Epstein (ed.), *Challenging Gay and Lesbian Inequalities in Education*, Buckingham, Open University Press.

Epstein, D. and Johnson, R. (1998) *Schooling Sexualities*, Buckingham, Open University Press.

Epstein, D., Elwood, J., Hey, V. and Maw, J. (eds) (1998) *Failing Boys? Issues of Gender and Achievement*, Buckingham, Open University Press.

Foucault, M. (1979) *The History of Sexuality*, Vol. 1, trans. R. Hurley, London, Allen Lane.

Francis, B. (1998) *Power Plays*, Stoke-on-Trent, Trentham Books.

Frosh, S., Phoenix, A. and Pattman, R. (2002) *Young Masculinities*, Basingstoke, Palgrave.

Gilbert, R. and Gilbert, P. (1998) *Masculinity Goes to School*, London, Routledge.

Gordon, T., Holland, J. and Lahelma, E. (2000) *Making Spaces: Citizenship and Difference in Schools*, London, Macmillan.

Griffin, C. (1985) *Typical Girls? Young Women from School to the Job Market*, London, Routledge.

Hammersley, M. and Woods, P. (eds) (1976) *The Process of Schooling: a Sociological Reader*, London, Routledge and Kegan Paul.

Hey, V. (1997) *The company She Keeps: an Ethnography of Girls' Friendships*, Buckingham, Open University Press.

Holland, J., Ramazanoglu, C., Sharpe, S. and Thomson, R. (1998) *The Male in the Head*, London, Tufnell Press.

Hollway, W. (1989) *Subjectivity and Method in Psychology*, London, Sage.

Hollway, W. and Jefferson, T. (2000) *Doing Qualitative Research Differently*, London, Sage.

Kehily, M.J. (2002) *Sexuality, Gender and Schooling: Shifting Agendas in Social Learning*, London, Routledge.

Kehily. M. and Nayak, A. (1996) 'The Christmas kiss: sexuality, story-telling and schooling', *Curriculum Studies*, 4(2): 211–227.

Kehily, M.J., Mac an Ghaill, M., Epstein, D. and Redman, P. (2002) 'Private girls and public worlds: producing femininities in the primary school', *Discourse*, 23(2): 167–177.

Kenway, J. and Willis, S. with Blackmore, J. and Rennie, L. (1998) *Answering Back: Girls, Boys and Feminism in Schools*, London, Routledge.

Lees, S. (1986) *Losing Out: Sexuality and Adolescent Girls*, London, Hutchinson.

Lees, S. (1993) *Sugar and Spice, Sexuality and Adolescent Girls*, Harmondsworth, Penguin.

Lingard, B. and Douglas, P. (1999) *Men Engaging Feminisms, Profeminisms, Backlashes and Schooling*, Buckingham, Open University Press.

Mac an Ghaill, M. (1994) *The Making of Men: Masculinities, Sexualities and Schooling*, Buckingham, Open University Press.

McRobbie, A. (1978) 'Working class girls and the culture of femininity', in Women's Study Group, *Women Take Issue: Aspects of Women's Subordination*, London, HarperCollins.

McRobbie, A. and Garber, J. (1976) 'Girls and subcultures: an exploration', in S. Hall and T. Jefferson, *Resistance through Rituals*, London, HarperCollins.

Nayak, A. and Kehily, M.J. (1996) 'Playing it straight: masculinities, homophobia and schooling', *Journal of Gender Studies*, 5(2): 211–230.

Pattman, R., Frosh, S. and Phoenix, A. (1998) 'Lads, machos and others: developing "boy-centred" research', *Journal of Youth Studies*, 1(2): 125–142.

Prendergast, S. and Forrest, S. (1997) 'Hieroglyphs of the heterosexual: learning about gender in school', in L. Segal (ed.), *New Sexual Agendas*, Basingstoke, Macmillan.

Rich, A. (1980) 'Compulsory heterosexuality and lesbian existence', *Signs*, 5(4): 631–660.

Rosser, E. and Harré, R. (1976) 'The meaning of trouble', in M. Hammersley and P. Woods (eds), *The Process of Schooling, a Sociological Reader*, London, Routledge and Kegan Paul.

Salisbury, J. and Jackson, D. (1996) *Challenging Macho Values*, London, Falmer Press.

Sears, J. (ed.) (1992) *Sexuality and the Curriculum: the Politics and Practices of Sexuality Education*, New York, Teachers' College Press.

Spender, D. (1982) *Invisible Women*, London, The Women's Press.

Stanley, L. and Wise, S. (1983) *Breaking Out: Feminist Consciousness and Feminist Research*, London, Routledge and Kegan Paul.

Thorne, B. (1993) *Gender Play: Girls and Boys in School*, Buckingham, Open University Press.

Trenchard, L. and Warren, H. (1984) *Something to Tell You: the Experiences and Needs of Young Lesbians and Gay Men in London*, London, Gay Teenage Group.

Walkerdine, V., Lucey, H. and Melody, J. (2000) *Growing Up Girl: Psychological Explorations of Gender and Class*, London, Macmillan.

Weiner, G. and Arnot, M. (eds) (1987) *Gender under Scrutiny: New Inquiries in Education*, London, Hutchinson.

Whitty, G. (1985) *Sociology and School Knowledge, Curriculum Theory, Research and Politics*, London, Methuen.

Willis, P. (1972) 'Pop music and youth groups', PhD., Centre for Contemporary Cultural Studies, University of Birmingham.

Willis, P. (1977) *Learning to Labour: How Working Class Kids Get Working Class Jobs*, Aldershot, Saxon House.

SECTION 3 DIVERSITY

10 Early Childhood
ANN LANGSTON, LESLEY ABBOTT, VICKY LEWIS AND MARY KELLETT

In this chapter we are taking the period of early childhood to cover birth to five years. Although this is not a vast period in terms of years it presents unique difficulties for researchers because of the huge changes which occur. Over these five years, the newborn baby develops from being entirely dependent on adults for his or her every need into a child who can take care of many personal needs independently of adults, can express desires, create imaginary situations, perhaps write his or her own name, communicate and interact socially with a range of people and so on. Nevertheless, there are vast individual differences which are especially apparent during this period of enormous development, with some children being extremely independent from a very young age, whereas others may remain highly dependent throughout this period. In addition, particularly in the minority world, by the age of five years many children will have already made a move away from their home environment through attending some sort of pre-school provision and will be embarking on the beginning of a lengthy period of formal education. Thus, it is a period of great change and variability. In this chapter we consider a number of issues which arise when carrying out research with children under five years old. However, it is first important to consider the status of knowledge in this area and the kinds of research that are undertaken with this age group of children.

The status of early childhood research

Those who live and work closely with young children, such as parents, playgroup staff or reception class teachers, have a wealth of knowledge about young children's capabilities and yet most research is carried out by people who are not in regular day to day contact with the children, for example researchers working within universities. This has led to two sorts of tension. The first concerns our understanding of the capabilities of young children. The second, related tension concerns the status which is afforded to different findings depending on who originated them.

Historically, much research evidence, often from within the discipline of developmental psychology, has suggested that young children are not capable of very much. This is despite reports of the competence of young children from those who know them best, namely families and practitioners. Thus, in 2002, in a report focusing on under-threes, the Department of Education and Skills commented:

> Families and practitioners who work with babies and young children have a fund of anecdotal evidence...demonstrating their amazing capabilities. Yet for too long perhaps, researchers thought that children under three could not do very much. This may be due in part to the ways in which research used to be carried out (DeLoache and Brown, 1987), since laboratory-based experimental research was considered the only reputable and scientific method and only a few researchers were brave enough to try to break this mould in order to provide more 'real-life' evidence. (DfES, 2002a)

This report points to the second tension, between laboratory-based research and more 'real-life' evidence which, while evident in much research with children and young people of all ages, is particularly clear when research in the early years is considered. This tension, often seen as a tension between quantitative and qualitative research, has been reflected on by Sylva (1995). She refers to a 'medieval banquet' attended by 'barons...from the quantitative alliance...and troubadours specialising in the rich vein of human discourse known as narrative...minstrels as well, singing passionately of childhood and its many different voices'. She argues that in this collection of researchers 'it's difficult to describe the contribution of each person let alone decide who should sit at high table or drink mead'. The implication of Sylva's argument is that guests at high table or invited to drink mead are more likely to be those whose research is considered 'credible'.

The question of credibility is key here. For many years academic research was the preserve of a predominantly male workforce in universities and laboratories. Such research has acquired a reputation for objectivity and credibility. However, even within academic psychology different topics were afforded more or less status. Thus, Gopnik, Professor of Psychology at the University of California at Berkeley, points out that prior to 1973 there were no women in the Berkeley psychology department, and she comments 'So long as men dominated academia, developmental psychology was' itself 'marginalised' (Gopnik et al., 2001). Clearly, power relations have been institutionally unequal between males and females and, perhaps not surprisingly, children who 'were part of women's realm' were in the past 'deemed unworthy of serious scientific interest' (ibid.).

However, recently there has been a growth in early years practitioner research. Such research, based in a largely female profession, is in its infancy both in terms of the funding it receives and the credibility attached to it. The current reality is that practitioner research is often viewed as subjective, reliant on anecdote and based on unproven hunches. The researchers involved may be workers from a nursery, playgroup or crèche. The research which they carry out may be extremely valid and worthwhile.

Nevertheless, what is published or valued and counts as 'real' research tends to be from well-established sources, such as that of a university-based research team.

As a consequence, there is a predictable imbalance between the relative status of different types of published research. 'Real-life' research, conducted in the course of familiar activities by those who know the child and the context well, such as practitioners, has traditionally been undervalued compared with laboratory-based research, which takes the child out of his or her usual context. This is gradually changing mainly because of a growing recognition that laboratory research, while useful for physical and scientific purposes, has less validity when making deductions about human behaviour or ideas. In addition, an expansion in education and vocational training has led to a more 'hands on' approach, where practitioners have been required to undertake research in the course of their work, in order to be able to reflect upon their own practice. In universities this has been mirrored by an increase in the numbers of academic posts in Early Childhood Education and Care, particularly at professorial level, most of which (six between 1998 and 2003) have been conferred on women emerging from a strong tradition of teaching and working in the early years sector.

There is a growing body of 'strategic' early childhood research. Young children have become high profile in the present economic climate. A great deal of money has been invested in the development of services for children and families and inevitably the government requires evidence that this is well spent. The importance of research and evaluation as key contributors to the government's childcare strategy is not disputed. In fact, research and evaluation undertaken in the UK and abroad, e.g. Headstart (Lazar and Darlington, 1982) and High/Scope (Schweinhart and Weikart, 1994), which showed unequivocally the long term and social importance of investing in high quality early childhood services.

Staying with government agendas, the introduction of the National Curriculum exerted a downward pressure on early years education (David, 1998) and generated polarised debate about developmentally appropriate learning experiences for young children (Owens, 1997). Researchers like Blenkin and Kelly (1994) argued that National Curriculum style programmes were the most alienating form of curriculum for young children. They advocated curricula that 'provide for and nurture the child's development through a range of symbolizing activities' (Blenkin, 1994: 28) where social context and a play environment were vital. Blenkin described a 'head-on-clash' (1994: 37) between *target-driven, formalised* learning and the *process* of learning, responding to young children according to what they are to become rather than what they are in the here and now.

In the remainder of this chapter we examine a number of methodological issues which arise when carrying out research with children between birth and five years.

Methodological issues

In addition to the question of who carries out the research there are many methodological issues which arise when carrying out research with young children. In this section we shall consider issues concerning who carries out the research, access, consent, where the research is located, the methods that are used and how the data are interpreted.

Who does the research?

Parallels may be drawn between the relative status of male and female work and pay in the childcare sector, and the relative status of practitioner and university research in the early years. As already indicated, this situation is gradually changing partly as a consequence of the expansion in education and vocational training. This has led to a more 'hands on' approach, in which practitioners have been required to undertake research in the course of their work, in order to reflect upon their own practice.

Nevertheless, since the vast majority of staff in childcare settings are female, practitioner research is equally gendered, raising the question as to whether the focus of research is skewed accordingly or whether, when males undertake research in such settings, they face particular problems. The first issue is itself worthy of research since feminist researchers would argue that gender is a significant factor in both what is studied and what is concluded when persons of either gender undertake research. The second issue is also important since, as we shall discuss later, if young children are involved in research in unfamiliar contexts, they may behave differently. Since the majority of children in the minority world, especially in their early years, still spend a larger proportion of their time with women than with men, the presence of a male researcher in their home or pre-school setting may well be an unfamiliar event and affect their behaviour.

A further concern is that of safety. In what has been described as a 'heavily gendered division of…labour' (Cameron et al., 1999) it is small wonder that the issue of 'safety' emerges in undertaking research with young children. Perceived threats to children's safety usually relate to perceptions about the motives of males in childcare, which link to their alleged propensity to being abusive to children and violent to both women and children. This follows on from a view that 'childcare' is 'naturally' women's work, whereas men childcare workers, being 'not women', are seen as 'unnatural' (ibid.). Reeves (2001) argues that having abolished myths that barred women from male professions, 'It is time to drop the similarly short-sighted prejudices about men's ability to care, to cuddle, to teach, to play' and, we would add, 'to research'. However, it is important that researchers, of either gender, safeguard children (and themselves), and ensure that their presence and purpose in the setting is transparent and supervised at all times so that safety is never compromised.

Access to children under five

Access to children under five has become increasingly complex. The rapid expansion of childcare and early education provision in recent years has meant that more young children are spending increasing lengths of time in out-of-home settings. Few research studies at the present time focus on the child in isolation. New initiatives such as Early Excellence Centres and Sure Start have opened up opportunities for young children and their families to access integrated care, education, training and support from a range of professionals, including those involved in health, social work, education and community care.

The traditional forms of pre-school provision, i.e. childminding, private and voluntary sector nurseries and playgroups, have also benefited from increased funding. This has meant, for some settings, changes in the type of service they offer and the length of time they are able to open in order to meet the needs of working parents. The provision of high quality services for children and families is a key priority for the government, whose 'vision' is that every parent will be able to access affordable, good quality childcare (DfES, 2002b). By March 2006, an extra 300,000 children will access children's centre services, including childcare. The Inter-Departmental Childcare Review provided strong evidence of significant benefits to children when good quality childcare is delivered alongside early years education, family support and health services. These kinds of initiative mean that access to children under five frequently has to go through several layers of 'gatekeepers'. In the past, consent from a parent was all that was needed for most research with young children. In integrated care settings additional consent may be required from health workers, social workers and educators with increased levels of ethical clearance and child protection checks. While these measures are clearly intended to protect children from unscrupulous or harmful research, there is also the possibility that the presence of additional gatekeeping layers introduces other 'agendas' into the research studies.

However, the fact that certain types of provision exist because they are responding to a particular set of community needs can make it easier for a researcher to identify the kind of provision, location and cultural context they require. For example, although there are considerable regional variations in the ways in which the Sure Start programme is delivered, the clear aims and principles to which each programme must adhere mean that representative samples can be located within that particular programme. It may be less easy to locate a representative sample for the researcher whose focus requires that very specific criteria are met. Nevertheless the variety of settings in the UK in which young children can be found makes this search much easier for researchers than it was prior to government changes since 1997.

Consent

Young children, and sometimes their parents, are especially vulnerable and it is important that researchers ensure that their health, safety and protection are safeguarded. Access to certain groups of particularly vulnerable children may be denied and where access is allowed researchers must behave in sensitive and ethical ways.

For those wanting to carry out research with very young children the consent of the parent or guardian is crucial, whether this is obtained directly from the parent or through an intermediary such as the head of some pre-school provision. Parents and others involved need to be informed clearly about the nature of the research and what will be involved. Sometimes the particular research questions being addressed may mean that parents cannot be fully informed of the aims of the research because such knowledge might influence the outcome, as in studies involving parents and children interacting with one another. In such cases it is important that parents are told as much as possible before the study and are fully debriefed about the study afterwards, including being told why they could not be fully informed at the outset and being given the option for their data to be destroyed. When research is of a potentially sensitive nature, for example the study of factors influencing educational achievement, care should be taken with how parents are informed to ensure that they take away positive, rather than negative messages which might impact adversely on how they behave towards their child. Parents should be told that they have the right to withdraw their child at any point, without this having any negative impact on how their child may or may not be treated subsequently. For example, in health research, parents might be concerned that if they do not agree to their child taking part in a research study their child's subsequent treatment outside of the study might be jeopardised. If it is not possible for parents to be present throughout the research study they need to be informed about the circumstances under which the researchers would terminate the research.

Very young children who are not yet verbal obviously cannot give their consent. However, they may indicate their like or dislike of taking part in a research study in a number of different ways. They may turn away, cry, refuse to engage with materials or the researcher and so on. It is crucial that the child's best interests are always paramount in the mind of the researcher. The child's responses should be monitored during the course of the research, preferably by someone outside the research team, such as a parent, carer or practitioner. Researchers need to be aware of the body language of babies and young children and show sensitivity to children and the messages they convey with regard to their consent or otherwise to taking part in research. Even very young babies can signal their dislike of a research procedure. In acknowledging that 'Birth to Three Matters' (DfES, 2002a), the government's framework of effective practice urges all those who work with young children to 'look, listen and note the body language of babies', in order to increase their skill and sensitivity in responding to them.

Researchers also need to be aware that children may hide their dislike of taking part in a research study. Children quickly become skilled in giving adults what they want and for very young children feelings of discomfort in being 'researched' may be masked by their desire to please. As Hatch (1995) reminds us, 'Children learn to manage their feelings and emotional expressions to correspond with adult expectations – that is, to deny their feelings and emotional expressions to correspond with adults' expectations'.

Context

We have already alluded to the fact that research with young children which is carried out in an environment that is familiar to them may be of greater value in terms of the validity of the findings than studying the children in an unfamiliar setting. A difficulty with laboratory-based research is that when a child is confronted with a task which is disembedded from his or her experience, it can have a marked effect on his or her performance.

Consider the following example. Under-twos were given four tasks to assess their developing skills: point to different facial features; put on and take off a pair of shoes; stack a pile of coloured bricks; draw lines and circles (rather than scribbles) on a piece of paper (Feinstein, 1999). These tasks were administered to the children in a research laboratory in a university. It was found that children with parents of middle class professional backgrounds were more successful at completing the tasks than children of working class parents, and this was interpreted as highlighting a socio-economic attainment gap.

These findings attracted the attention of the media and were headlined in *The Observer* in November 2002 as 'Britain's class divide starts even before nursery school' (Ahmed, 2002). Children, it was reported, were observed to be greatly different even at 22 months, illustrating, *we are informed*, that unless the class divide is tackled head on, only 14 per cent of young people from lower class backgrounds in the current child population will go on to university, compared with 75 per cent of those from advantaged backgrounds. In response to such shocking findings the government was said to have set up a special unit to look at how parents of working class children can be helped to close the divide.

So what might be going on here? Do these findings demonstrate a real class divide or can they be attributed to the context in which the research was carried out? Support for the latter view comes from a seminal study carried out by Tizard and Hughes (1984). They studied two groups of four-year-old girls who all attended the same nursery. One group of girls came from a middle class background; the other group had parents classified as working class. The girls were observed both at nursery and in their own homes. At nursery the two groups of girls behaved very differently. The girls with middle class backgrounds were more likely to engage in table-top activities, to interact with the staff, to produce longer and more complex sentences, etc. In effect, the middle class girls appeared more competent. However, when the two groups of girls were observed at home with their mothers the differences disappeared. The children of working class parents were just as fluent, played just as imaginatively, etc. In this study the comparison was not between a laboratory and a familiar context but between two familiar contexts. So why should there be this difference in how the children of working class parents behaved in these two contexts? Tizard and Hughes argue that the nursery environment more closely resembled the home environments of the girls from middle class homes in terms of the décor, the toys and materials, what was expected of them, and the ways in which the adults talked and behaved.

Given Tizard and Hughes's findings, it seems very plausible that Feinstein's results could be due to the children from working class backgrounds being more affected by the nature of the testing set-up, the researchers and the university environment than the children from middle class backgrounds. These factors alone could explain the results, rather than any underlying differences in ability.

It is therefore crucial that researchers working with young children take account of the children's familiarity with the building in which the research takes place, their familiarity with the people carrying out the research, and their familiarity with the language and resources used. In support of this, childcare workers and those involved with young children frequently comment upon the differences in children's behaviour both at the setting and between home and the setting. There may even be differences within one setting. In a study of four-year-olds a child was described

> who said nothing inside his nursery but, when he was tape-recorded in conversation with the [nursery] caretaker in the garden, he stood next to him and explained some of the most complicated details about the scaffolding he could see around a building. (Cousins, 1999: 29).

Similarly, close family members also know that their children may be 'shy' or 'show off' in the presence of certain people. Children, including young babies, respond to a number of contextual factors and for this reason, research in children's homes may be more representative of their 'normal' behaviour than in an out-of-home setting, with which they are less familiar. Conducting research in the home may nevertheless be fraught with difficulties, particularly since it is likely to be undertaken by researchers with whom the child is unfamiliar. This raises issues connected with 'observer effects', that is, the situation being changed as a consequence of the researcher's presence in the home. This is likely to be emphasised when the accommodation is small or when the researcher is focusing on a single aspect of experience, such as a child's play choices, where the researcher's intervention may influence the child's usual routines or activity. In addition, familiarity with the people carrying out the research may be particularly significant when very young children are involved, since there is evidence that at between six and nine months of age babies become less confident with strangers, 'sometimes showing stranger fear' (Bruce and Meggitt, 2002: 71). This fear may continue for a considerable time, emerging and disappearing throughout the early years.

Appropriate methods

The aim of empirical research is to clarify understanding. However, very often the way in which we set about research is coloured by our current view of things. This is especially evident in research with young children. As we saw in Chapter 3, for a number of years the prevailing scientific view of young children, particularly among developmental psychologists, was one of incompetence. To an extent this was consistent with the view in the minority world of young children as dependent and perhaps because of this it remained unchallenged for some time. However, it was at odds with experiences in the majority world, where young children are often invested with responsibility for the care of even younger siblings, or for contributing to the family's subsistence, by working either in or outside of the home. In addition, since the development in the 1980s of children's rights legislation (UN, 1989; Children Act, 1989), listening to children and taking their views and wishes into account has become increasingly important. Thus, researchers, particularly those working with young children, need to consider how to elicit competence, rather than being influenced by their own, and others', preconceived notions of what young children can and cannot do.

The influential work of Bell (1979) heralded a turning point in our understanding of early social communication. Until then the infant had been regarded as a passive individual. Bell signalled the infant's potential as a sophisticated communicator. There followed a rapid growth in research relating to caregiver–infant interaction (e.g. Schaffer, 1977; Brazelton, 1979; Stern, 1985). Bruner (1977: 273) examined the relationship between early social interaction and language acquisition, maintaining that 'many of the organising features of syntax, semantics, pragmatics, and even phonology may have important precursors and prerequisites in the pre-speech communicative acts of infants'. Sameroff (1975) and Hodapp and Goldfield (1983) developed the concept of social development occurring as a result of the infant interacting with his or her social environment. Research also grew in the areas of intentionality (Newson, 1979) where the attribution of intention to infant acts facilitated *proto-conversations* (Bateson, 1975) and assisted the infant's progress through three distinct phases of communication: *perlocutionary* (non-directive), *illocutionary* (directive communicative acts) and *locutionary* (representational communicative acts).

The onus, then, is upon researchers to determine the fitness for purpose of any methods used in their endeavours to find out about babies and young children. Adapting methods to meet the purpose of research is essential if young children are to be represented fairly. Some early research by Kaye (1977) used the burst-pause (sucking-scanning) sequences of breast-feeding babies to explore the importance of synchronised rhythms and timings in effective interpersonal interaction.

Successful research with young children has often involved the design of specialised methods. Take, for example, the question of whether children in their first year have any understanding of simple addition and subtraction. These arithmetical operations are characteristically associated with formal education and therefore outside the province of the age group considered in this chapter, let alone those under one year of age. However, Wynn (1992) has argued that babies of less than six months do show an understanding of these operations. Using a 'looking-time procedure' infants aged between $4\frac{1}{2}$ and $5\frac{1}{2}$ months were presented with a Mickey Mouse on a platform in front of them. Then a screen was raised between the baby and the toy and the baby saw the experimenter place a further toy behind the screen. The screen was then removed, exposing two toys or only one. For the subtraction task, two toys were presented initially, the experimenter removed one while the screen was in place, and either one or two toys remained when the screen was removed. The infants looked longer when the outcome was incorrect. Thus, they looked longer when there was only one Mickey Mouse although a second had been added and when there were two toys when one had been removed. This suggests that infants under six months of age have an understanding of simple addition and subtraction.

This task is ingenious in several ways. It overcomes the fact that infants cannot verbalise an answer and it utilises a behaviour that they do have, namely looking. It also contrasts an unexpected outcome with an expected outcome and therefore allows the possibility of a differential response. Nevertheless, Wynn's findings have not been without their critiques and Wakeley, Rivera and Langer (2000a, 2000b) failed to replicate her findings. However, although the original findings have not been replicated, the important point her study demonstrates is that researchers need to think creatively about how to adapt methods in order to address particular questions and not be restricted by previous findings and theories.

Wynn's study is a good example of how developmental psychologists have developed methods which utilise the behaviours of very young children as a way of examining competence. However, as pointed out earlier in this chapter, one of the problems with such research is that it commonly takes place in a context which is unfamiliar to the child. A further limitation is that conclusions are often based on a single task or variations of a task.

In contrast, a number of researchers have developed a more participatory and multi-method approach in which the perspectives of children, families, siblings and practitioners are represented. One such study, based on the pedagogical documentation of Reggio Emilia pre-schools, is the Mosaic approach (Clark and Moss, 2001), an iterative process in which data derive from multiple sources. Clark (2004) describes how she used a variety of different methods to explore what three- to four-year-olds felt about the early childhood centre they attended. She set out to 'find methodologies which played to young children's strengths rather than weaknesses' and which allowed her 'as the adult recorder to be the "inexpert" who is there to listen and learn from the children'. Clark used a variety of tools including the familiar methods of observing the children and interviewing the parents, staff and children. However, she also gave these young children single use cameras to take photographs of important things, invited the children to take her on a tour of the site and tell her about it, and asked the children to create maps of the site using their photographs and drawings.

The use of this type of approach, together with increasing technological advances, has resulted in evidence supporting our belief in the young baby as sentient, participatory and intelligent. This reiterates the views expressed by DeLoache and Brown (1987; 1998 edn: 163) who have pointed out that 'much research carried out in the past treated *young children as deficient* rather than exploring the ways in which *the research model might be deficient*' (our italics). The result is that we now have an understanding that from birth children are social beings, skilful at communicating, competent at learning and able to 'say' (if others learn to 'listen') something about their lived experiences.

Interpreting findings

The question of interpretation is especially relevant when young children are the research participants. This can be illustrated by exploring further some of the findings described in the previous section. One of the possible ways that the conclusion drawn from Wynn's study could be criticised is that the incorrect outcome (which the babies looked at most) was always the same as the starting point. Thus, in the addition task they started with one Mickey Mouse and ended with one. Perhaps therefore they looked longer because they expected a change rather than because they had carried out the addition or subtraction and realised the number was wrong. This difficulty was acknowledged by Wynn, who therefore revised the addition task so that when the screen was removed after the addition of one toy there were either two or three toys: i.e. in both cases there had been a change. The babies still looked longer at the incorrect number of dolls. So perhaps they can add 1 plus 1 after all.

However, there is at least one further complication to be resolved before we can accept this interpretation. In the revised addition task the babies looked longer when they saw three toys than when there were two toys. It is therefore possible that they looked longer at three toys just because there were more to look at and maybe this took them longer to process. So, the result may have nothing to do with any ability to add 1 plus 1 but may simply reflect how much there is to look at. This criticism was made by Wakeley et al. and in order to explore it they carried out the equivalent subtraction task. In this task the baby first saw three toys, then, while the screen was in place one toy was removed and when the screen was removed either two toys or one toy remained. Thus, if babies of this age can do simple subtraction they should look more when only one toy remained than when there were two. In fact, Wakeley et al. found no differences in looking times. This finding seriously undermines the original findings and raises questions about whether or not babies under six months have any appreciation of mathematical operations. Nevertheless, what is important about this example for our current purposes is that it illustrates the care that researchers need to take to ensure that their findings have only one interpretation. As we have seen in this example, it is crucial that alternative explanations are eliminated. Of course, this is true of all research but it is especially marked when carrying out research with very young children or others whose responses may be limited. Further discussion of this issue can be found in Chapter 13 on Disability.

The problems associated with data interpretation are not restricted to the study of children whose communication is limited. In an earlier section we suggested that some of the differences which have been reported between the behaviour of children from different social classes could be explained by differences in how familiar the context of the study was to the different groups of children. However, this may not be the only reason. For example, Tizard and Hughes found differences in how the teachers in their study talked to the girls, depending on the girls' background. When the teachers were talking to the girls from a working class background they used simpler language, began more conversations with a question, asked more closed questions and provided more limited information than when they were talking to the girls from a middle class background. These differences could explain the differences observed in the children's behaviour at school.

Conclusions

The early years until the age of five represent a time of rapid change for the developing child and present great challenges to the researcher both in the scope and methods of study. We have moved a long way from the laboratory-type experiments of early developmental psychologists for whom young children were helpless, malleable organisms ready to be shaped by their environment. Current research recognises the importance of studying young children in their familiar environment and of involving adults who co-exist with them in a social context. Methods that facilitate non-verbal responses are enabling greater exploration into the natural world of very young children. Despite the tension between practitioner-based and academic research, new partnerships and collaborative practice are beginning to take root. More attention is being afforded to ethical concerns, children's rights agendas, consent and there is increased sensitivity to context and access.

The constraints on both academics and practitioners as researchers are many, whether in relation to entry to the setting for a university researcher, or lack of time for a practitioner researcher. A partial solution to the differences between the two types of research may lie somewhere in the middle. It could be argued that improvements in technological tools, such as digital video recording and Magnetic Resonance Imaging (MRI scanning) of the human brain, assist and add weight to the common-sense beliefs and anecdotal evidence that practitioners have frequently held, yet were perhaps unable to prove, suggesting that both methods have something valid to contribute to the sum of knowledge about babies and young children.

The complete solution to their shared problems may be to undertake collaborative research, as early childhood practitioners and academics in universities in many areas have already begun to do. Where such research is conducted (e.g. Abbott and Gillen, 1999), some of the problems faced by both groups can be reduced since collaboration may require less rather than more time and the benefits of working with others towards shared ends will result in the research focus being examined from multiple perspectives, rather than from that of either one or other group.

References

Abbott, L. and Gillen, J. (1999) 'Revelations through research partnerships', *Early Years*, 20(1): 43–51.

Ahmed, K. (2002) 'Britain's class divide starts even before nursery school', *The Observer*, 10 November.

Bateson, M. (1975) 'Mother–infant exchanges: the epigenesis of conversational interaction', *Annals of the New York Academy of Sciences*, 263: 101–113.

Bell, R.Q. (1979) 'Parent, child and reciprocal influences', *American Psychologist*, 34(10): 821–826.

Blenkin, G. M. (1994) 'Early learning and a developmentally appropriate curriculum: some lessons from research', in G.M. Blenkin and A.V. Kelly (eds), *The National Curriculum and Early Learning: An Evaluation*, London, Paul Chapman.

Blenkin, G.M. and Kelly, A.V. (eds) (1994) *The National Curriculum and Early Learning: An Evaluation*, London, Paul Chapman.

Brazelton, T.B. (1979) 'Evidence of communication during neonatal behavioural assessment', in M. Bullowa (ed.), *Before Speech*, Cambridge, Cambridge University Press.

Bruce, T. and Meggitt, C. (2002) *Child Care and Education*, 3rd edn, London, Hodder and Stoughton.

Bruner, J. (1977) 'Early social interaction and language acquisition', in H.R. Schaffer (ed.), *Studies in Mother–Infant Interaction*, London, Academic Press.

Cameron, C., Moss, P. and Owen, C. (1999) *Men in the Nursery: Gender and Caring Work*, London, Paul Chapman.

Children Act (The) (1989) London, HMSO.

Clark, A. (2004) 'The Mosaic approach and research with young children', in V. Lewis, M. Kellett, C. Robinson, S. Fraser and S. Ding (eds), *The Reality of Research with Children and Young People*, London, Sage.

Clark, A. and Moss, P. (2001) *Listening to Young Children: The Mosaic Approach*, London, National Children's Bureau.

Cousins, J. (1999) *Listening to Four-year-olds: How They Can Help Us Plan Their Education and Care*, London, National Early Years Network.

David, T. (1998) 'Issues in early childhood education in Europe', *European Early Childhood Education Research Journal*, 6(2): 5–17.

DeLoache, J.S. and Brown, A.L. (1987) 'The early emergence of planning skills in young children', in T. David (ed.), *Researching Early Childhood Education: European Perspectives*, London, Paul Chapman, 1998.

Department for Education and Skills (DfES) (2002a) *Birth to Three Matters: A Framework to Support Children in their Earliest Years*, London: DfES Publications.

Department for Education and Skills (DfES) (2002b) *Delivering Sure Start, Early Years and Childcare – The Way Ahead*, London, DfES Publications.

Feinstein, L. (1999) *Pre-school Educational Inequality? British Children in the 1970 Cohort*, London School of Economics and Political Science.

Gopnik, A., Meltzoff, A. and Kuhl, P. (2001) *How Babies Think: The Science of Childhood*, London, Phoenix.

Hatch, J.A. (ed.) (1995) *Qualitative Research in Early Childhood Settings*, London, Praeger.

Hodapp, R.M. and Goldfield, E. (1983) 'The use of mother–infant games as therapy with delayed children', *Early Child Development and Care*, 13: 17–32.

Kaye, K. (1977) 'Towards the origins of dialogue', in H.R. Schaffer (ed.), *Studies in Mother–Infant Interaction*, London, Academic Press.

Lazar, L. and Darlington, R. (1982) *The Lasting Effects of Early Education: A Report from the Consortium of Longitudinal Studies*, Monographs of the Society for Research in Child Development 47, 2–3 Serial no. 195.

Newson, J. (1979) 'The growth of shared understanding between infant and caregiver', in M. Bullowa (ed.), *Before Speech*, Cambridge, Cambridge University Press.

Owens, P. (1997) *Early Childhood, Education and Care*, London, Trentham.

Reeves, R. (2001) 'What's wrong with men working in childcare?' *The Guardian*, 6 March.

Sameroff, A. (1975) 'Transactional models in early social interactions', *Human Development*, 18: 65–79.

Schaffer, H.R. (ed.) (1977) *Studies in Mother–Infant Interaction*, London, Academic Press.

Schweinhart, L.J. and Weikart, D.P. (1994) 'A summary of significant benefits: the High Scope Perry pre-school study through age 2–7', in C. Ball, *Start Right: The Importance of Early Learning*, London, Royal Society for the Encouragement of Arts, Manufactures and Commerce.

Stern, D.N. (1985) *The Interpersonal World of the Infant*, New York, Basic Books.

Sylva, K. (1995) 'Research as a medieval banquet – barons, troubadours and minstrels'. Paper presented at RSA 'Start Right' Conference, London, September.

Tizard, B. and Hughes, M. (1984) *Young Children Learning: Talking and Thinking at Home and at School*, London, Fontana.

UN *Convention on the Rights of the Child* (CRC) (1989).

Wakeley, A., Rivera, S. and Langer, J. (2000a) 'Can young infants add and subtract?' *Child Development*, 71: 1525–1534.

Wakeley, A., Rivera, S. and Langer, J. (2000b) 'Not proved: reply to Wynn', *Child Development*, 71: 1537–1539.

Wynn, K. (1992) 'Addition and subtraction by human infants', *Nature*, 358: 749–750.

Middle Childhood
MARY KELLETT AND SHARON DING

How children must tire of adult introductions prefaced with 'And how old are you?' For it would appear a child cannot belong to a gender or ethnic group, be a keen footballer, a fan of Westlife, have ginger hair, dimples or adore sticky toffee pudding until he or she is first 'aged'. And once 'aged' there is a seemingly endless conveyor belt of comparisons to endure: 'she's rather small for eight'; 'he doesn't eat much for ten'; 'she's a marvellous reader for six'; 'gosh hasn't he got big feet – and only five!'

This preoccupation with age labelling is particularly noticeable in 'middle childhood', the period sandwiched between 'early years' and 'youth' that is generally associated with the primary school years. 'Middle childhood', as we have opted to name it, has been relatively neglected by researchers outside the field of developmental psychology. Until the 1990s the focus of sociological research tended to be on the pre-school and teenage years when it was assumed that more rapid changes and adjustments were being made (Hill, Laybourn and Borland, 1996). It is only recently that anthropological research has challenged the bedrock of age as a structuring principle in society by showing how conceptions of age and maturity vary significantly across cultures (James and Prout, 1997).

For much of the twentieth century research with this age group has been the domain of developmental psychology and it seems appropriate to begin this chapter by examining the main contributions from that discipline. We then explore how middle childhood research has expanded out from the developmental centre to embrace sociological, anthropological and emancipatory perspectives, shifting the focus away from children as 'objects' of research to children as active participants. We examine a number of issues that this increased participation raises for researchers, including the need to adapt methodologies and grapple with the flexibility of research design. Finally we consider the issues surrounding the role of the adult researcher in children's worlds.

The influence of developmental psychology

As a discipline, psychology drew many of its methodologies from the natural sciences, particularly in the early days. Principles of experimental design, objectivity and laboratory work were given a high priority, and still permeate the vast majority of work carried out by developmental psychologists.

One of the most influential developmental psychologists was Jean Piaget. His main aim was to develop an epistemological theory (one concerning the *nature* of knowledge), rather than a theory which explains how children *develop*, i.e. how they move towards an 'adult' way of thinking. In order to discover what the nature of knowledge is, he traced the origins of reasoning ability in infants, and its progression through childhood. Because of this, he embarked on a programme of research aimed at discovering and explaining the changes in how children think as they get older. This emphasis set the tone for viewing children as developing gradually from incompetence to competence. The way in which Piaget has been interpreted has led to notions of children *lacking* various skills. His theories (and those of others who have followed in his tradition) have been described as constructivist. This is because he claimed that children are active *constructors* of their own knowledge, in that their actions on their environment lead them to discover certain logical truths about objects and concepts. Piaget asserted that all children develop through the same sequence of stages before achieving mature, logical thought. The structure of children's thinking at each stage is distinctive and different from that of adults and children at different stages, and the same as other children of the same age. Much of his work was concerned with discovering the nature of the different types of reasoning children were engaged in during a particular developmental stage, and the approximate age when they moved on to the next stage.

Piaget argued that some important changes happened in middle childhood. Because of this, and the impact of Piagetian theory, there is now a large body of psychological research focusing on this age group of children. Piaget proposed that a major change occurs in children's thinking around the age of seven years. We shall use examples of this to illustrate the type of work undertaken by Piaget, and the criticisms of it.

Children aged below around six are in what Piaget termed a pre-operational stage of reasoning. He designed what is now a series of classic tasks to establish this. In one of these, he presented a child with two rows of counters, arranged in one-to-one correspondence (see Figure 11.1). After the child had agreed that both rows of counters were the same, Piaget would move the positions of the counters on one of the rows (see Figure 11.2).

When a five-year-old child sees the two rows of counters laid out in the new position, s/he is likely to say that the top row of counters has more. This is because length has been taken as an indicator of number. The child has not noticed that the relative length of the top row of counters has been 'compensated' for by the relative density of the bottom row. In other words, s/he cannot co-ordinate two changes that happen simultaneously. Piaget argued that this was because the child was acting on what s/he was currently observing, rather than operating systems of thought to co-ordinate

O O O O O O
X X X X X X

Figure 11.1 *First arrangement of counters*

OOOOOO
X X X X X X

Figure 11.2 *Second arrangement of counters*

two changes. Once children are able to succeed at this task (generally by age seven) they move from the pre-operational to the concrete operational stage.

Piaget's theory was appealing and powerful because of its generality – it explains why, in many different situations, a seven-year-old thinks differently from younger children.

However, many people were critical of Piagetian theory. They argued that the tasks used by Piaget meant that he underestimated the nature of children's thinking. These dissenters have produced many accounts of children who were 'too young' in Piagetian terms.

Researchers have drawn attention to problems with Piagetian tasks in three main areas.

Use of language

The researcher has to communicate the nature of the problem to the child. If, however, the child does not share the experimenter's understanding of the words being used, then a failure to complete the task might well be due to a breakdown in communication rather than the child's inability to reason appropriately.

Making sense of the questions

In the task we have described above (Figures 11.1 and 11.2) the child was asked the same question twice. S/he was asked whether the two rows were the same or different both before and after the spacing between the counters in the second row was changed. In everyday interaction, the repetition of a question by an adult to a child usually indicates that the first answer the child gave was wrong or somehow inappropriate. It therefore follows that the child in the Piagetian task may well be thrown by what he or she assumes the adult is implicitly indicating, rather than thinking about the logical aspects of the problem.

Understanding the task

Perhaps the most influential criticism is that Piaget's research involved tasks which are artificial and unfamiliar to children. They therefore made errors because the tasks did not make 'human sense' (Donaldson, 1978). In the 1970s Donaldson and her colleagues designed some experimental tasks which, they argued, tested the same types of reasoning as classic Piagetian research, but were more meaningful to the children. Instead of asking children to answer questions about a very odd situation in which they (the experimenters) moved counters around (as in Figure 11.2) they introduced 'Naughty Teddy' to the children. He was rather careless, and so accidentally rearranged the counters into position 2. Now that the situation is familiar and meaningful, children well below the age of seven years are quite happy to explain that the two rows of counters are still equivalent in terms of number.

These critiques of Piaget led many developmental psychologists to conclude that children's true competencies were masked in Piagetian tasks, as the tasks were not 'child-friendly'. Piaget, however, was not just concerned with whether or not the children could answer his questions correctly. He was more interested in their understanding of the situation, and to explore this he asked the children to give reasons for their answers. If a child could not give a rational explanation for her/his answer, then Piaget would argue that her/his thinking was still pre-operational.

Nonetheless, Piagetian tasks do place additional demands on language and on social understanding and interaction. Many researchers (e.g. Harris, 1983) have suggested that children's 'incorrect' responses should actually be construed as ingenious attempts to make sense of what are to them strange and incomprehensible contexts. Following in the footsteps of Vygotsky, more recent work has been carried out with children which emphasises their skills as social actors and communicators, continually trying to make sense of their social world. They do this with a great deal of support from the adults and older children around them.

Research in the Vygotskian tradition tended to focus on observing children as they live their lives. Rogoff, working in the 1980s and 1990s, was interested in learning how children increase their skills and intellect by participating with more able others. Working from the starting point that learning is a social rather than an individual process, she observed children learning how to participate in culturally relevant activities. She showed how adults and older children structured the child's environment, using their knowledge of the child's past experience (Rogoff, 1990).

Undoubtedly developmental psychology has made a major contribution to research in the middle childhood years. Critiques of this type of research contributed to the emergence of new perspectives from anthropology and sociology (for detailed expositions of these perspectives see e.g. Harkness, 1996; Corsaro, 1997; James, Jenks and Prout, 1998) and new methodological challenges.

Methodological challenges

Children are themselves the best source of information about matters that concern them, so collecting data directly from children is preferred as secondary sources may not be able to orient sufficiently to the children's perspectives. In this section we address some of the methodological challenges of research with children in the middle years of childhood. We seek answers to some key questions including the relationship between age and competence, whether some methods are more suitable for this age range than others and whether 'less suitable' methods can be adapted for use with children of this age.

Competence

Judgements about age, maturity and competence are difficult to make. Some lines are already defined for us, 10 as the age of criminal responsibility in England and Wales, for example. Yet there is a vast range of maturity among 10-year-olds, as there is among seven-year-olds or any other specific age one might choose, so drawing boundaries is always going to be controversial. Waksler (1991) suggested that it is more helpful to think in terms of children's competence as being 'different' not 'lesser'. Children in these middle years are generally credited with being able to read, write and make themselves understood, but in research terms they still carry 'reliability health warnings' such as 'children can't tell fact from fiction', 'they say what the interviewer wants them to say', 'they don't have enough knowledge and understanding to relate their experiences'. Recent studies have challenged these claims (Scott, 2000). Adults are just as likely to blur truth and fiction as children because truth is itself a personal construct. Children can and do provide reliable responses if questioned in a manner they can understand and about events that are meaningful to them. The challenge is to find appropriate techniques that neither exclude nor patronise children. Notions of children's incompetence are reinforced by methods that oversimplify and 'talk down' to them, thus preventing them from responding at anything other than a superficial level (Alderson, 2000). Alderson gives a poignant example of how misguided our preconceptions about children's competence can be from her research into children's consent to surgery (1993). She asked a 10-year-old girl, 'So you're having your legs made longer?' and the girl replied, 'I suffer from achondroplasia and I am having my femurs lengthened' (cited in Alderson, 2000: 244). The '*Gillick*-competence' ruling (1985) emphasised that it is not just chronological age which determines competence but sufficient understanding and intelligence to comprehend what is being proposed and sufficient discretion to make a wise choice in one's own interests.

Adults' attitudes to children's levels of competence are also reflected in their approach to consent procedures. All too often it is assumed that children are not competent enough to give their informed consent, that this needs to be gained from a 'more competent adult' and the simpler level of 'assent' (agreement to participate) is sufficient from the child. No one would contest the desirability of an adult gatekeeper being involved in the consent process but this is not to assume that a child is not also capable of giving his or her informed consent (Cree, Kay and Tidsall, 2002). An issue associated with that of consent is whether or not children should be paid for participating in research. Some bodies advocate this (e.g. National Children's Bureau, 1993) whereas others oppose it, including an EU directive issued in April 2001 (Cree, Kay and Tidsall, 2002).

Interviewing children

How appropriate is the interview as a research tool with children? Mauthner (1997) considers individual interviews and self-completed instruments to be more suited to older children and small group discussions to be more appropriate for younger children. Middle childhood spans them both and so particular attention needs to be given to the interview techniques employed. The 'conditioning' to which children are exposed in many primary schools may prompt children to respond to adult questioning even when they don't know the answer (to answer 'I don't know' risks being thought cheeky, awkward or inattentive). This has implications for individual interviews where the power imbalance is acute. If a researcher's role becomes blurred with that of a teaching role children may expect more guidance and direction in their responses and not be as forthcoming. Researchers with little or no experience of talking to children may also underestimate the length of time children commonly take to answer a question. This can lead to the collection of inaccurate and incomplete data. Listening skills are crucial (Roberts, 2000).

The rapport that develops between researcher and child is important for encouraging more forthcoming responses and trust with regard to confidentiality. Interviewers who are intimidating or impatient may inhibit children's responses. 'Walkman-type' interviews, where children listen to questions on a personal audio cassette and pause the tape or rewind it as needed, can have advantages although they are obviously more time consuming to administer. Adult-style questionnaires can be problematic if the questions are complex or the number of response choices too extensive. Short concentration spans may incline children to lose interest if the list is long and they may pick a response from those that appear early in a given list. Conversely, memory limitation may cause children to forget some early choices and pick from those that appear late in a list. Standard biases that affect adult respondents may differ slightly for children. For instance, acquiescence bias may be greater because of the power imbalance but social desirability bias less because of the relatively lowly status of children.

Group discussions – sometimes referred to as 'focus' groups – originally designed for adults, have been successfully adapted for children (e.g. Hill,

Laybourn and Borland, 1996; and Jones, Atkin and Ahmad, 2001). 'Groups give children space to raise issues that they want to discuss' (Mauthner, 1997: 23). Different dynamics arise depending on whether children know each other well or are strangers, and researchers need to consider how the composition of groups e.g. friendship groups, mixed age or gender groups, is likely to affect the quality of data. Peers can be supportive of each other but also hurtful. Hill et al. (1996) give an example of one child in a focus group interview who suggested 'bashing' someone as a solution to the problem that was being posed. Single sex groups may raise issues that mixed gender groups would be inhibited about raising but mixed sex groups can address gender differences in the topics discussed. Many writers acknowledge that it is less intimidating to speak in a group than in a one-to-one interview with a stranger. Focus groups can be organised around 'themes' so that the interviewer gets to find out information without necessarily using a question and answer format. Gender issues arising in interviews are discussed in more detail in Chapter 9.

Adapting interview methods

Increasingly interview methods are being adapted to meet the needs of different groups of children. Techniques such as brainstorming, ranking exercises and visual prompts are used to engage children with the questions. Hill et al. (1996) used pictorial faces to show different expressions to help stimulate discussion about feelings. They also used a mask to role-play 'Mr Numb' as a character who had no feelings and to whom children would explain what certain feelings were. Other researchers have used *pictorial vignettes* (one or more pictures portraying a situation with an emotional connotation), role play and drawings to similar effect. Sentence completion can also be an effective adaptation of interview method, for instance '*I am sad when...*', or '*When I am sad I tell...*'. Other techniques include *fantasy wishes* (listing three things that would make the child really happy). Word prompts can be helpful in enabling children to express feelings that might otherwise be difficult (Hill, 1997).

It has been common for researchers to consider children below the age of seven or eight years old as not viable as interviewees, partly because of Piagetian ideas about children's 'concrete' thinking at this stage (Hill, 1997). However, many writers (e.g. Alderson, 2000; Aldgate and Bradley, 1999) and professional associations (e.g. British Educational Research Association; Social Research Association) are now challenging this notion, maintaining that poor data are not necessarily a product of the young age of the child but of inappropriate interview techniques. Many good examples of studies with interview data from young children are emerging (Lewis, 2002). Flexible participatory techniques that engage young children's interest are also proving to be successful, such as the Mosaic approach pioneered by Clark and Moss (Clark, 2004).

Children as active participants in research

Methodological issues such as access, consent, confidentiality and ownership of data are not unique to research with children. Difficulties frequently arise with adult population groups. What makes the situation more acute with children is the unequal power relations between adult researcher and child (Mayall, 1994; Mauthner, 1997). Encouragingly, the number of research studies using child participatory approaches is growing and verbal communication is often superseded by activities such as drawing, songs and story writing to elicit children's views. This not only optimises their abilities but also enables them to set the agenda, have greater control and participate on their own terms (James, 1995). In participatory research studies the role of the researcher is that of a facilitator of the activities.

Thomas and O'Kane's (1998) study used a variety of participatory techniques to facilitate children's views about decision-making processes and how these affected them. Box 11.1 shows an example of a 'decision-making' chart completed by a 12-year-old boy in foster care.

Box 11.1 Example of a decision-making chart

	When I see my mum	What time I have to be in	What I should do	Who I should live with	Going into foster care	My room
12-year-old boy in foster care	∇	•	∅	∅	•	∅
My social worker	∅	•	∅	∅	∅	•
My mum	∅	•	∇	∅	•	•
My foster carers	∅	∅	∅	∅	∅	∅
My teacher	•	•	∅	•	•	•

Key • = no say   ∇ = some say   ∅ = a lot of say

Source: O'Kane, 2000: 144

The Diamond Ranking exercise was another participatory technique Thomas and O'Kane used to elicit children's views about issues that were the most important in decision making. Nine statements were identified from individual interviews and the children then had to work in groups to rank them according to order of importance, in a diamond shape, so that the most and least important statements formed the tip and base of the diamond, as illustrated in Box 11.2.

Box 11.2 Example of a diamond ranking exercise: Important issues in decision making

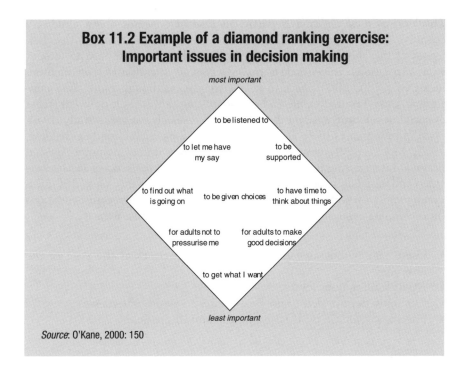

Source: O'Kane, 2000: 150

Another technique used in the same study to ascertain children's views about participation levels in review meetings was the Pots and Beans Activity. This used six differently labelled pots: (1) preparation before the meeting; (2) support; (3) how much you speak; (4) how much you are listened to; (5) how much influence you have and (6) how much you like meetings. Children could put between 0 and 3 beans in each pot to express the strength of their feelings about that particular topic. This is a way of using an attitude scale in a proactive way that engages children.

The challenge of quantitative methods

In large-scale, general population, social survey research children have been traditionally excluded.

Much of the research that does take children into account is concerned with the impact of children on adult lives, rather than focusing on children as social actors in their own right. Panel studies of households, for example, are conducted as if children are auxiliary members. Even studies on the costs of children have tended to view children as items on the parent's budget, rather than as economic actors who exercise considerable clout in family expenditure on food and consumer durables. (Scott, 2000: 99–100)

This exclusion of children is partly because of concerns about children's cognitive ability to process and respond to structured questions but the challenges of this should not necessarily exclude them and we need to look at what adaptations can be made to make large-scale quantitative research more inclusive (Scott, 2000). Face-to-face interviews, although more time consuming, can be more flexible and can adapt questions to suit different stages of social development. Some health-related research has successfully developed questionnaires to elicit views from school-aged children (e.g. Balding, 1987). More recently, new interviewing techniques using Computer Assisted Personal Interviewing (CAPI) have greatly simplified the process and include video and visual and auditory stimuli to reduce over-reliance on verbal questioning and answering. Spencer and Flin (1990) have four recommendations for optimising responses from children in quantitative research:

- Use unambiguous and comprehensive instructions at the start of the interview.
- Avoid leading questions.
- Explicitly permit 'don't know' responses to avoid best guesses.
- Interview children on their home territory if possible.

Issues of context and location

We have already alluded to power relations in Chapter 6 and the difficulties that arise in interview situations when the researcher's role mimics that of a teacher or other adult in a position of power. The context and location of a study involving children can have an equally significant impact on the research. The most common location for such research is the primary school, where there are inherent dangers that participation could verge on coercion if children interpret it as schoolwork (David, Edwards and Alldred, 2001). David et al. ask whether this is 'informed consent' or 'educated consent' and comment that 'the high pupil response rates achieved in school-based studies [are] rooted in this hidden pressure, and researchers need to consider the ethics of their practice in this respect' (p. 352). It is now widely acknowledged that informed consent should incorporate the facility for 'informed dissent'.

School locations require researchers to negotiate multiple layers of gate-keeping, work around the limitations of timetables and accommodate the agendas of senior managers.

> The school secretary was an important gatekeeper for the headteacher who in turn acted as gatekeeper for the class teacher. The headteacher was concerned that the research should have some educational value to the children and so complement the perceived function of the organization...Thus our study presented a potential threat to the organization if it did not parallel the school's perceived function as educator of children. The exclusion of children as participants in feedback

suggested that children had low status as active acquirers of knowledge within the school setting. (Hood, Kelly and Mayall, 1996: 120)

An alternative location is to access children in their own home, but here too there can be difficulties. Parents, as gatekeepers, may want to be present in interviews and may exert influence and control over children's responses (Brannen, 1994).

> The home is hung about with ideologies as well as emotions…The privacy of the home has high value – those negotiations are meant to take place out of the sight, and outside the concerns of the public worlds that surround it. For researchers, who are also strangers, to enter the home and ask questions, however sympathetic, is an invasion and a crossing of traditional boundaries between the public and the private. (Hood et al., 1996: 119)
>
> As a guest in the family home, the researcher's social position does not have clearly established parameters; it has to be negotiated. There is a triangle of conventions and negotiations. As an adult, and a guest, the researcher may feel obliged to accept what conditions are offered by the adult, the parent. But as a guest of the child too, the researcher must take account of what the child sees as appropriate (Mayall, 2000: 127).

The adult researcher in children's worlds

What role does an adult need to adopt to gain access to children's worlds? This requires a shift to a more equal distribution of power between the adult and child. There are several roles that a researcher might adopt with children, ranging from the friend to the authoritarian teacher figure. The type of role is affected by the nature of the research, the location and the context and plays a significant part in the power relation dynamics. Some advocate minimising the power difference by attempting to become 'one of the children' but others maintain that this is a naïve and unachievable goal and that the power of adults will always be omnipresent despite all our attempts to nullify it. Mayall (2000) suggests that a more realistic way forward is to invite children to help us to understand their perspective rather than pretend that we do not have any power over them.

Some researchers take on multiple roles, particularly in ethnographic studies.

> [If] there were a number of different children's cultures present in the research setting then ethnographers not only may have to bridge the cultural gap between themselves (as adults) and the children but also have to understand the differences within and between different groups of children and different groups of adults. (Davis, Watson and Cunningham-Burley, 2000: 213)

It is difficult for an adult ethnographic researcher to pretend he or she is not an adult, particularly in a classroom setting where children expect adults to be in positions of authority (see Thorne, 1993; Punch, 2004). In Davis et al.'s study (2000) the researcher's eight weeks in the classroom resulted in him adopting the roles of friend, mediator, entertainer, authoritarian adult, non-authoritarian adult and helper at various times throughout the life of the study.

Conclusion

The shifting horizons of research with children in the middle years of childhood are linked to many issues, not least changing attitudes to children's 'competence' and acceptance of their status as social actors. New perspectives of sociology, anthropology and emancipatory rights agendas are occupying a position once dominated by developmental psychology. Questions are beginning to be asked about how capable adults are of interpreting and writing about children's lives. Several writers are advocating that children themselves should be more involved in this process (Morrow and Richards, 1996; Thomas and O'Kane, 1998; Scott, 2000) and that the best way adults can gain access to children's worlds is by fostering greater participation of children and young people themselves. The more children are given a primary research voice, the less adults will be required to 'interpret' their worlds. Increased participation of 'middle years' children in the research process brings with it new methodological and ethical challenges. Facilitating participation by child-friendly adaptations to adult methodologies is an important, although only partial, solution – some would argue that this merely reinforces adult methods as the norm and patronises children. Research *with* children in the middle years requires more than a little tinkering around the methodological edges.

References

Alderson, P. (1993) *Children's Consent to Surgery*, Buckingham, Open University Press.

Alderson, P. (2000) 'Children as researchers: the effects of participation rights on research methodology', in P.H. Christensen and A. James (eds), *Research with Children: Perspectives and Practices*, London, Routledge Falmer, pp. 241–257.

Aldgate, J. and Bradley, M. (1999) *Supporting Children through Short Term Fostering*, London, The Stationery Office.

Balding, J.W. (1987) *General Health-Related Behaviour Questionnaire* (Version 11), Exeter, Exeter University, HEA Schools Health Education Unit.

Brannen, J. (1994) *Young People, Health and Family Life*, Buckingham, Open University Press.

Clark, A. (2004) 'The Mosaic approach and research with young children', in V. Lewis, S. Fraser, M. Kellett, C. Robinson and S. Ding (eds), *The Reality of Research with Children and Young People*, London, Sage.

Corsaro, W. (1997) *The Sociology of Childhood*, Thousand Oaks, CA, Pine Forge Press.

Cree, V.E., Kay, H. and Tidsall, K. (2002) 'Research with children: sharing the dilemmas', *Child and Family Social Work*, 7: 47–56.

David, M., Edwards, R. and Alldred, P. (2001) 'Children and school-based research: "informed consent" or "educated consent"?' *British Education Research Journal*, 27(3): 347–365.

Davis, J., Watson, N. and Cunningham-Burley, S. (2000) 'Learning the lives of disabled children: developing a reflexive approach', in P.H. Christensen and A. James (eds), *Research with Children: Perspectives and Practices*, London, Routledge Falmer, pp. 201–224.

Donaldson, M. (1978) *Children's Minds*, London, Fontana.

Harkness, S. (1996) 'Anthropological images of childhood', in C.P. Hwang, M.E. Lamb and I.E. Sigel (eds), *Images of Childhood*, Hillsdale, NJ, Lawrence Erlbaum.

Harris, P.L. (1983) 'Children's understanding of the link between situation and emotion', *Journal of Experimental Child Psychology*, 36: 490–509.

Hill, M. (1997) 'Participatory research with children', *Child and Family Social Work*, 2: 171–183.

Hill, M., Laybourn, A. and Borland, M. (1996) 'Engaging with primary-aged children about their emotions and well-being: methodological considerations', *Children and Society*, 10: 129–144.

Hood, S., Kelley, P. and Mayall, B. (1996) 'Children as research subjects: a risky enterprise', *Children and Society*, 10: 117–128.

James, A. (1995) 'On being a child: the self, the group and the category', in A.P. Cohen and N. Rapport (eds), *Questions of Consciousness*, London, Routledge.

James, A. and Prout, A. (1997) 'Re-presenting childhood: time and transition in the study of childhood', in A. James and A. Prout (eds), *Constructing and Reconstructing Childhood*, London, Routledge Falmer.

James, A., Jenks, C. and Prout, A. (1998) *Theorizing Childhood*, Cambridge, Polity Press.

Jones, L., Atkin, K. and Ahmad, W. (2001) 'Supporting Asian deaf young people and their families: the role of professionals and services', *Disability and Society*, 16(1): 51–70.

Lewis, A. (2002) 'Accessing through research interviews, the views of children with difficulties in learning', *Support for Learning*, 17(3): 110–116.

Mauthner, M. (1997) 'Methodological aspects of collecting data from children: lessons from three research projects', *Children and Society*, 11: 16–28.

Mayall, B. (1994) *Children's Childhoods: Observed and Experienced*, London, Falmer Press.

Mayall (2000) 'Conversations with children: working with generational issues', in P.H. Christensen and A. James (eds), *Research with Children: Perspectives and Practices*, London, Routledge Falmer.

Morrow, V. and Richards, M. (1996) 'The ethics of social research with children: an overview', *Children and Society*, 10: 90–105.

National Children's Bureau (1993) *Guidelines for Research*, London, National Children's Bureau.

O'Kane, C. (2000) 'The development of participatory techniques: facilitating children's views about decisions which affect them', in P.H. Christensen and A. James (eds), *Research with Children: Perspectives and Practices*, pp. 136–159, London, Routledge Falmer.

Punch, S. (2004) 'Negotiating autonomy: children's use of time and space in rural Bolivia', in V. Lewis, M. Kellett, C. Robinson, S. Fraser and S. Ding (eds), *The Reality of Research with Children and Young People*, London, Sage.

Roberts, H. (2000) 'Listening to children: and hearing them', in P.H. Christensen and A. James (eds), *Research with Children: Perspectives and Practices*, pp. 225–240, London, Routledge Falmer.

Rogoff, B. (1990) *Apprenticeship in Thinking: Cognitive Development in Social Context*, New York, Oxford University Press.

Scott, J. (2000) 'Children as respondents: the challenge for quantitative methods', in P.H. Christensen and A. James (eds), *Research with Children: Perspectives and Practices*, pp. 98–117, London, Routledge Falmer.

Spencer, J. and Flin, R. (1990) *The Evidence of Children*, London, Blackstone.

Thomas, N. and O'Kane, C. (1998) *Children and Decision-Making: A Summary Report*, University of Wales, Swansea, International Centre for Childhood Studies.

Thorne, B. (1993) *Gender Play: Girls and Boys in School*, New Brunswick, NJ, Rutgers University Press.

Waksler, F.C. (1991) *Studying the Social Worlds of Children: Sociological Readings*, London, Falmer.

Young People
ALAN FRANCE

This chapter is concerned with researching youth issues. Its core objective is to highlight some of the theoretical and pragmatic challenges that emerge when trying to research issues related to young people. While there is much debate over when the youth phase starts and finishes (Jones and Wallace, 1992) this chapter is focused specifically on researching those young people under the age of 18. Doing social research with this age group is full of methodological and ethical tensions that need to be overcome if we are to gain a greater understanding of their lives, attitudes and actions. In the discussion that follows I will start by outlining some of the substantive historical and contemporary challenges that impact upon how we might approach the study of 'youth'. Recognising this context is critical if we are to undertake research that has a positive contribution to make to debates about what it might mean to be young. In the second part of the chapter I will discuss more pragmatic issues that impact on how we might 'do research with young people'. These relate to ethical and legal questions of 'informed consent' and 'protection from harm'. I will argue that both are critical factors that can be empowering to young people themselves but they need detailed attention at all stages of the research process. Without such focus we are at risk of, at best failing to implement research, at worst of undertaking unethical research. Getting it right requires having a reflective and flexible approach to doing research with young people.

The political context of doing 'youth research'

Youth as a social problem

Researching youth and youth related issues has recently become a major growth area for social research. In an historical context youth has always been of interest to academics and policy makers because of its problematic nature (Muncie, 1999a; Griffin, 1993). Over the centuries focus on youth has been dominated by middle class anxieties about 'dangerous or undeserving youth (Pearson, 1983). More recently concern about the 'youth problem' has increased (MacDonald, 1998; Colley and Hodkinson, 2001). For example, the Social Exclusion Unit argued that major problems exist for young people's transition into adulthood (SEU, 1998) and that although much is known about the 'youth problem' more research is needed if intervention policies are to be effective. In response to this concern with the youth problem there has been an avalanche of policy and practice initiatives that aim to target both those most vulnerable and those most at risk of being future problems. For example, the Children's Fund, the Connexions Programme and the Youth Inclusion Programme all aim to target and assess 'problem youth' and find ways of improving their transition into adulthood or to reduce their future problem behaviour. Such an approach is built up from a deficit model where youth are seen as being bad: 'Overwhelmingly, they are portrayed [in *Bridging the Gap*] as deficient, delinquent, or a combination of the two, as are dysfunctional families and communities' (Colley and Hodkinson, 2001: 340).

Such a context greatly influences how we engage with 'youth issues'. It underpins the objectives of many funders (finding solutions to the 'youth problem') and shapes the way in which our work is disseminated. This clearly sets us all substantial challenges for doing research with young people (Griffin, 1993; France, 2000).

Understanding youth

In thinking about how we might research youth and related issues it is also important to recognise the complexities and problems surrounding the boundaries of what we mean by the term 'youth'. In much of the academic literature youth is associated with the notion of adolescence and with stages of development linked to puberty (Thompson, 1992; Griffin, 1993). Youth is therefore defined by the notion of 'growing up' and has linkages to physical and psychological development rather than more cultural forms and norms (France, 2000). As a result youth is understood as a universal experience that is seen as linear and transitional, moving young people from childhood to adulthood. This phase is also seen as a critical stage in the formation of identities and rational thought and behaviour (see, e.g. Jessor, 1984; Hendry et al., 1993). While there is much debate over questions of individual difference, diversity and the role of the social context (Heaven, 1996), these factors remain important in shaping what is understood as adolescence (France, 2000).

This is the dominant discourse that influences how policy is shaped. In much legislation youth does not officially exist. For example, in the Children Act (1989) all young people under the age of 18 are defined as children. Yet in reality policy has recognised difference, suggesting that at different age stages young people go through certain 'rites of passage' that move them towards adulthood. But inconstancies and contradictions exist within policy over what these 'rites of passage' are and how the law can and should support them (Jones and Wallace, 1992). Many are greatly influenced by psychological notions of competence and responsibility and focus on beliefs that young people have major problems with puberty (France, 2000). The classic example is the right at the age of 16 to get married (with parental consent), start work, ride a motorbike, and smoke cigarettes, yet a young person cannot legally vote until s/he is 18. As we will see, this complexity and the different understandings of what youth means can create all sorts of problems for the researcher doing youth research, a point I shall return to later in the discussion on competency.

It is important to acknowledge that there is little recognition within the policy framework that our understanding of youth is greatly influenced by social and cultural factors. For example, Pilcher (1995) suggests that in understanding young people's lives we need to have a greater awareness of the cultural and historical context of what it means to be young:

> Context is central to the conceptualisation of the human life span as a life course, in the sense of structural contexts as well as historical contexts. The life course approach allows us to see that 'ages and stages', and transitions between them, have culturally determined institutional bases, which may vary by historical context. (Pilcher, 1995: 20)

Such a position suggests that youth policy (and also research) has to be more aware of the cultural context of human behaviour (Hollands, 2002). Relying upon psychological theorising and models of social development creates a narrow focus on what is a complex set of relationships and lives (France, 2000).

Understanding and including 'voice'

While there remains continuity in the research agenda (Colley and Hodkinson, 2001; Muncie, 1999b) there are also differences and new opportunities. This relates to the emergence of a new orthodoxy that encourages us to listen to the voices of young people. Historically, research has marginalised the 'voice' of young people. Up until the mid-1980s most research was focused *on* rather than *with* young people. In other words the dominant paradigm of social research treated young people (and children) as objects of study and something for academics to theorise about. For example, the Birmingham CCCS research unit gave little time and space to the voice of young people.[1] Even when young people were given voice in the research process they were not allowed to speak for themselves (Widdicombe and Woolfitt, 1995). As a result they tend to be portrayed as 'cultural dupes' and not as competent to explain or theorise about their own social worlds.

In more recent times youth research has started to pay more attention to the need to listen to young people and has recognised them as competent and reliable witnesses to their own lives. Three major developments have been at work. Firstly, there has been a growing interest within childhood studies in the contribution children can make to our understanding of childhood. Writers such as James and Prout (1998) have argued that not only should children be given a voice in research but also that they have a critical role to play in providing us with an insight into what childhood means. Children are seen as capable and competent participants in social research. In much of this work children and young people are not differentiated, being seen as suffering from the same forms of exclusion within social research. As a result of this new emerging paradigm methodological and theoretical support to listening to the voice of children has grown.

Secondly, over the past 20 years there has been a growth of legislation that supports and values the voice of children and young people. In a UK context the most important development has been the incorporation of the European Convention on Human Rights into English domestic law through the new Human Rights Act. This has created an opportunity for the enshrinement of children's rights in practice. While there remains uncertainty about its possible impact (Muncie, 1999b; Jeffs, 2002) opportunities for establishing a rights framework for children within constitutional law now exist (Franklin, 2002). While problems may remain, children have been given the right to be heard as a fundamental right of childhood (Fortin, 2002). This builds on other historical developments. For example, the 1989 Children Act (England and Wales) was a critical piece of English legislation that created an opportunity to involve and listen to children in social care services (Roche, 2002).

Finally, since 1997 with the election of New Labour there has been a growing interest in listening to children and young people and while some may argue this is symbolic rather than real, policy developments have opened doors towards an approach that wants to hear what children and young people have to say. For example, Quality Protects, the Children's Fund, and the development of the Connexions Service have all built into them requirements to listen to children and young people in the development of services, something unheard of seven years ago.

Such developments are positive and create new opportunities to increase the contribution young people can make to understanding what it means to be young. It would seem that a new orthodoxy is emerging that puts young people's voice at the centre of the research agenda. This being said, such idealism and commitment do not guarantee that young people will be listened to or that they will influence the political process.

Understanding voice is also a fundamental objective of much social science research (May, 2000). It is at the core of approaches that prioritise qualitative methodologies. Listening and reflecting the meanings and significance of what people have to say about their lives is a critical aspect of social research and has a long history (Silverman, 2001). Little has been written that deals directly with how we might engage with and encourage the voice of young people. A strong theoretical and methodological position has been developed in childhood studies about listening to children. In many cases the disciplinary boundaries between this and youth studies have been blurred, suggesting that there is significant overlap. For example, many writing in childhood studies reflect on the 'youth phase' as 'late childhood' (see for example, Brannan and O'Brien, 1996 which discusses children's lives in families. However, it is clear that this talks about young people, not children). Methodologically this can be problematic, as the youth experience can be substantially different.

Childhood studies does give us a route into thinking about the importance of young people's voices to the research process. As James and Prout (1998) have argued, we need to recognise that when children are positioned as a 'social subject' rather than object of study they can start to give us insights into the complex world of what it means to be a child. The sociology of the family has assigned very little relevance to children's contribution, suggesting that they are not competent or able to provide reliable data. James and Prout (1996) argue that such an approach is built upon a social developmental model and relies on adult definitions of what is competent and reliable in terms of social knowledge.

We also need to acknowledge that 'voice' and the production of 'voice' is an interpretive process and involves an interaction between the researcher and the researched (Silverman, 2001; Clough and Nutbrown, 2003). For example, Clough (2002) argues that it is impossible to separate out the voice and influence of the researcher – given that they have selected the topic, designed the questions and constructed the final report. To see 'giving voice' as a valueless project is to deny the politics of doing research.

But there are dangers in listening to 'voice' in isolation and without understanding the broader context of events. While listening to young people and their perspectives is important, others may also have an important contribution to make: for example, parents and professionals may have an alternative perspective that adds to our understanding of the broader social and cultural processes that help shape and impact upon the lives of young people (MacDonald and Marsh, 2001). Including these in analysis is essential if we are to have a more detailed understanding of what it means to be young.

The challenge of informed consent

So far I have highlighted the historical the contemporary processes that make researching youth issues both difficult and challenging. But other more pragmatic challenges also exist. In this section I want to turn to more pragmatic issues, focusing on 'informed consent' and 'protection from harm' as critical challenges we have to address in the implementation of research.

In much social research young people under the age of 18 are not the main givers of consent. It is traditional that parents or guardians make the final decision on whether a young person should or should not be involved in research (Alderson, 1995). Yet such a position creates substantial difficulties and uncertainty. Not only does it deny young people the right to make their own decisions about involvement but it gives control over the research process to others. There is much debate over young people having the right to make the decisions for themselves (Masson, 2000; Lindsay, 2000; Alderson, 1995).

The legal framework

When we are trying to get access to young people under 18 we are normally confronted by the requirement to get parental consent. Differences exist in practice but it is generally argued that parents should have the final say. As Masson (2004) outlines, such a position is not actually legally correct. The law supports young people being able to make their own decisions about their life and in most cases it can allow the rights of young people to override parental rights:

> Parental responsibility is not the determining factor for a child's participation in research where a child is mature. A child who has the capacity to understand fully decisions affecting his or her life automatically has the capacity to make that decision. (Masson, 2000: 39)

Requiring parental consent can also be seen as a denial of young people's right to be heard or to make decisions for themselves (Masson, 2004). While the legal context of this is debated (Franklin, 2002) there has been a growth in English legislation that encourages and supports young people being involved in making decisions for themselves. For example, the 1989 Children Act established that children are legal subjects who have rights in how they are treated and about their involvement in decisions concerning the welfare services they receive (Roche, 2002). Similarly, the 1985 *Gillick* ruling established that young women (if deemed to be 'mature') have the right to make decisions about their own health needs. These, and other more recent developments (for example, Quality Protects legislation, and developments in the Children's Fund – see www.cypu.gov.uk last accessed 01/09/03) give a strong statutory framework and support to young people making decisions about being involved in social research. Of course problems arise over the notion of maturity. The legal framework for young people's rights tends to hinge on the decision by others as to whether a young person is mature enough to make his or her own decisions, a point I discuss further in the section on competence.

Ethical considerations and consent

Of course the law is not always ethical; nor can it give us clear ethical guidance on what is right and wrong in all situations (Beyleveld and Brownsword, 1986). So what is the ethical position in terms of parental consent? As Homan (1991: 1) points out, 'Ethics is the science of morality; those who engage in it determine values for the regulation of human behaviour'. Getting agreement on what is ethical is a matter of moral judgement greatly influenced by other factors. As a result what is ethical (or unethical) is problematic, being a process of social construction linked to moral arguments and positions. Firstly, this creates problems in that ethics are contested and much debated. In other words there is no definitive agreement on what might, or might not be ethical. Secondly, as highlighted by Lindsay (2000), different professions have different ethical frameworks and little agreement has been achieved between or even within professions over what the ethical principles should be. Finally, even where some agreement can be made, for example in terms of broad principles (i.e. subjects not to be harmed), there is no hierarchy of ethical principles that can deal with conflicts, contradictions or disagreements. So professional organisations can only give very broad guidance as a framework for researchers to work within (Lindsay, 2000). Ethics cannot always help us make a decision about parent versus young person's consent. What is unethical to one person may be ethical to another. Different situations will require different responses. Once again it is a matter of definition and position.

Competence as a social construct

Both legal and ethical frameworks rely upon the notion of competence but such a concept is problematic. Many professionals working with children and young people are, by law and statute, given the power to define who is competent and who is not. For example, doctors have the power and responsibility to judge if a young woman, under the age of 16 is competent to make her own decisions about sexual health matters (Gillick, 1985). Similar powers exist within education over the definition of 'special needs' and 'learning difficulties'. Educational psychologists and education authorities have the legal power and responsibility to define if a child is in need of specialised intervention as a result of their level of competence and need. While many of these decisions are determined by policy and resource factors, professionals are in a strong position to determine how a young person (or child) is defined and described. This process of labelling by others, especially those with power and influence, has a long history of debate (Becker, 1973). It is widely recognised that professional action and processes of definition can and do shape those being labelled (Lemert, 1951).

This issue is especially relevant for understanding how competence is defined in relation to children and young people. Christensen (1998), for example, writing about how competence is defined in medical treatment, shows that discussions that try to match age stages with levels of competence miss the point. Competence is variable and very much determined by processes of social interaction and negotiation. Christensen goes on to argue that if there is a *presumption of competence* rather than incompetence, children can be very capable of understanding and making decisions about their lives. Competence therefore has to be recognised as a contested term that is open to these types of process.

From a research point of view this issue is important because we should be careful about accepting professional definitions of incompetence as a reason for excluding a young person from research. The danger of relying upon others to define who should and should not be involved can have an impact on what voices we listen to. An alternative way of looking at this question is to focus on those who are excluded and defined as incompetent as a means of understanding how such labels and actions affect their identities and sense of self. For example, in a research project on young people's attitudes and experiences of risk taking[2] I was told by teaching staff that a certain young man should be excluded from my sampling because he was 'mentally retarded' and could not be relied upon as a competent research subject. I ignored this advice and interviewed the young man concerned. His story was illuminating and showed that he knew he was defined by others as different. He was also able to discuss what impact these labels and definitions had on him and his own behaviour and identity. Hearing his story enhanced the quality of my understanding of the social processes at work.

From theory to practice

Given the discussion so far it would seem that there is a case for arguing that young people should be the sole givers of consent. But I now want to turn to the issue of trying to implement such a position, highlighting some of the difficulties we may encounter. Getting access to young people in the first place is complex and difficult, as usually we must rely upon a number of different gatekeepers (Butler and Williamson, 1996). For example, Oakley (2000), writing about her attempts to access young people in care, notes that she had to pass through a whole range of gatekeepers before agreement to allow access to a young person could be reached. These can range from powerful institutional guardians such as Directors of Education down to teachers, secretarial staff and even classroom assistants. As May (2000) argues, getting agreement and acceptance of ethical positions on consent is a process of complex negotiation between researchers, multiple gatekeepers and the research funders. All may have different ethical positions and beliefs and all will have a position on access. Gatekeepers (or funders) may demand that we get parental permission before we are allowed to involve a young person within a research project. Without it we may lose funding, co-operation or access. For example, in my experience schools are usually very keen to get parental permission and normally insist that parents are given the right to stop their teenage son or daughter participating in research.

Similarly, organisations that have protective or welfare responsibilities, such as social services, may require us to get consent from parents because they are concerned that parents may complain or feel they have not been consulted. As researchers our way of dealing with this is usually not to challenge the school or agency by trying to insist that it is not necessary but to argue for 'passive consent' (France et al., 2000). This usually takes the form of a letter that requires a response if the parents wish to object. If no response is made it is assumed that parents have agreed. Having to implement such a position is inevitable if the school or agency demands it. Researchers have no power over the gatekeeper institution and its ethical position.

This being said, there are strategies we might want to use to try to ensure it is young people who are the key decision makers in this process. Firstly, we could encourage the agency to word the letter to suggest parents contact either the researchers or the agency for further details. This will create a situation of dialogue and allow further discussion to take place before parents make a final decision. Similarly, we could propose that our letter is sent out by the agency,[3] and that any questions from parents are targeted at us. Of course this may not resolve the issue, as parents may still demand that their child is withdrawn. Not having permission has to be accepted in these situations if we wish to continue with the research. To oppose parents' wishes may cause problems for the school, and of course for the young person too – something we as researchers would want to avoid.

The importance of 'informed' consent

One of the problems about the debate over parental rights and young people's choice is that it detracts us from the main issue – that of getting *informed* consent from young people. In our need to satisfy others we tend to give limited attention to young people themselves. If we think again about the school setting, we tend to feel relieved once the passive consent of parents has been achieved and our focus turns to the process of implementing our work in the classroom. Again other gatekeepers, such as teachers, become our focus. Getting agreement over how we implement our programme of research and how it fits into the curriculum (or not) becomes central. Limited attention is then given to informed consent with young people.

But if we are committed to listening to young people's voice we need to give them detailed information about the research so that they can make an informed decision. Doing this requires us to enter into a dialogue with them about the aims and objectives of the research and about our practice. This will require us to provide accessible and readable material (Butler and Williamson, 1996) that explains: the reasons for the research; what it is trying to achieve; what rights they have in this process and most importantly that they have the right to withdraw from the research at any time (Stanley and Sieber, 1992). It should also provide information about the research team, how to get in contact with them for further information and how, if necessary, someone can complain about their experience. Details on confidentiality and autonomy and about storage of data and their right to have access to it if they wish (which are requirements under the Data Protection Act) should also be included. It is not appropriate for us to assume that once we have passive consent from others or access as a result of negotiation we should not give this detailed attention.

Ensuring informed consent may also require us to deal with structural difficulties that may block young people making a choice (Weithorn and Scherer, 1994). The classic example for me is the school. Even if we go through the detailed process of giving information about choice, how much choice might a young person have to opt out of the research in practice? One critical issue that can facilitate choice is the availability within the school of an alternative to taking part in the research (Butler and Williamson, 1996; France et al., 2000). This might mean negotiating with the school or teacher about allowing young people to leave the room or sit in another classroom. Similar issues may exist in other settings or environments and it may be that in designing our consent procedures we will need to consider the type of pressure young people might be under or the constraints on their being able to act upon their decision not to be involved in the research. We also need to continually keep talking and asking young people about their willingness to be involved. Good practice should include a continual review of consent to ensure that young people remain happy with their involvement. The right to withdrawal has to be emphasised regardless of how uneasy we might feel about losing our cohort.

Protection from harm

I now want to turn my attention to the second issue that I think is important in doing research with young people: our responsibility to protect them from harm. While we might wish to debate whether or not young people are a 'special case' (Butler and Williamson, 1996, Pollard, 1987), the reality is that we have a responsibility to protect any research participant from harm. Harm reduction is a critical component of any research practice (BSA, 2003). For example, the British Sociological Association ethical guidelines state that:

> Sociologists have a responsibility to ensure that the physical, social and psychological well-being of research participants is not adversely affected by the research. (BSA, 2003: 2)

Similarly:

> When it comes to young people some of these responsibilities are not only covered by ethical frameworks but are also set down within a legislative framework and policy. (Department of Health et al., 1999)

When working with young people we need to make a detailed reflection on how we might implement a policy in practice to reduce risk and harm to participants. It is impossible to construct a planned strategy that fits all situations, as each research project will have its own challenges, but good practice would be to plan and think through any situations within a research project that might be seen as harmful. To help in this process there are certain legal and legislative frameworks (Masson, 2000) that can guide us on how we might implement a strategy that protects young people from serious harm.

Risky environments

As social researchers, our work with young people will, in the majority of cases, not put them into high-risk situations. We are not conducting experiments or trying to cure them of illnesses and physical problems. We are exploring understandings and meanings through conversation and discussion, therefore it is unlikely that we will put young people into physical danger. Yet we do need to think about physical spaces and places. Questions are raised for us about the types of venue and place we invite them to. We need to make sure we are not requiring young people to walk through dangerous neighbourhoods to get to a site where the research will be conducted. We also need to be confident that young people have the resources to get home and do not have to travel using risky means and methods. It might also be worth encouraging them to travel in pairs with friends to ensure they are not vulnerable on their way to and from the research project. For example, we may feel that it is important to undertake interviews with young people 'in their own communities' at a local youth centre. It may be assumed that this is safe but it might be that such resources are controlled informally by other groups of young people and going inside will be a risk. We have to recognise that our responsibility for risk reduction goes beyond the interview or survey work to cover travel to and from the research.

Risk to emotional health and well being

Risk reduction and protection from harm also requires us to think about 'emotional' harm. Measuring the potential for this is massively problematic.

For example, the United States Department of Health and Human Sciences argued that the acceptable threshold is that no risk should be greater than those experienced in normal everyday life (Koocher and Keith-Spiegel, 1994). Measuring and identifying what this might be in reality remains both contentious and problematic; yet it is not unreasonable for us to think through our own research proposals and identify areas that might create emotional upsets and difficulties. For example, in a project looking at family relationships and divorce it is likely that the sensitivity of the subject will cause emotional upset and difficulties. Taking a sensitive approach to interviewing and data collection is therefore essential. Being prepared for areas of distress that might emerge will help us to identify at an early stage whether a problem exists (Butler and Williamson, 1996). Of course research is not counselling; neither should it be. But being sympathetic and offering personal support is a responsibility that we should all take seriously. A good practice tip is to carry information with you about local support services for young people. Having up to date information about counselling, health, relationship and personal advice organisations is a useful way of directing young people to services better equipped to help with these matters.

Protection from harm by adults

Working with young people in any context, we have to think about how to protect them from adults who may wish to do them harm. This issue may arise because they decide to disclose to us that they are being abused or in danger. But there is also the potential for us to put young people at risk by employing people who have a history of child abuse. Building into research projects a clear policy and practice for dealing with these issues is critical.

Under the 1989 Children Act (England and Wales) and more recently in the Department of Health et al. (1999) publication and supporting documentation (Department of Health, 2001/2), professionals and adults who come into contact with children and young people[4] in either a professional or an informal context have a responsibility to protect them from harm. Government guidelines give the clear message that it is not appropriate to withhold information if a child or young person is identified as being in danger. While this is not legally enforceable, it is seen as immoral and unacceptable practice for professionals not to report incidents of suspected abuse.

This requirement sets down clear challenges for us as researchers with young people. Firstly, it requires us to acknowledge that confidentiality has limits. While we might debate what these are and what the threshold might be, we still have to recognise that boundaries exist over what we can promise around confidentiality (France et al., 2000). The consequence is that in terms of informed consent we have a responsibility to tell young people that this is the case and that if they decide to disclose abuse to us we have a responsibility to pass this information on to the relevant authorities. On all my research projects researchers have to explain the existence of these limits to young people. This allows them to make their own decisions around what they disclose knowing that if they do raise this in an interview with the researcher, it will have to be acted upon. This is not to say that as researchers we do this without involving the young person; only that we have a clear duty to be proactive in this area.

A second issue is that, as required under the *Inter-agency Inspection of Safeguards for Children* (Department of Health, 2001/2), we have a clear policy on how we are going to deal with this issue if it arises. As researchers and as organisations that run research projects we need to have clarity about our processes of dealing with this issue. Understanding the local context and developing a policy in advance of the event is for me good practice. In one research project I managed, (the National Evaluation of On Track 1998–2002) I was on-call to researchers to give advice and guidance if such an incident arose. If it was felt, by the researchers and myself, that further action was needed, staff had managerial support to take action immediately. Building such a strategy into the project work is critical if we are to respond with speed and efficiency.

Finally, I think we have a responsibility to ensure that all researchers who work with young people undergo a police check prior to undertaking fieldwork. Under the Police Act 1997 prospective employees are able to obtain criminal record certificates. With the setting up of the Criminal Records Bureau we are now in a position to insist that researchers have police checks. Historically, this issue has been given little attention within social research organisation but there is no rationale for researchers to see themselves as exempt from this requirement.

Building these kinds of practice into our research projects with young people not only ensures that we will be undertaking our core responsibilities but also brings reassurance to agencies and gatekeepers who will be making judgements about our suitability. They want to know that they are not putting young people that they are responsible for at risk by letting agencies and researchers become involved with them without showing they are responsible organisations.

Conclusion

In this chapter I have highlighted the complex influences and pressures that are at work in shaping the agenda when researching youth. Youth as a social problem remains a core focus of the research agenda and the lack of attention in the policy framework to the influence of culture and history in understanding what it means to be youth sets us all many challenges. But new opportunities are emerging, which encourage the importance of acknowledging 'voice', that should allow some of these issues to be addressed.

In the second part of this chapter I argued that in terms of pragmatics two key issues are fundamental to 'doing research' with young people. Informal consent shapes not only questions of access but also how we perceive young people themselves. In taking a less risky approach to consent (relying on gatekeepers and parents as key decision makers) we are making a statement about young people themselves. While pragmatic difficulties remain, approaching consent through a rights-based approach should allow us a more empowering methodology to doing research with young people. Such an approach advocates the importance of rights and choice of young people over others.

I also strongly believe that we also have, as social researchers, major responsibilities in our work with young people. It is critical that we recognise they can be vulnerable and at risk of harm. We need to be proactive in our planning and design, ensuring that we provide a safe and supportive environment. At the same time we have a legal duty not to put young people at risk from adults who may wish to exploit or harm young people. Building in procedures and practices that stop this from happening is essential.

Notes

1 The Birmingham Centre for Contemporary Cultural Studies made a major contribution to the development of youth research in the 1970s and 1980s. A good critical review of this work can be found in Wyn and White, 1997.

2 Funded by the National Health Executive under the South Thames Mother and Child Health Programme, 1996–98.

3 Under Data Protection an agency cannot release a person's details until they have agreed to it. So the first point of contact must be made by the gatekeepers, not the research team.

4 Defined as agencies within the public, private or voluntary sector whose staff (including volunteers) have contact with children and/or families in any capacity.

References

Alderson, P. (1995) *Listening to Children*, London, Barnardo's.

Becker, H. (1973) *Outsiders: Studies in the Sociology of Deviance*, New York, Free Press.

Bell, R. and Jones, G. (2000) *Youth Policies in the UK: A Chronological Map*, www.keele.ac.uk/departs/so/youthchron.

Beyleveld, D. and Brownsword, R. (1986) *Law as a Moral Judgment*, London, Sweet and Maxwell.

Brannen, J. and O'Brien, M. (1996) *Children in Families: Research and Policy*, London, Falmer Press.

British Sociological Association (2003) *Ethical Guidelines for Social Research*, Durham, BSA.

Butler, I. and Williamson, H. (1996) *Children Speak: Children, Trauma and Social Work*, London, NSPCC.

Christensen, P.H. (1998) 'Difference and similarity: how children's competence is constituted in illness and its treatment', in I. Huchby and J. Moran-Ellis (eds), *Children and Social Competence*, Arenas of Action, London, Falmer Press.

Clough, P. (2002) *Narratives and Fictions in Educational Research*, Buckingham, Open University Press.

Clough, P. and Nutbrown, C. (2003) *A Students' Guide to Methodology*, London, Sage.

Colley, H. and Hodkinson, P. (2001) 'Problems with bridging the gap: the reversal of structure and agency in addressing social exclusion', *Critical Social Policy*, 21(3): 335–361.

Cull, L. (2002) 'Parental responsibility', in P. Foley, J. Roche and S. Tucker (eds), *Children in Society*, Buckingham, Open University Press.

Department of Health, Home Office and Department for Education and Employment (1999) *Working Together to Safeguard Children: a Guide to Inter-agency Working to Safeguard and Promote the Welfare of Children*, London, DOH.

Department of Health (2001/2) *Interagency Inspection of Safeguards for Children: Standards and Criteria*, London, DOH.

Fortin, J. (2002) 'The Human Rights Act 1998: human rights for children too', in B. Franklin (ed.), *The New Handbook of Children's Rights*, London, Routledge.

France, A. (2000) 'Towards a sociological understanding of youth and their risk taking', *Journal of Youth Studies*, 3(3): 317–331.

France, A., Bendelow, G. and Williams, S. (2000) 'A "risky" business: researching the health beliefs of children and young people', in A. Lewis and G. Lindsay (eds), *Researching Children's Perspectives*, Buckingham, Open University Press.

Franklin, B. (ed.) (2002) *The New Handbook of Children's Rights*, London, Routledge.

Gillick versus West Norfolk and Wisbech Health Authority (1985) 3, ALL ER 402 (HL).

Griffin, C. (1993) *Representations of Youth*, Cambridge, Polity Press.

Hamilton, C. (2002) *Offering Children Confidentiality: Law and Guidance*, London, The Children's Legal Centre.

Heaven, P. (1996) *Adolescent Health*, London, Routledge.

Hendry, L., Shucksmith, J., Love, J. and Glendinning, A. (1993) *Young People's Leisure and Lifestyles*, London, Routledge.

Hollands, R. (2002) 'Divisions in the dark: youth cultures, transitions and segmented consumption spaces in the night time economy', *Journal of Youth Studies*, 5(2): 152–171.

Homan, R. (1991) *The Ethics of Social Research*, Harlow, Longman.

James, A. and Prout, A. (1996) 'Strategies and structures: towards a new perspective on children's experiences of family life', in J. Brannen and M. O'Brien (eds), *Children in Families: Research and Policy*, London, Falmer Press.

James, A. and Prout, A. (1998) *Constructing and Reconstructing Childhood*, London, Falmer Press.

Jeffs, T. (2002) 'Schooling, education and children's rights', in B. Franklin (ed.) *The New Handbook of Children's Rights*, London, Routledge.

Jessor, R. (1984) 'Adolescent development and behavioral health', in J. Matarazzo, S. Weiss, J. Herd, N. Miller and S. Weiss (eds), *Behavioral Health: A Handbook of Health and Enhancement and Disease Prevention*, New York, John Wiley and Sons.

Jones, G. and Wallace, C. (1992) *Youth, Family and Citizenship*, Milton Keynes, Open University Press.

Koocher, G.P. and Keith-Spiegel, P. (1994) 'Scientific issues in psychological and educational research with children', in M.A. Grodin and L.H. Glantz (eds), *Children as Research Subjects*, Oxford, Oxford University Press.

Lemert, E. (1951) *Social Pathology*, New York, McGraw-Hill.

Lewis, A. and Lindsay, G. (eds) (2000) *Researching Children's Perspectives*, Buckingham, Open University Press.

Lindsay, G. (2000) 'Researching children's perspectives: ethical issues', in A. Lewis and G. Lindsay (eds), *Researching Children's Perspectives*, Buckingham, Open University Press.

MacDonald, R. (ed.) (1998) *Youth, the 'Underclass' and Social Exclusion*, London, Routledge.

MacDonald, R. and Marsh, J. (2001) 'Disconnected youth', *Journal of Youth Studies*, 4(4): 373–391.

Masson, J. (2000) 'Researching children's perspectives: legal issues', in A. Lewis and G. Lindsay (eds), *Researching Children's Perspectives*, Buckingham, Open University Press.

Masson, J. (2004) 'The legal context', in S. Fraser, V. Lewis, S. Ding, M. Kellett and C. Robinson (eds), *Doing Research with Children and Young People*, London, Sage, pp. 43–58.

May, T. (2000) *Social Research: Issues, Methods and Process*, Buckingham, Open University Press.

Muncie, J. (1999a) *Youth and Crime*, London, Sage.

Muncie, J. (1999b) 'Institutionalised intolerance: youth justice and the 1998 Crime and Disorder Act', *Critical Social Policy*, 19(2):147–177.

Oakley, M. (2000) 'Children and young people in the care proceedings', in A. Lewis and G. Lindsay (eds), *Researching Children's Perspectives*, Buckingham, Open University Press.

Pearson, G. (1983) *Hooligan: A History of Respectable Fears*, Buckingham, Open University Press.

Pilcher, J. (1995) *Age and Generation in Modern Britain*, Oxford, Oxford University Press.

Pollard, A. (1987) 'Studying children's perspectives – a collaborative approach', in G. Walford (ed.), *Doing Sociology of Education*, London, Falmer Press.

Roche, J. (2002) 'The Children Act 1989 and children's rights: a critical reassessment', in B. Franklin (ed.), *The New Handbook of Children's Rights*, London, Routledge.

Silverman, D. (2001) *Interpreting Qualitative Data: Methods for Analysing Talk, Text and Interaction*, 2nd edn, London, Sage.

Social Exclusion Unit (1998) *Bridging the Gap*, London, HMSO.

Stanley, B. and Sieber, J.E. (eds) (1992) *Social Research on Children and Adolescents*, Newbury Park, CA, Sage.

Thompson, R.A. (1992) 'Developmental changes', in B. Stanley and J.E. Sieber (eds), *Social Research on Children and Adolescents*, Newbury Park, CA, Sage.

Weithorn, L.A. and Scherer, D.G. (1994) 'Children's involvement in research participation decisions', in M.A. Grodin and L.H. Glanz (eds), *Children as Research Subjects*, Oxford, Oxford University Press.

Widdicombe, S. and Woolfitt, R. (1995) *The Language of Youth Subcultures*, London, Harvester Wheatsheaf.

Wyn, J. and White, R. (1997) *Rethinking Youth*, London, Sage.

13 Disability
VICKY LEWIS AND MARY KELLETT

A relatively recent and welcome change has been a willingness to expand traditional research that has focused on what disability can teach us about child development to a wider agenda that explores the 'lived experiences' of disabled children in a socially inclusive era (Gillman et al., 1997). In this chapter we discuss some of the issues and controversies associated with research in this area: methodological and ethical difficulties of developmental research when disabled children and young people are included; the challenges of engaging with children who have profound and multiple learning difficulties; the desirability of involving disabled children as active research partners and the undesirability of a 'labelling culture' that pathologises disability. But first we examine some of the issues that arise from the terminology that is associated with disability.

Terminology

The terminology that is used when referring to disabled children and young people is important for several reasons. Terminology is a shorthand for indicating to others what or whom we are talking about. But terminology is more than this. The words used to describe people with disabilities often convey a particular attitude towards these people and in turn this can result in expectations which may or may not be justified. To take an extreme and now defunct example, people with learning difficulties were described as idiots, imbeciles and feeble minded (Mental Deficiency Act 1913) based on their assessed performance on intelligence tests. Such terms are especially derogatory and convey a very negative and narrow view of the person. It is important that as researchers we think carefully about how we talk about disabled people, because of how the terms we use may be perceived by others, including those with disabilities.

The use of a particular term, such as Down's Syndrome, Attention Deficit Hyperactivity Disorder, or Blind, implies a degree of similarity between individuals with that disability. However, this may be far from the truth and increasingly, professionals and academics, as well as parents and families, have emphasised the need to see the child or young person first and foremost, rather than the disability, hence the adopted convention is to refer to 'children/young people with spina bifida' rather than 'spina bifida children/young people'. This is especially important in research where it is crucial that we pay attention to differences between individuals rather than assuming that just because people have the same disability they will behave in the same way and have the same needs.

Nevertheless, although the strategy of putting the child first is widely accepted, in many situations it is not straightforward. Consider blindness. Should we say 'children who are blind', 'children with visual impairments' or 'blind children'? Most children, who for educational purposes are considered blind, can see something and for this reason the term 'visual impairment' is often used in preference to blind since the latter implies that the children cannot see. However, within this group we must distinguish between those who cannot see anything or only shades of light and dark and those who have enough vision to make out the shape and form of objects in their environment. The former are often described as children with profound visual impairments; the latter as children with severe visual impairments.

Like blindness, hearing loss is rarely total but varies from mild to profound. In addition, about 10 per cent of deaf children have at least one deaf parent and a significant proportion of these families will be part of a cultural minority with their own distinct language – a sign language. The preference of this group is to be described as Deaf, with a capital D, just like any other cultural group label. In addition, this group perceive their deafness as a significant aspect of their identity and therefore argue that it should be given prominence. Thus, children with hearing impairments born to Deaf parents would be most appropriately described as Deaf children. However, children with hearing impairments born to hearing parents are not born into Deaf culture, although they may become part of it as they get older. It is therefore more appropriate to describe these children as deaf children.

There is also an issue of how to refer to children who do not have any disabilities, particularly when their development is being compared to that of children with specific disabilities. Obviously such children can be described as children without any disability. Some researchers refer to them as normal children. However, use of the term normal implies that disabled children are not normal whereas in reality many aspects of their development may be very similar to those of children without a disability. As a result the term 'typically developing' is often adopted.

Disabled children also have other identities and belong to other social groupings. For example, a child with muscular dystrophy also belongs to a family, a gender group, an age group and an ethnicity group. The disability label should not suffocate these multiple identities. Society must afford disabled people ample opportunity to explore the plural aspects of their identity and we, as researchers, must be sensitive to the complexities of the interrelationship between these pluralities. How a child relates to being severally black, female and having a diagnosis of autism is likely to vary over time as the different aspects of her identity fluctuate in importance.

Disability research and child development

Any account of development needs to be able to explain how individual children without any disability develop and how, when there is a disability, the developmental process may be altered. An understanding of how a particular disability may change the course of development in individual children can also illuminate our understanding of what may be going on in typically developing children; for example, it may alter the emphasis any explanation places on certain experiences, may help to clarify the relationship between different areas of development and may throw light on prerequisites for particular developments. Thus, children who have had no more than light perception (the ability to distinguish light from dark but inability to make out any forms or shapes) from birth can develop much like sighted children, provided they have no other disabilities (e.g. Lewis, 2003). Clearly these children must be relying on information through modalities other than vision and theories of development must take account of this.

However, there is a problem with drawing implications about developmental processes from studies of disabled children which was pointed out by Urwin (1983). Urwin, writing about the development of communication in blind children, argued that we need to consider the development of disabled children with care. If their development is underestimated, the role of disability in their development may be overestimated. In studies of disabled children it is important to be sure that what we are looking at is genuine development and not an artefact of the situation or of our expectations of how a disability may influence the course of development. We also need to be certain that any conclusions we reach as to the role of a disability in development cannot be attributed to some other problem or difficulty.

Including disabled children and young people in developmental research

The very fact that particular children and young people are grouped together and labelled as blind, or deaf or as having Down's Syndrome suggests that the individuals in each group share certain characteristics. It is obviously true that they will have certain features in common, but the nature of the disabilities of individuals who might be ascribed the same label may be very different. Indeed, the notion of autism as part of a spectrum of disabilities, rather than as a distinct disorder, points to the variability observed in individuals with autism. This problem is particularly relevant for individuals with profound and multiple learning difficulties. The severity and multiplicity of impairment renders it highly improbable that a homogeneous group can be found from within this population. The same is true of any group of children and young people who happen to be given the same label as a result of sharing a specific characteristic such as the additional chromosome 21 of Down's Syndrome.

Children and young people who have a disability in common will be different from one another in many ways. Knowing the pathology of the disability is not enough, since each individual will have a unique genetic makeup and have been exposed to different experiences and these together will influence the effect of the disability on that individual's development. Every child or young person is an individual, and this applies as much to those who have a disability as to those who do not.

Another problem, which arises when we begin to explore the consequences of a particular disability for development, is the question of whether any different behaviours or developments we observe are primary or secondary to the disability. Sometimes the primacy of the disability can eclipse other factors; for example problems faced by disabled children are often attributed to the disability rather than other variables such as teaching methods, social environment or type of school. We need to address the question of whether the disability caused the behaviour directly or the behaviour is the result of some secondary effect of the disability. Thus, if a disabled child or young person lives away from his or her family in some form of residential care and language development is delayed, the delay may not be a direct consequence of the disability: rather it may be due to some aspect of the residential environment.

In many developmental psychology studies of disabled children and young people two or more groups are compared. Often this is with the intention of finding out how the disability has affected development. A difficulty here is to select a group against whom to compare the development of the disabled individuals. Such comparative research which relies on control groups may be especially difficult to undertake with children with profound and multiple learning difficulties due to their heterogeneity (Hogg and Sebba, 1986). However, even when children can be grouped in terms of a shared feature, such as the additional chromosome 21 of Down's Syndrome, the choice of comparison group is not straightforward since group membership should not be taken to imply homogeneity. Thus, children with Down's Syndrome could be judged to be similar in some sense to all of the following: children with learning difficulties but not Down's Syndrome of the same chronological and mental ages; typically developing younger children at a similar stage of development; typically developing children of the same chronological age; older children with Down's Syndrome; their typically developing siblings. Any or all of these comparisons could be justified and yet none of them is ideal.

A further problem occurs in studies of children with sensory or motor difficulties. Take blind children. Many studies of blind children have involved comparisons between the performance of blind children and the performance of sighted children who have been blindfolded. However, blindfolding sighted children may disadvantage them because they will have to carry out the task in a different way from how they would normally do it. This raises questions about the value of such comparisons.

Researchers interested in the development of disabled children often want to study how a process or development observed in typically developing children is affected by the disability. This very often leads to the use of methods with disabled children which have been employed to study the phenomenon in typically developing children. Such methods may be inappropriate for children with particular disabilities. Conversely, it may be inappropriate to draw conclusions when a phenomenon has been studied in two groups of children using different methods.

Related to all this is the problem of how to interpret any differences, or for that matter similarities, in the behaviours of children with and without a particular disability. Does a difference indicate that a process, which is presumed to underpin the behaviour in a typically developing child, is missing in the disabled child? Or does it mean that the disabled child is processing the information differently? Or what?

There are no satisfactory answers to these sorts of question. However, research with disabled children and young people can make significant contributions to understanding their lives and experiences. It is crucial that researchers acknowledge and address the problems raised in this section.

Implications for developmental research

A key question for researchers working with disabled children and young people is whether it is appropriate to group children with a particular disability together, either based on a shared cause or similar behaviour, given that such an approach will mask individual differences. The tendency to view disabled children as a homogeneous group has been criticised (Shakespeare and Watson, 1998; Priestley, 1998). It does not acknowledge diversity such as gender and ethnicity and fails to appreciate their capacities to develop complex and multiple identities (Davis et al., 2000). An alternative is to study individuals. It is clear that much can be learned from individual case studies. However, as Pérez-Pereira and Conti-Ramsden (1999) point out with respect to blind children, if small numbers of children are studied, it is important that they are studied in depth and that sufficient data are collected and analysed both quantitatively and qualitatively to justify any conclusions. It is also important that understanding which comes from studying individuals is replicated. Unfortunately, replication research is often seen as a 'poor relation' of original research and as a result there is a little such research involving disabled children. This situation is unlikely to change until replication research is viewed more positively.

Although case studies may have many advantages they can be costly and time-consuming, especially if longitudinal. It seems likely therefore that many researchers will continue to make group comparisons. In this case careful thought must be given to the basis on which children with a particular disability are included and how different groups of children are matched. As we have already argued, children who have the same disability often differ greatly from one another in developmental terms. It is crucial that if a group of children are studied the group is as homogeneous as possible.

Matching groups of children is not straightforward and two specific difficulties are illustrated well when children with Down's Syndrome are considered. The first is that assessments on developmental scales, such as the Bayley Scales, early in infancy are not correlated with later cognitive development (e.g. Wagner et al., 1990). This raises questions about the meaningfulness of matching infants for developmental age given that the rationale for such matching is that the groups will be of similar cognitive ability.

The second issue concerns the nature of the matching. Most developmental scales employed with young children assess a range of abilities, including cognitive, perceptual, motor, language and social skills. To take a specific example, children with Down's Syndrome have particular difficulties in the area of language and consequently they are more likely to fail language items than, say, items assessing social development. Therefore, if a child with Down's Syndrome is matched with a typically developing child for overall performance on a developmental scale, the child with Down's Syndrome is likely to do relatively well on social items and less well on language items whereas the typically developing child is more likely to perform at a similar level on both language and social items. Thus, although the children have been matched overall the matching procedure itself hides underlying differences. This becomes a problem if the research question to be addressed in a study assumes that the children have been matched for particular skills. Ideally the children should be matched on specific aspects of development which are relevant to the research questions being addressed. For example, if expressive and receptive language abilities of children with Down's Syndrome and typically developing children are being examined, it would make more sense to match the children on expressive language and to compare their receptive language abilities than to match the children for overall developmental age and examine both expressive and receptive language.

Research focusing on group comparisons raises the question of the composition of the comparison group. Mervis and Robinson (1999) suggest that for Down's Syndrome the most informative comparison is with children who only differ from the child with Down's Syndrome in terms of not having Down's Syndrome, that is, monozygotic twins discordant for Down's Syndrome. However, such an approach is not possible in the case of Down's Syndrome since both monozygotic twins would have Down's Syndrome and is hardly realistic for any disability. In most studies, unrelated typically developing children will make up the comparison group and such comparisons can be informative provided that some of the issues identified above are addressed.

An alternative experimental design to control groups in research with children with learning difficulties and other disabilities is the use of 'reverse phase' intervention. Such a design is effectively a within-subjects design in which each child first experiences some form of intervention and then experiences a phase in which the intervention is withdrawn. However, such a design has serious ethical implications, particularly if the 'reverse phase' involves withdrawing a beneficial intervention in order to prove its efficacy (Kellett, 2000). Inevitably, therefore, much research with children who have severe learning difficulties has relied on case study design.

Great care must be taken to design tasks which assess the specific process under consideration. Unless this is achieved any differences could be due to something other than the process which was supposedly being examined. This difficulty has been illustrated well for studies of emotional understanding in children with autism by Hobson (1991) and is also particularly evident when studies of blind children and deaf children are examined. For children with motor disabilities it is obviously crucial that tasks which are assessing processes other than motor skills do not have a motor component (e.g. Wilson and McKenzie, 1998). In line with this Fletcher et al. (1996) suggested using tasks presented on computer for children with spina bifida, rather than paper and pencil tasks.

If research does rely on group comparisons particular attention should be paid to what data are collected and how the results are examined. For example, it is often difficult to make comparisons across studies because data have been collected and coded in different ways. In terms of results we need to know whether or not the range of scores of two groups overlap, rather than just that the means are significantly different. In other words, do all the disabled children behave in the same way as the group means suggest? This matters because whether or not there is overlap between the behaviour of different groups can address questions of universality (a characteristic is shown by all children with the disability) and uniqueness (a characteristic that occurs only in children with the disability).

A further implication for research concerns how behaviour is interpreted. The behaviour of disabled and typically developing children may look the same but the processes underlying the behaviour may differ. For example, Wright (1998) has shown that the performance of children with Down's Syndrome on object permanence tasks may simply reflect their ability to imitate the hiding action, rather than reflect an underlying representation of the hidden object. Similarities in behaviour must not be taken to mean that the processes underlying the behaviour are necessarily the same. In a related way it is also important that care is taken when interpreting failures on particular tasks. Again, children with Down's Syndrome are reported to be more likely than typically developing children to avoid certain tasks. While such avoidance may reflect an underlying inability, it may also be due to other problems such as inattention or lack of motivation. Researchers, and practitioners, need to be aware of this and to ensure, as far as possible, that such alternative explanations cannot account for the behaviour observed. One way around this particular problem is to repeat tasks in different settings and on different occasions. If the child succeeds on some occasions but not on others it is unlikely that the failures reflect a lack of the ability being tested.

Children and young people with severe learning difficulties

Children with severe learning difficulties present many challenges to the researcher. Those who cannot speak or sign may be considered too difficult to include and left on the fringes of the research arena. Including children with the most profound learning difficulties involves making considerable adaptations to research designs and methodologies that may compromise scientific rigour and increase the 'messiness' of the data. However, such compromises are balanced by increased social validity and real world relevance (Kellett and Nind, 2001). If disability research is to become ethically purer and more socially inclusive then methodological design has to become more flexible and creative. Detheridge (2000) discusses some of the innovations in information communication technology and iconic communication systems that are opening up opportunities for more children with profound learning difficulties to respond and make choices.

> In the research context, part of empowering children with learning difficulties is ensuring that we develop and use the tools whereby they can communicate; thereby research respondents include these children…The freedom to communicate will depend not only on the availability of appropriate communication mechanisms and sensitive interpretation, but also on the power relationships in the exchange and attitudes established over time. (Detheridge, 2000: 114)

Davis's ethnographic account (Davis et al., 2000) of his attempts to get close to a group of children with multiple impairments is very informative about the cultural preconceptions that can inhibit communication. Because of his relative inexperience with children who had such severe disabilities, Davis found himself relying on adult staff to interpret for him. He felt immense pressure to conform to their view:

> It was as if his permission to enter the research setting was granted on the grounds that he accept the staff's view that communication with these children would be troublesome due to their cognitive difficulties. These experiences revealed an immense gulf between the staff's view of the children and the research team's preconceptions that children should be treated as competent social actors and that understanding these children would be a task involving reflexivity and hermeneutical exchange (Davis et al., 2000: 209).

It was by being reflexive that Davis realised he had allowed his own gender to affect his interaction with some of the children. His lack of success with the girls compared to the boys was down to a failure to address gender nuances and see beyond the homogeneous disability label. Subsequently, his role play as 'fashion commentator' did much to improve the nature of his interaction with the girls. Davis also learned much about the assumptions we commonly make about the communicative ability of disabled children through our persistent failure to appreciate their diversity. For example it was some time before he realised that lack of communication did not necessarily equate with *inability* to communicate – it might mean that the individual child *chose* not to communicate.

> John [Davis] realised that Scott had chosen not to speak to him and that he had previously mistakenly interpreted Scott's behaviour as meaning Scott could not communicate...He had failed to recognize the children's social ability to withhold access to their world; he had ignored the concept that children are the final gatekeepers to their worlds. (Davis et al., 2000: 210)

As well as the reflexive approach advocated by Davis, a flexible approach is also needed. While interviews might be a suitable approach with young people without learning difficulties, Booth and Booth (1996) discuss four problems of interviewing young people with learning difficulties: inarticulateness, unresponsiveness, lack of a concrete frame of reference and difficulties with the concept of time. They argue that 'the challenge of interviewing inarticulate subjects calls for unorthodox methods, the only way of collecting their stories may be to loan them the words' (Booth and Booth, 1996: 65). The idea of 'putting words into mouths', as it were, rings all sorts of ethical alarm bells. However, it can be argued that 'constructing' a narrative via sensitive interpretation may be more valid than some insensitive and often naïve observations of able-bodied researchers about disabled individuals or the inappropriate use of assessment and measurement tests that have been developed with typically developing children. Ownership of 'constructed narratives' and the manner in which these are disseminated also have ethical implications, particularly in relation to informed consent.

The broadening arena

Children and young people are a vulnerable population group, easily exploited by researchers. When disability is added into the equation the level of vulnerability increases and issues of power relations become more acute. Greater ethical sensitivity and increased layers of gatekeeping have done much to protect disabled children from becoming easy prey to unscrupulous researchers.

The reorientation of disability thinking away from the medical model (where the 'problem' is seen as within the child) to a social model of disability (where society is disabling, not the child) has encouraged research that focuses on the social environment of disabled children, notably the responsiveness of that environment as a focus for communication (see Ware, 1996). There has also been a growth in educational research that places more emphasis on the quality and flexibility of teaching approaches and less emphasis on pupil disability. This has resulted in the development of a research base for interactive teaching approaches with children with learning difficulties replacing much of the behaviourist research that had dominated this field until the mid-1980s (Coupe O'Kane and Goldbart, 1998).

There is also an issue with regard to what type of disability research is chosen and, more contentiously, what gets funded. Gillman, Swain and Heyman (1997) claimed that in the area of learning difficulties research tended to privilege studies relating to IQ and medical diagnosis rather than lived experiences. This pathologises and objectifies the way children with learning difficulties are perceived. A willingness to adapt research designs has resulted in some explorations of these kinds of 'lived experiences'. Begley and Lewis's (1998) study of self-perception in children with Down's Syndrome is one such example. The recent rise in 'narrative' techniques described earlier is opening more participatory doors to young people with learning difficulties.

There are a number of controversies surrounding areas of validity and reliability in research involving children and young people with learning difficulties. Validity concerns whether the findings are really about what they appear to be about (Robson, 2002). The interview is an approach commonly adopted in research with children who have learning difficulties and some of the problems associated with this were raised earlier in relation to children with severe learning difficulties. The use of a question and answer technique is seen by some as a reflection of adult – child power relations (Edwards and Westgate, 1994). Statements and prompts are a preferred means of eliciting views. A new approach using cue cards to structure narratives is being evaluated by Lewis (2002) with primary aged children who have moderate learning difficulties. The cue cards act as prompts and contain carefully selected symbol pictures that convey meaning in a neutral way.

> The cards were presented in succession with minimum talk (if needed – 'Does this remind you of something else?') from the interviewer so that the child's narrative was prompted but not substantially interrupted. After practice in the use of the cards, the children became adept at retelling a series of events or an incident, including significant and correct details…The advantage of the prompted (using cue cards) version in eliciting a more detailed and accurate account over unprompted accounts was sustained across a range of children and events. (Lewis, 2002: 114)

A valid research design needs to be able to demonstrate that responses are not being misinterpreted, questions misunderstood or responses fashioned to the researcher's expectations. Traditional methods of triangulation may not be possible and sustained contact with respondents over a longer period of time may be necessary in order to establish whether their interpretations are valid. This also has implications for young people with learning difficulties acting as co-researchers. An example is Crozier's research (2000) with Tracey, a young woman with learning difficulties. In this research Crozier empowers Tracey to tell her own story about her disaffection and her schooling experiences. By adopting a methodology that utilised a sustained period of contact, Crozier was able to incorporate several validity checks into the process:

> a process of enabling Tracey to give her account, to have time to reflect on what she has said and to modify it in the light of her reflections, to select what she wishes to include or leave out and to check the accuracy of the representation of her thoughts. The process we used was to tape record an interview loosely structured by questions and prompts, meet subsequently to discuss thoughts and memories that had been stirred up, look at the transcript and raise new areas or emphases from reflections on the material. (Crozier and Tracey, 2000: 174)

Emancipatory disability research

Increased participant research by disabled individuals is giving rise to a new impetus of emancipatory research by disabled young people. Similar to the discourse that has grown up around white researchers exploring black issues, questions are being asked about whether able-bodied researchers should be undertaking disability research at all (Shakespeare, 1996; Stalker, 1998). This challenge is based on the premise that research techniques emerge from a theoretical position reflecting the researcher's beliefs, values and dispositions towards the social world (Gray and Denicolo, 1998). Gray and Denicolo illustrate this with an example in which hearing researchers falsely hypothesised that the deaf children they were studying were incapable of certain behaviours characteristic of typically developing children. It was not until months of protest from the children's deaf teacher that the researchers agreed to view their video data with the sound turned off. Only then did they notice a level of non-verbal activity similar to that of hearing children. Some would argue that the inability of able-bodied researchers to orient their perspective to one of disability compromises the validity of their research. Others maintain that disabled people cannot effectively represent all populations of disabled people and that there is a danger that those with the severest disabilities might become disenfranchised by power shifting to the less disabled. Perhaps a solution to the dilemma lies in increased participation of disabled people in research councils and other initiatives that foster greater collaboration.

Stalker (1998: 6) identifies three main characteristics of the emancipatory approach:

First, that conventional research relationships, whereby the researcher is the 'expert' and the researched merely the object of investigation, are inequitable; secondly, that people have the right to be consulted about and involved in research which is concerned with issues affecting their lives; and thirdly, that the quality and relevance of research is improved when disabled people are closely involved in the process.

Disabled writers such as Aspis (2002) and Zarb (1992) set out criteria for an 'emancipatory research paradigm' that require changes in the social and material relations of research production. This includes giving control of research funding to disabled people because real power lies in having control over what research gets commissioned. Oliver (1997) goes further by claiming that some research by able-bodied people is a violation of the experiences of disabled people, irrelevant to their needs, fails to improve their quality of life and sometimes even makes it worse. Foundations like the Joseph Rowntree aim to empower disabled people by ensuring that those central to the projects the Foundation funds are involved at every stage – including the dissemination stage. They launched their *Plain Facts* initiative whereby information from Joseph Rowntree projects is produced in accessible formats for individuals with learning disabilities. Organisations such as People First, a self-advocacy group of disabled people, have several branches nationally, control their own funds and decide what research projects to become involved with and whether or not to allow able-bodied researchers to be research partners. Clement (2002) points to a paradox in that this brings increased emancipation on the one hand but reduced diversity on the other. He writes about the dilemmas of his position as an able-bodied researcher working with a steering group of young people with learning difficulties from People First Birmingham:

> I have found the 'would-should dilemma', a concept associated with Carl Rogers Humanist Psychology, a useful way of understanding the conflict I have been feeling. As a researcher either I have to or I would like to research in a certain way, but feel that I should research in another. For example, in this research I wanted to use ideas about 'organisational culture' to frame my study, but I felt like I should use the social model of disability…

Whether or not emancipatory disability research is achievable in the form that writers such as Oliver and Aspis advocate is still open to debate. However, there is much that able-bodied researchers can do by expanding the range of methods to facilitate greater participation by disabled young people and much that funding bodies can do to encourage this.

Conclusions

Research with disabled children and young people presents many ethical and methodological challenges. Much has changed in recent years. The shift from a positivist to an interpretive paradigm is opening up new opportunities for disability research through the value now being placed on biographical and 'lived experience' methods. We are entering a research era that values disabled children and young people as individuals first, prizing their humanity and childhood ahead of the disability 'label'. The move away from 'normalisation' and towards treating 'difference' with greater respect is propelling disability research towards a human rights platform. More creative and flexible research designs are broadening the remit, beginning to foster participatory research with disabled young people and to invite them on to research advisory councils. An emancipatory impetus is building towards greater self-advocacy. Perhaps this will lead to greater inclusion of disabled young people as *active* researchers. Whatever the future holds, research with disabled children and young people will continue to provide us with many challenges.

References

Aspis, S. (2002) 'How valid is your research project?' *Community Living*, 15(4): 17–18.

Begley, A. and Lewis, A. (1998) 'Methodological issues in the assessment of the self-concept of children and Down Syndrome', *Child Psychology and Psychiatry Review*, 3: 33–40.

Booth, T. and Booth, W (1996) 'Sound of silence: narrative research with inarticulate subjects', *Disability & Society*, 11(1): 55–69.

Clement, T. (2002) 'There's no progress without struggle: views on doing disability research'. Paper given at The Open University School of Health and Welfare Research Seminar Programme.

Coupe O'Kane, J. and Goldbart, J. (1998) *Communication before Speech*, 2nd edn, London, David Fulton.

Crozier, J. and Tracey (2000) 'Falling out of school: a young woman's reflections on her chequered experience of schooling', in A. Lewis and G. Lindsay (eds), *Researching Children's Perspectives*, pp. 173–184, Buckingham, Open University Press.

Davis, J., Watson, N. and Cunningham-Burley, S. (2000) 'Learning the lives of disabled children', in P. Christensen and A. James (eds), *Research with Children: Perspectives and Practices*, London, Routledge Falmer.

Detheridge, T. (2000) 'Research involving children with severe learning difficulties', in A. Lewis and G. Lindsay (eds), *Researching Children's Perspectives*, Buckingham, Open University Press.

Edwards, A.D. and Westgate, D.P.G. (1994) *Investigating Classroom Talk*, Lewes, Falmer Press.

Fletcher, J.M., Brookshire, B.L., Landry, S.H., Bohan, T.P., Davidson, K.C., Francis, D.J., Levin, H.S., Brandt, M.E., Kramer, L.A. and Morris, R.D. (1996) 'Attentional skills and executive functions in children with early hydrocephalus', *Developmental Neuropsychology*, 12(1): 53–76.

Gillman, M., Swain, J. and Heyman, B. (1997) 'Life history of "case" history: the objectification of people with learning difficulties through the tyranny of professional discourses', *Disability & Society*, 12(5): 675–693.

Gray, D.E. and Denicolo, P. (1998) 'Research in special needs education: objectivity or ideology?' *British Journal of Special Education*, 25(3): 140–145.

Hobson, R.P. (1991) 'Methodological issues for experiments on autistic individuals' perception and understanding of emotion', *Journal of Child Psychology and Psychiatry*, 32(7): 1135–1158.

Hogg, J. and Sebba, J. (1986) *Profound Retardation and Multiple Impairment. Vol. 1: Development and Learning*, London, Croom Helm.

Kellett, M. (2000) 'Sam's Story: evaluating Intensive Interaction in terms of its effect on the social and communicative ability of a young child with severe learning difficulties', *Support for Learning*, 15(4): 165–171.

Kellett, M. and Nind, M. (2001) 'What do we compromise? Ethics in quasi-experimental research', *British Journal of Learning Disabilities*, 29: 51–55.

Lewis, A. (2002) 'Accessing, through research interviews, the views of children with difficulties in learning', *Support for Learning*, 17(3): 110–116.

Lewis, V. (2003) *Disability and Development*, Oxford, Blackwell.

Mervis, C.B. and Robinson, B.F. (1999) 'Methodological issues in cross-syndrome comparisons: matching procedures, sensitivity (Se), and specificity (Sp)', *Monographs of the Society for Research in Child Development*, 64(1): 115–130.

Norgate, S.H. (1998) 'Research methods for studying the language of blind children', in N. Hornberger and D. Corson (eds), *The Encyclopaedia of Language and Education* Vol. 8, pp. 165–173, The Netherlands, Kluwer Academic Publishers.

Oliver, M. (1997) 'Emancipatory research: realistic goal or impossible dream', in C. Barnes and G. Mercer (eds), *Doing Disability Research*, pp. 15–31, Leeds, The Disability Press.

Pérez-Pereira, M. (1999) 'Deixis, personal reference, and the use of pronouns by blind children', *Journal of Child Language*, 26: 655–680.

Pérez-Pereira, M. and Conti-Ramsden, G. (1999) *Language Development and Social Interaction in Blind Children*. Hove, Sussex, Psychology Press.

Priestley, M. (1998) 'Childhood disability and disabled childhoods: agendas for research', *Childhood*, 5(2): 207–223.

Robson, C. (2002) *Real World Research*, 2nd edn, Oxford, Blackwell.

Shakespeare, T. (1996) 'Rules of engagement: doing disability research', *Disability & Society*, 11(1): 115–119.

Shakespeare, T. and Watson, N. (1998) 'Theoretical perspectives on research with disabled children', in C. Robinson and K. Stalker (eds), *Growing Up with Disability*, London, Jessica Kinglsey.

Stalker, K. (1998) 'Some ethical and methodological issues in research with people with learning difficulties', *Disability & Society*, 13(1): 5–19.

Urwin, C. (1983) 'Dialogue and cognitive functioning in the early language development of three blind children', in A.E. Mills (ed.), *Language Acquisition in the Blind Child*, London, Croom Helm.

Wagner, S., Ganiban, J. and Cicchetti, D. (1990) 'Attention, memory, and perception in infants with Down syndrome: a review and commentary', in D. Cicchetti and M. Beeghly (eds), *Children with Down Syndrome: A Developmental Perspective*. Cambridge, Cambridge University Press.

Ware, J. (1996) *Creating a Responsive Environment*, London, David Fulton.

Wilson, P.H. and McKenzie, B.E. (1998) 'Information processing deficits associated with developmental coordination disorder: a meta-analysis of research findings', *Journal of Child Psychology and Psychiatry*, 39(6): 829–840.

Wode, H. (1983) 'Precursors and the study of the impaired language learner', in A.E. Mills (ed.), *Language Acquisition in the Blind Child: Normal and Deficient*, London, Croom Helm.

Wright, I. (1998) 'The development of representation in children with Down's syndrome', Doctoral dissertation, University of Warwick.

Zarb, G. (1992) 'On the road to Damascus: first steps towards changing the relations of disability research production', *Disability, Handicap and Society*, 7(2): 125–138.

14 Participatory Action Research in the Majority World
OLGA NIEUWENHUYS

When thinking of children (aged under 18) in the majority world, images of malnutrition, illiteracy, homelessness, abandonment, exploitation, sexual abuse and violence tend to come to mind. These images are in stark contrast with the qualities we commonly associate with the word *childhood*: a healthy and safe environment, a protective, loving family, a comfortable home, access to high quality education and plenty of time to play. These qualities are but rarely found in the majority world. The main reason is not simply parental poverty, but inadequate governmental outlays for health, education and child welfare services as well. No serious agency or institution would today claim that it realistically aims at endowing the majority world's children with the kind of childhood experienced by those in the minority world. The focus is rather on strengthening other qualities, deemed more relevant in the context of these children's lives. It is not easy, however, to know what these qualities are and how they can best be strengthened. The countries of the majority world do not have an elaborated, uniform conception of childhood endorsed by the vast majority of the population as is common in the minority world. Legal systems and family laws have been either simply inherited from colonial administrations or copied from the minority world. They fail to reflect local customs, beliefs and practices as they evolve under the impact of current events.

Strengthening the qualities of childhood in the majority world will need to rely on low-cost, locally adapted and creative approaches, a challenge that heavily indebted national governments cannot possibly carry out on their own. They have therefore sought support from the private sector, most notably from both local and international non-governmental organisations (NGOs) that seek to address development issues by working at a micro or local level directly with the people concerned. Typically NGO-notions such as *empowerment, participation* and *self-reliance* are in agreement with the idea of a low-cost, locally adapted, creative approach. Recent debates about children's right to participation have lent support to the idea that the NGO approach would be relevant to addressing children's issues. Contemporary critiques of pedagogy and social work theory that take issue with treating children as passive recipients of expert knowledge and stress the need to acknowledge their *agency* have given additional credit to NGOs' new role in addressing children's issues (Wyness, 1996; Nieuwenhuys, 2001).

This new role has revived interest in using Participatory Action Research (PAR) methods with children. PAR aims at encouraging children's exploration, reflection and action upon their social and natural environment with the aim of strengthening their capacity for self-determination. PAR is particularly well suited to make up for a lack of relevant expertise in situations where interventions are bound to be small-scale, local and of an experimental character. PAR can help children construct their everyday experiences into knowledge, gain self-confidence in their abilities and influence decisions that are taken about their lives.

Obviously, there is a world of difference between intended and actual participation, and this is particularly true of PAR. The method presupposes a fair capacity for independent thinking and collective action, something we might expect to find among active members of co-operatives or trade unions rather than among children. But children who face situations of crisis are likely to be much more actively engaged in negotiating their place in society than common opinion may suppose. The chapter briefly reviews the majority world's experiences of childhood and the theoretical assumptions of PAR, then addresses the three main implications of PAR with children: taking responsibility; balancing participation with facilitation; and negotiating spaces for children's agency. The chapter is based on personal experience with PAR notably in Ethiopia and South India and on a review of relevant literature and case studies.

Child welfare in the majority world

The involvement of vulnerable children in research can be traced back to, firstly, budgetary constraints that have led to a crisis in government services and family support networks; secondly, political concern arising from fear and unfamiliarity with how children respond to the crisis; and, finally, a perceived lack of specialist knowledge to address the crisis. These problems support the choice of research methods that are cheap, easy to grasp and apply, and deliver information that can be used for direct, local intervention.

The early 1980s saw an increasing number of majority world countries introducing severe cuts in social spending as a corollary to SAPs (Structural Adjustment Programmes) and economic reforms deemed necessary to foster economic growth. The result has been a marked decrease in the standard of living of majority world children and rising levels of malnutrition, child mortality and illiteracy (Bradshaw, 1993). The situation has become particularly severe in the countryside, but cities too increasingly lack facilities and services for the fast growing urban population. Many city authorities do not have sufficient finances for piped water, schools, feeding programmes and day care facilities, housing, clinics, playgrounds, etc. in the sprawling slum areas. Facing the failure to provide these services, both governments and NGOs are increasingly critical of ideals of childhood which they see as failing to reflect the reality of their country. These ideals are grounded in a minority world's vision of childhood happiness as a matter of public concern requiring a vast array of institutions, services and specialist knowledge. When set against these ideals, the reality of children in the majority world appears as a mere *lack*. Governments and NGOs now find it more fruitful to take a positive approach that respects children's integrity and recognises the precious coping mechanisms on which their livelihood depends (Connolly and Ennew, 1996; Bemak, 1996). The aim is to devise interventions that build on this reality and involve children as full participants (Wyness, 2001; Woodhead, 1999; Chawla, 2002).

The lack of services for poor children manifests itself, secondly, in a heightened presence of children in the streets. This causes public anxiety and reflects a feeling that the state is failing in its task of controlling social tensions. The result is a burgeoning of NGO initiatives that seek to come up with original approaches in which the children themselves have a part to play. International donor agencies are particularly interested in funding this type of private initiative in the majority world.

Thirdly, not only resources but also specialist knowledge to help develop and improve intervention policies and school curricula, set up day care centres, address the situation of street and working children etc., is inadequate. Institutions that impart this type of knowledge are in many countries either non-existent or hardly up to the task of delivering professionals with the necessary frame of mind and creative skills. Where career prospects are minimal, there is little incentive for young intellectuals to devote their talents to poor children's needs. Even those who find a calling in this type of work or are particularly dutiful, as is the case with many school teachers and social workers, may find it in the end hard to develop their professional skills in the absence of sufficient response from the local academic community. Still very much imbued with minority world paradigms of child development, this community has lacked both the motivation and the means to provide insights into the problems faced by vulnerable children.

These insights will have to rely on a substantial new shift in the ways research into children's issues is organised. Conventional research is often felt to be inopportune because it is costly and time consuming both in terms of the generation of results and of the structure it requires for implementation. But quite apart from that, conventional methods may be intrusive and distanced and engender 'top-down' types of intervention which may be difficult to implement not only because of the modesty of outlays but also because support among the people concerned may be lacking. There are three major reasons for this: the position of the conventional researcher, the kind of knowledge that s/he generates, and his/her hidden values and presuppositions.

Firstly, when speaking of 'conventional researchers' local governments and NGOs clearly have in mind the type of researcher who has little practical understanding of the day to day experiences of the people s/he researches. As an example one could take the many surveys undertaken to count children on the streets. This counting is generally done on the basis of an *a priori* definition of what a 'street child' would be, without the researcher needing to know first-hand the reality in which these children live. When invited to define him/herself no child would probably say that s/he is a 'street child', a term experienced as insulting. It is more likely that s/he will see him/herself as a working child or dutiful son or daughter (Lucchini, 1996: 167).

Secondly, the knowledge produced in this type of research tends to justify rather than challenge domination. The ways the problem of 'street children' is defined in Brazil, for example, already contain a form of stereotyping that puts the blame on the children themselves, their parents or their poverty. The political pressure of rural elites who wish to control the migration of youngsters fleeing from conditions of semi-slavery in the countryside to the cities, is left out of consideration. These elites, with strong ties to government and ruling parties, influence the representation of street children as children 'out of place' (Hecht, 1998: 155–156).

Thirdly, in spite of apparent objectivity, there are, in all research, hidden values and presuppositions that influence the outcome. This outcome may be quite different if one starts, as in the Brazil case, from the presupposition that the problem to be addressed is not the children but the power that rural elites wield over their former slaves. If the values and presuppositions underlying research on 'street children' are made more explicit, results often find little support among the ruling elite. But because this type of conventional research positions itself as being value-free, it also fails to provide room for alternative views, and particularly of the powerless who are all too often its 'objects' of inquiry.

The allegations against 'conventional' research must be treated with a degree of caution. There is also another type of influential research that uses qualitative methods of inquiry and is strongly oriented towards critical reflection – including on the researcher's own presuppositions. Drawing inspiration from the 'new sociology of childhood' (Prout, 2000; James and James, 2001; Morss, 2002), this type of research has evinced children's active role in shaping their own lives, lending support to the involvement of children in planning and designing local interventions (O' Kane, 2000).

In short, both governments and NGOs are receptive to the idea that they need the feedback of children if they want to come up with the kind of innovative and low-cost interventions that may count on the support of the children and their parents. To get this feedback they often turn to unconventional research methods such as PAR.

Participative action research with children

PAR is more of an inspiring and challenging philosophy of research than a clear method. It is born out of a critique of the scientific outlook adopted by some forms of 'conventional' research that:

values public testing, but at the same time places the researcher firmly outside and separate from the subject of his or her research, seeking for an objective knowledge and for one separate truth. (Reason, 1998: 261–262)

PAR belongs to the school of qualitative research that sees people:

> as cocreating their reality through participation: through their experience, their imagination and intuition, their thinking and their action (Reason, 1998: 262).

PAR is a form of participative research that emphasises the political aspect of knowledge production. It has a double objective. One aim is to produce knowledge and action directly useful to a group of people – through research, adult education and socio-political action. The second aim is to empower people at a deeper level through the process of constructing and using their own knowledge. PAR researchers take a critical stand against the ways in which the elite monopolises the production and use of knowledge for its own benefits. This is what Paolo Freire has termed *conscientisation*. An additional aspect is commitment. The academic knowledge of formally trained people works in dialectical tension with the practical knowledge of the people to produce a more profound understanding of the situation (Reason, 1998: 269–270). The researcher has therefore to accept a much more humble role than s/he may have in conventional research and engage in a mutually enriching dialogue during all the phases of doing research, from the formulation of the problem and the framework of analysis to the use and presentation of data. S/he is an *intellectual mediator* in the process of transformation of society so that:

> those who are currently poor and oppressed will progressively transform their environment by their own praxis. In this process others may play a catalytic or supportive role, but will not dominate. (Rahman, 1993: 82)

PAR works from the belief that social oppression is rooted not only in material conditions but in the means of knowledge production. To challenge the ways knowledge is currently used to justify domination, oppressed people need to develop *their own processes of knowledge generation* and acquire the means to assert this knowledge *vis-à-vis* the knowledge of the dominant class (Rahman, 1993: 83). Though this requires the support of a mass movement, even micro-level experiments can help develop this type of self-reliant knowledge.

Being committed to genuine collaboration in knowledge generation starts with defining problems and concepts so that they reflect the experiences of the people concerned. But crucial in PAR is to address the logical system of analysis of social research that implicitly favours dominant knowledge. Consider for instance how the practical knowledge that children acquire of their environment and how to cope in it is currently interpreted within the framework of dominant developmental psychology. Growing up is, in this framework, a process divided into phases that correspond to a certain level and intensity of both physical and emotional experience. Many of children's coping mechanisms in the majority world do not fit in this framework. Even if their coping mechanisms are effective and conducive to the development of their identity, the implicit reference to a dominant logical system of analysis translates into a belief that, however competent, the children still miss out on a normal childhood. The frequent references to *stolen child-hoods* and to *giving a childhood* to the poor that one encounters in much writing on children in the majority world are cases in point. PAR cannot undermine overnight dominant knowledge on which this kind of judgement is passed, but it can start building countervailing knowledge that values the active role of people in co-creating the real-life childhood of the majority world.

PAR cannot also do away with hidden values and presuppositions, but it can make them explicit and help open a dialogue between different players. Taking children really seriously appears in practice infinitely more difficult when this clashes with the values of the elites than when it does not. As an example one could take Montgomery's research on children who work as prostitutes in Thailand. Using empathic methods of anthropological research, Montgomery comes to the conclusion that even young children are aware of the risks involved in their occupation. They have both economic and moral reasons to engage in prostitution because it is the best way for them to fulfil their filial duties (Montgomery, 2001: 257) – a conclusion that challenges the moral values of both urban elites in Thai society and some NGOs that address these children's plight. PAR would in this case be helpful to start a dialogue in which various positions are mapped and confronted and action is undertaken that recognises children's emphatic desire to fulfil their filial obligations.

By its very nature, PAR does not have, as conventional research does, a distinct set of self-contained methods. Conventional research methods work from the separation of subject (the researcher) and object (the researched), in which the researched is assigned a role of passivity and incompetence. Because it wants to undermine what is essentially a power relation in the production of knowledge, PAR seeks to actively develop tools of research conducive to the type of dialogue that is sought after. Preference is given to methods and techniques of inquiry that allow for the expression of different values, views and interpretations. Creative tools such as drawings, games, drama, songs, photographs, role play, map making, etc., are techniques believed to allow not only for a maximum of participation but also for a maximum of sharing in the knowledge generated during PAR (see for the use of photographs for example Young and Barrett, 2001).

PAR has been used to designate all kinds of applied research that to some extent do not suit the paradigm of value-free, positivistic research carried out by expert researchers independently from the people they research. It has been particularly ill used in cases in which the intended beneficiaries have been consulted by the researcher or enrolled at some stages of the data gathering, without this consultation leading to a genuine sharing of power at the decision-making level. This type of research is more correctly referred to as *policy oriented* and is not the subject of this chapter. What PAR is also not about is the reflexive qualitative type of research discussed in the previous section that recognises the unique, creative individuals who influence their own life and the society in which it is embedded, but remains impartial when it comes to action. Other types of participative inquiry such as *co-operative inquiry* (based on co-operation as a way to achieve self-determination) and *action inquiry* (seeking to understand how action improves the nature of organisations) also have less clear political aims than PAR (Reason, 1998: 262, 272). The distinction between PRA (Participatory Rural Appraisal), now popular among development NGOs, and PAR is less evident, as both aim at tilting the balance of power in favour of disadvantaged groups in society (Chambers, 1997). PRA has been criticised for consulting 'the grassroots' without challenging the political power relationships underlying their oppression (Harriss, 2002). This is not the intention of PAR.

While the problems a researcher may expect to encounter when undertaking PAR with children are probably similar to those encountered with adults, they are certainly, as I will now turn to argue, more difficult to solve. This is not only because social differences based on age complicate the nature of power between researcher and researched, but also because society regards children, unlike even the most wretched of adults, as essentially unable to take responsibility for their own actions. PAR takes issue with the general belief that children are passive. But it has also to deal with a number of dilemmas: firstly, the need to take direct responsibility for the children who are the intended actors in research; secondly, the difficulty of balancing the role of the facilitator with the need to allow for a maximum of participation; and, thirdly, the necessity to protect and negotiate the needs of children whom society perceives as deviant. I will discuss them in the following three sections by pointing out the main problems that have to be addressed and providing examples along the way.

Taking responsibility

Children's dependency on adults for the fulfilment of even simple needs is so great that one can hardly expect them to co-operate in a research programme that does not from the outset address these needs seriously. Baker, Panter-Brick and Todd (1996) give us telling insight into how the apparently innocuous collection of anthropometrical data in Nepal, though carefully planned and explained, resulted in street children expecting medicines shortly thereafter – an experience undoubtedly common to anybody who has tried to collect data from poor children without linking this activity to a direct intervention. The alternative is in no way simple. In the example above, any straightforward distribution of medicines in connection with the research would have increased dependency at least at the cognitive level, resulting in, to put it bluntly, children trading their personal information for medicines.

In her clinic AMMOR (Atendimento Médico aos Meninos e Meninas de Rua) in Belo Horizonte (Brazil), Doctor Adams has been addressing this problem with what she calls the method of the *liberating plaster*. Inspired by Paolo Freire's approach (1996), she sought to avoid the problem of expert medical knowledge making children dependent or increasing their feeling of worthlessness by using a method based on dialogical learning. The process starts right in the clinic's waiting room, where the doctor explains to the children that they need to wait for their turn, not only for the doctor's sake, but also because it is in their own interest to get private care. The doctor however also accepts that the children have other than purely physical complaints, and takes care to accompany her explanations in the waiting room with immediate comfort, talking with children who seem upset, hugging them, looking at their wounds, listening to their complaints.

During the medical consultation the AMMOR doctor asks the children not only about their complaints but also for additional information about what treatment they have already taken. By being asked why s/he has neglected a wound the child is not only taught that s/he has to care for his/her body, that it is important to stay healthy and that s/he can consult a doctor, but is also invited to communicate how s/he feels about the treatment. So the doctor, instead of condemning the child for carelessness or apathy, and reinforcing feelings of inferiority or lack of self-respect, learns about health problems connected with life on the streets. This is how putting on a plaster becomes an act of liberation for children who struggle to value themselves. Gradually a very personal and intimate relation develops that often leads to the child requesting a full medical check-up. The medical findings are discussed with the child in detail, the child receiving a copy of the photo taken by the doctor as well as free access to his/her mediscal file, which from then on can also function as a storage place for his/her personal history. Consent is asked also for an HIV test, with full explanation of what this can entail. The result is a very thorough documentation of each individual case. Data on HIV infection and risk factors are not only highly reliable, they are also directly linked to preventing the spread of the disease. This example illustrates that delivering immediate support need not be postponed until after the results of a research project are analysed, but has advantages, both in terms of quality of data and impact, when compared with the traditional separation of the process of data gathering from intervention.

Working with children who are on an NGO-project is no guarantee of mutual understanding and respect. After a PAR on topics chosen with the children and their families, social workers of several NGOs based in Addis Ababa admitted to having become aware of prejudices they had unconsciously been harbouring. They discovered that the children, contrary to their presupposition, had extensive supportive networks both among kin and in the neighbourhood. Neglecting these networks had not only made the social workers' job unduly stressful but had predisposed them to think negatively of the children's future. This example highlights that though PAR with children should preferably be carried out in contexts in which the direct needs of children are taken care of, the reverse is also true. Taking responsibility for vulnerable children needs to be continuously supported by knowledge generated in close collaboration with the children and their caregivers.

Balancing participation and facilitation

As said, participation is a crucial ingredient of PAR. But differences between the facilitator and children not only in power, wealth and knowledge but also in age, make participation particularly problematic. Though it may not be difficult to avoid overt paternalism, it is hardly possible, and not even desirable, to treat the children as if they were adults. In addition to establishing a tension between academic and practical knowledge, the facilitator has a pedagogical role to fulfil.

It does make quite a difference if a facilitator understands participation as granting children a voice in research (a situation in which s/he remains in full control of the process) or seeks to define the conditions of research in such way that children obtain a voice. The second option has clear consequences at all the levels at which knowledge is generated and precludes the use of pre-set categories and formalised instruments of research. Obtaining a voice means facilitating the research process in such a way that children learn how to use cognitive instruments that can capture and give meaning to their lifeworlds.

During writers' workshops in Soweto children were encouraged to make a collective book containing stories, poems and drawings about themselves and their lives:

> The boys would read each other's stories (and often re-read their own). They could not believe that strangers coming into the room were interested in reading their stories…What all of my students seemed to enjoy the most was getting their stories back from me, typed on the computer but still in rough form, with questions for them, asking for more details, clearing up confusion on meaning… (Hirsch, 1993: 1)

There are many examples of this type of intervention from deprived areas – particularly schools – in the minority world, but experiences in the majority world are far less common. In overcrowded schools and NGO-projects the tendency is to give precedence to basic skills training and to treat alternative approaches as an unaffordable luxury. The work of a large international NGO, Environmental Development Action, known as ENDA, in Francophone Africa with youths aged 15 to 18 shows that PAR experiences tend to be pragmatically oriented towards income generation. In Rwanda, a laborious exercise under the guidance of an educator led the youngsters to identify *clothing* as their main need. From there they investigated possibilities to add to their meagre income from porterage at the local market place and decided to take up a collective project to make and sell charcoal. They planned the research on a day-to-day basis, according to what was achieved the previous day and not according to a predetermined time schedule. Problems regarding the choice and use of research instruments to collect data were likewise solved, the youths finding it counterproductive to separate observation and interviewing, preferring the more informal *chatting, walking* and *visiting* instead (ENDA-JEUDA 1995: 166).

In another ENDA experience, this time with young female domestics in Dakar, the girls discovered the advantage of representing abstract categories in ways that made sense, for instance by using the image of *the one who delivers children* to explain the concept of the independent variable (Punch, 1998: 53–54). To devise a method of time planning the girls likewise represented activities in sequence and frequently evaluated whether they had collected enough information to proceed to the execution of the next sequence (ENDA-JEUDA, 1995: 193ff.).

These experiences also illuminate the central role of the PAR facilitator as *instrument of research*. S/he is not a person skilled in applying sets of procedures and techniques but a *reflecting actor*, a responsible person who is thinking and rethinking constantly what s/he is doing and is sharing this process of knowledge generation with the youngsters with whom PAR is carried out. The dividing line between what a social worker does in his/her daily practice and PAR is thin, the difference lying essentially in the planning of moments of conscious reflection and documentation (Nieuwenhuys, 1995: 63). In other words, what makes the ENDA experiences into PAR is their being undertaken with the intention not only of constructing children's needs and wishes into knowledge, but also of reflecting upon each step and documenting the process.

Documentation should certainly not be limited to recording and reporting but should produce *texts* that voice different meanings and feelings (*multi-vocality*). Figure 14.1 is an example of such a text, the product of an exercise in which the Dakar domestics were asked to prioritise the variables that influenced their lack of training opportunities.

The text, graphically representing a father who is wielding a large club against a running girl, suggests the existence of conflicting interests between the girls and their fathers, an aspect which both the social worker and the girls disregarded in the analysis. But the text remains important for later: if the activities undertaken do not work out as expected one can return to them to ask why so little importance was given to crucial

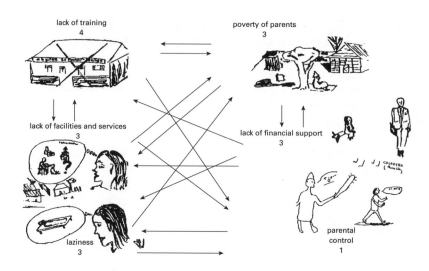

Figure 14.1   Prioritization: lack of training

Source: ENDA-JEUDA (1995), translation by author

information on the girls' powerlessness, how this problem could have been acknowledged and addressed, how it relates to the lack of professional training, etc.

In other words, what happens to results is crucial. Are they generating categories, concepts and criteria for understanding and changing the lives of the children involved or are they 'translated' into research data that must primarily convince sceptical donors or feed the authorities' thirst for sensitive information (Mohan, 2001: 161)? As I shall argue next, the facilitator has a responsibility to protect information from eroding, in the process of translation, the chosen self-representation of children.

Spaces for children's agency

The third difficulty of PAR with children is about negotiating spaces in which children can legitimately act upon their environment. It may be useful, in this connection, to go back to the AMMOR experience. Even if sensitive data on HIV infection, as in the case of AMMOR, is gathered primarily to enhance self-representation, there remains the problem that health authorities may also be interested in them, and may have interests in mind that do not necessarily coincide with those of the children. As the tragic news about the activities of death squads in Brazil has shown, negative representations of vulnerable children's lives can also inspire deeply antagonistic and violent responses. Doctor Adams had to find ways to manage her data with the utmost discretion, taking care to safeguard not only the interests of the individual patient but also those of the group as a whole. This latter point, she suggests, could best be done by linking children's health problems to the past history of slavery, economic crisis, famine, displacement, etc. (see also Hecht, 1998). Demonstrating their resourcefulness in facing these problems is a way to establish and safeguard public respect for these children.

An interesting example of how PAR can help create spaces for children comes from Bogotá. A team of researchers of the National University of Colombia sought to promote working children's self-organisation in the hope that this would make them less vulnerable to exploitation. From the outset, the research team was critical about the forms of knowledge it was to utilise and used different instruments (socio-drama, autobiographies, interviews and oral history) to encourage the children to share the knowledge they had about their families and their work situation (Salazar, 1991: 55–56).

The research team talked to the children of human rights and their cultural origins, strengthening the feeling that they could act upon their environment. The idea that working children could establish an organisation that furthered their rights was thus quickly established. The process was consolidated by the creation of *cultural meeting spaces* in which the children could deploy activities that helped them understand the need to contest the dominant value system that condemned them as child labourers. The initiative led a number of children to leave their demeaning jobs and start self-managed bakeries and carpentry shops.

The management of NGOs may see social workers as mere instruments for the delivery of goods and services and not appreciate their taking sides in favour of the children. An experience with the training of social workers through PAR in South Indian cities is illustrative. The training programme aimed primarily at developing professional skills to enable social workers to better understand and negotiate their own and poor children's place both in the NGO and in society at large. The programme wanted to impart competence not only in activating children but also in negotiating choices with the management. Dealing with the management appeared in the end far more difficult than working with the children. Though the social workers were making interesting and original contributions and developed innovative methods of intervention, many of them lost their jobs or were moved to other projects even before the end of the programme. Rather than as an important asset, the management apparently experienced the generation of countervailing knowledge by children as a threat (cf. for a similar experience Driskell et al., 2001).

In his discussion on children's participation Roger Hart has graphically represented the powerlessness of children in a ladder of participation (Figure 14.2).

Only the last four levels of the ladder are actually about genuine participation, while only the last one is useful at the level of interventions for children. Only when children initiate an intervention and share decisions

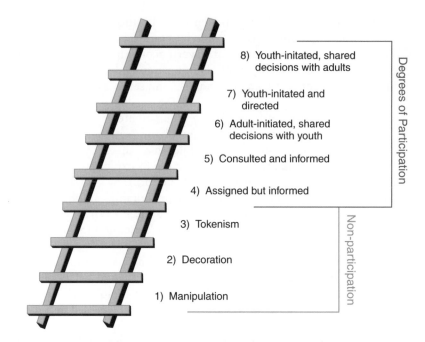

8) Youth-initated, shared
decisions with adults

7) Youth-initated and
directed

6) Adult-initiated, shared
decisions with youth

5) Consulted and informed

4) Assigned but informed

3) Tokenism

2) Decoration

1) Manipulation

Degrees of Participation

Non-participation

Figure 14.2   Ladder of participation

Source: Hart (1997)

with adults are they taken seriously at the level of political decision making. Unhappily, Hart recognises, this is the most difficult if not unlikely form of participation, since it requires caring adults who are attuned to the interests of children and have themselves the means to help them voice their needs and desires.

Parents, teachers, social workers or political activists in the majority world, though best equipped to realise the conditions for children's participation, are also the traditional vehicles of authority and control. Top-down political thinking all too often sees them as mere instruments of enforcement of policies as disparate as mass vaccination, HIV control, political indoctrination, cultural assimilation, control of truancy, etc. Often burdened by heavy responsibilities *vis-à-vis* their employers, difficult work circumstances and poor pay, one can hardly expect social workers or teachers to make additional efforts to create spaces that invite children's participation without a considerable improvement in their conditions of work. But this is certainly not enough, and, as suggested by the South Indian experience, those who work with children need also to understand their own position in society and how it is related to that of the children in their care. In other words, changing the balance in favour of oppressed children entails that the social worker too will agree to become the object of research (Schrijvers, 1995: 25).

Concluding remarks

PAR with children is no doubt a highly relevant and promising way of generating, with a minimum of means and expertise, knowledge that is respectful of local practices and reflects the everyday reality of children in the majority world. It can do so because its basic aim is to open a dialogue in which various ways of generating knowledge – both academic and practical – are given equal weight. PAR methods are devised to share power and this makes it possible to take oppressed children seriously as partners in research. The feedback of children is crucial for the success of innovative and low-cost interventions.

PAR can best be used within NGOs and social movements that ensure that results are put into action. Working with organisations reduces the risk of research disempowering desperately poor children by making them trade their personal information for a little food or a few coins. Very much depends however on the motivation and interpersonal skills of a facilitator capable of cleverly balancing a pedagogical role with that of listener and learner. If s/he is to succeed in this s/he must build upon experiences that allow for a maximum degree of creativity, diversity and local initiative. But his or her role is not limited to research and action that helps children gain self-respect and become aware of their rights. It has also to do with the attitude of those in positions of command – for example schools or NGO managements – the ways children are represented in the media, negative feelings of the public, etc. By strengthening self-representations of vulnerable children as people who can think, make choices and act, PAR can help further alternative visions of these children's futures. But producing such visions is not enough. Action based on an alternative self-representation must link up to organisations or movements challenging the existing power structure (Liebel et al., 2001). There is a real danger of raising expectations which cannot be satisfied and exposing already vulnerable children to more hostility and negative stereotyping.

The minority world's institutions for the protection of childhood are very unlikely to be replicated in the majority world not only because of their costliness but, more deeply, because they presuppose children to be subordinate and passive objects of care. Children's coping strategies in the majority world negate in practice this passivity. Participation is a low-cost alternative to the protection – but also control – of youngsters belonging to the popular classes. It can result in oppression if the balance of power remains unquestioned. It is from taking up this challenge that the payoffs of PAR with children may be expected.

Acknowledgements

An earlier version of this chapter originally appeared in *Environment and Urbanisation*, 9(1): 233–249, (1997) and, translated into Dutch, in

M. De Winter and M. Kroneman (eds) (2002) *Sociaal-wetenschappelijk onderzoek samen met kinderen en jongeren.* Assen: Van Gorcum. I wish to thank all those who have commented on the earlier version.

References

Baker, R., Panter-Brick, C. and Todd, A. (1996) 'PRA with children in Nepal', *Childhood, Children out of Place: Special Issue on Working and Street Children,* 3(2) May: 171–194.

Bemak, F. (1996) 'Street researchers: a new paradigm redefining future research with street children', *Childhood,* 3(2): 147–156.

Bradshaw, Y.W. (1993) 'New directions in international development: a focus on children', *Childhood,* 1: 134–142.

Chambers, R. (1997) *Whose Reality Counts? Putting the First Last,* London, IT Publications.

Chawla, L. (ed.) (2002) *Growing Up in an Urbanising World,* Paris, UNESCO.

Connolly, M. and Ennew, J. (1996) 'Introduction: children out of place', in *Childhood, Children out of Place: Special Issue on Working and Street Children,* 3(2): 131–146.

Driskell, D., Banerjee, K. and Chawla, L. (2001) 'Rhetoric, reality and resilience: overcoming obstacles to young people's participation in development', *Environment and Urbanization,* 13(1): 77–89.

ENDA-JEUDA (1995) *Enfants en recherche et en action, une alternative Africaine d'animation urbaine,* Dakar, Editions ENDA.

Freire, P. (1996) *Pedagogy of the Oppressed,* London, Penguin.

Harriss, J. (2002) *Depoliticizing Development: The World Bank and Social Capital,* London, Anthem.

Hart, R. (1997) *Children's Participation, The Theory and Practice of Involving Young Citizens in Community Development and Environmental Care,* London, Earthscan; New York, UNICEF.

Hecht, T. (1998) *At Home in the Streets: Street Children of Northeast Brazil,* Cambridge, Cambridge University Press.

Hirsch, R.V. (ed.) (1993) *A Day Like Any Other. Stories, Poetry and Art by Street Children in South Africa,* Johannesburg, COSAW Publ.

James, A. and James, A.L. (2001) 'Childhood: towards a theory of continuity and change', *ANNALS AAPSS,* 575: 25–37.

Liebel, M., Overwien, B. and Recknagel, A. (eds) (2001) *Working Children's Protagonism,* Frankfurt am Main, IKO.

Lucchini, R. (1996) 'Theory, method and triangulation in the study of street children', *Childhood, Children out of Place: Special Issue on Working and Street Children,* 3(2): 167–170.

Mohan, G. (2001) 'Beyond participation: strategies for deeper development', in B. Cooke and U. Kothari (eds), *Participation: The New Tyranny?* London, ZED.

Montgomery, H. (2001) *Modern Babylon? Prostituting Children in Thailand,* New York: Berghahn Books.

Morss, J. (2002) 'The several social constructions of Prout, James and Jenks: A Contribution to the Sociological Theorization of Childhood', *International Journal of Children's Rights,* 10: 39–54.

Nieuwenhuys, O. (ed.) (1995) *Drafting an Action Research Curriculum for Street Educators*, Workshop Report, University of Amsterdam, Institute for Development Research, Amsterdam.

Nieuwenhuys, O. (2001) 'By the sweat of their brow? Street children, NGOs and children's rights in Addis Ababa', *Africa*, 71(4): 539–557.

O'Kane, C. (2000) 'The Development of Participatory Techniques, Facilitating Children's Views about Decisions which Affect Them', in P. Christensen and A. James (eds) *Research with Children, Perspectives and Practices*, London, Falmer Press.

Prout, A. (2000) 'Representing Children: reflections on the Children 5–16 Programme, *Children and Society*, 15: 193–201.

Punch, K.F. (1998) *Introduction to Social Research: Quantitative and Qualitative Approaches*. London, Sage.

Rahman, M.A. (1993) *People's Self-development. Perspectives on Participatory Action Research: A Journey through Experience*, London, ZED.

Reason, P. (1998) 'Three approaches to participative inquiry', in N.K. Denzin and Y.S. Lincoln (eds), *Strategies of Qualitative Inquiry*, pp. 261–291, London, Sage.

Salazar, M.C. (1991) 'Young laborers in Bogotá: breaking authoritarian ramparts', in O. Fals-Borda and M. A. Rahman (eds), *Action and Knowledge, Breaking the Monopoly with Participatory Action Research*, pp. 54–64, New York, Apex Press; London, Intermediate Technology Publications.

Schrijvers, J. (1995) 'Participation and power: towards a transformative feminist research perspective', in N. Nelson and S. Wright (eds), *Power and Participatory Development: Theory and Practice*, London, IT Publications.

Woodhead M. (1999) 'Combating child labour: listen to what the children say', *Childhood*, 6(1): 27–49.

Wyness, M.G. (1996) 'Policy, protectionism and the competent child', *Childhood, A Global Journal of Child Research*, 3(4) 431–447.

Wyness, M.G. (2001) 'Children, childhood and political participation: case studies of young people's councils', *International Journal of Children's Rights*, 9: 193–212.

Young, L. and Barrett, H. (2001) 'Issues of access and identity: adapting research methods with Kampala street children', in *Childhood*, 8(3): 383–395.

15 Race and Ethnicity
MANI MANIAM, VIJAY PATEL, SATNAM SINGH AND CHRIS ROBINSON

Why do we need a specific chapter on issues of race and ethnicity in a book on research with children and young people? This chapter seeks to answer this question in a number of ways: by recognising that racism impacts upon research, from the choice of topics, to the experiences of researchers and that of children and young people from minority ethnic communities, and the ways in which research findings are disseminated. We begin with two important quotes, which acknowledge the historical context of our topic and the debates which have occurred within the social sciences.

> At the turn of the twenty first century...Socially structured racial inequality and disadvantage persist. Developments in a number of countries have highlighted the power of racial ideas in a number of countries, often with murderous consequences...But as we reach the eve of the next century hardly anybody needs to be reminded of the virulence of racism as a social phenomenon, or indeed the importance of understanding the origins and contemporary role of racial ideas and societies structured along racial lines. (Bulmer and Solomos, 1999: 3)

> There are not many areas within the social sciences that can equal research on 'race' and ethnicity in terms of the heated methodological debates and controversies that have been generated. Some of the more central points of conflict within the debate include: arguments surrounding the need for a more politicised research agenda, in particular the development of an anti-racist methodology, questions over racial identity and experience and who is best placed to do meaningful research on 'race' and ethnicity and finally which methods are most appropriate to the study of racism and racialised relations. (Connolly and Troyna, 1998: 1)

Within one chapter it is not possible to encompass fully the complexity of these debates but we will select and address key aspects which are relevant to research with children and young people and will indicate where interested readers can find more discussion.

There are four sections in this chapter. The first provides a brief historical perspective, which recognises the content and approach of some of the early studies of race and ethnicity. The second section explores research which reflects the multi-cultural view of race relations. Multi-culturalism failed to address issues of power and was replaced by the growth of an anti-racist perspective. This is explored in the third section. The fourth section discusses research methods and within the context of examples of recent research examines the current issues and tensions in research approaches with black and ethnic minority children and young people. But first we say something about our own backgrounds and discuss the meanings of certain terms which are widely used.

We came together to write this chapter for several reasons. We all work in Scotland in differing contexts with children and families. Mani, Vijay and Satnam also work as consultants on black issues and have published research in a number of areas relating to children and families (e.g. Singh et al., 2000; Robinson et al., 2001). Together with Chris we organised a major conference 'Putting Racism Back on the Agenda' in 1999 to mark the opening of the Scottish Parliament, and we have followed this up with a project to research the views of Scotland's minority ethnic communities on access to education in social work and social care. We write this chapter at the time of the second elections to the Scottish Parliament and reflect that despite the strong, vibrant and articulate minority ethnic community in Scotland not one member was elected to the first or second parliament.

Ideas about race have emerged in specific social and political environ-ments, and the development of racism needs to be situated in an historical perspective. A comprehensive account can be found in Bulmer and Solomos, 1999.

The growing influence of post-structuralism has led to a reassessment of the debates concerning racial identities and experience and within this there has been a growing critique of the term 'black'. Modood et al. (1997) argued that it is the product of the African Caribbean experience and does not address the real differences of South Asian people. Many commentators have argued that the term 'ethnicity' has become a euphemism for 'race' and weakens the struggle against racism. Modood et al. (1997: 13) defined ethnicity as 'a multi-faceted phenomenon based on physical appearance, subjective identification, cultural and religious affiliation, stereotyping and social exclusion'. There has been a debate within sociology about the meaning of these terms and readers who wish to explore the issues more fully are referred to Smith, 2002 and Modood, Berthoud and Nazroo (2002). The current discourse on 'institutional racism', following the publication of the Macpherson Report (1999), has again highlighted the importance of recognising the distinctive ways in which each of these competing terms is conceptualised and deployed in research and policy. The definition of racism which we will draw on, is: 'a belief that some races are superior to others, used to devise and justify actions that create inequality between racial groups' (Bhopal, 1998: 70). The Race Relations Act 1976, and its principal amendment in 2000, continue to make it unlawful to discriminate on 'racial grounds', defined as, 'colour, race, nationality or national and ethnic origins'. The Act refers to both direct and indirect racial discrimination. This has now been extended in the Amendment Bill to include 'institutional discrimination' defined in the Macpherson Report as:

The collective failure of an organisation to provide an appropriate and professional service to people because of their colour, culture and ethnic origin. It can be seen or detected in processes, attitudes and behaviour which amount to discrimination through unwitting prejudice, ignorance, thoughtlessness, racist stereo-typing which disadvantages minority ethnic people (Macpherson, 1999: 634).

Bourne (2001) has argued that while the Macpherson Report is important, it nevertheless overlooked state racism, which affects the lives of black and minority ethnic people, asylum-seekers, refugees, gypsies and travelling people. This chapter concentrates mainly on research with children and young people from black and minority ethnic families, as it is in research with this group that the key debates have taken place. We recognise the complexity and sensitivity of terminology and for the purposes of consistency within this chapter will refer to black and minority ethnic children and young people.

An historical perspective

The phenomenon of racism on a national scale has deep roots. The early studies of black and minority ethnic children and young people and their families to some extent mirrored what were then the current approaches towards race in Britain. The period of extensive African Caribbean migration to Britain, followed by people from South Asia in the 1950s and 1960s, has been characterised as assimilationist. The content and approach of some of the early work of mainly white researchers studied the education and health of black and minority ethnic children often with a view to understanding why they were not 'fitting in' to British society (e.g. Cheetham, 1972; Rex and Moore, 1967; Rex and Tomlinson, 1979). The serious consequences of the labelling of black children as 'educationally subnormal' was identified in Coard's work (1971) which showed that this processing resulted from low teacher expectations and racially biased systems of testing. Many of these studies reflected the belief that racism was caused by the 'strangeness' of the immigrants, and that with the acculturation and eventual assimilation of the immigrants – or their children – racism would disappear. The value of diversity was often unrecognised in favour of assimilation to the collective.

Early research in the USA in the 1960s tended to concentrate on children within the family context, a context which was seen as problematic. Thus, in *The Negro Family* (1965) Moynihan argued that the matriarchal structure of the black family inhibited the roles of boys and men in families: 'There is not one personality trait of the Negro the source of which cannot be traced to his living conditions. There are no exceptions to this rule. The final result is a wretched internal life' (quoted in Kardiner and Ovesey, 1972). The book was rapidly discredited by black writers but nevertheless held influence for some years (Dominelli, 1997). In Britain a paediatrician Lobo (1978) suggested in his book a similar stereotypical view of African-Caribbean families as less able than Asian or white ones: 'There is no tradition of the West Indian mother playing with her young child as a toddler' (Lobo, 1978: 36). Owusu-Bempah and Howitt (2000: 34) commented on this book that 'One shudders to think how historically it has affected the interactions of professionals with the black community, and their decisions concerning Afro-Caribbean children and their families'.

In America, the Civil Rights movement and the struggles for recognition of black people led to an assertion of black identities and the formation of professional groups. For example, the National Association of Black Psychologists was founded in America in 1968 and the *Journal of Black Psychology* was started in the same year. Mama (1995) described this period as a defensive one:

> Because of this onslaught of anti-black research, one finds black people who became professional psychologists during the 1970's did so with a somewhat defensive, problem solving orientation, rather than out of a proactive approach with the positive aspects of what it might mean to be black in America. (Mama, 1995: 55)

They did not challenge the premises of empiricist psychology which even more than other social sciences at this time concentrated on a narrow, dualistic explanation of human behaviour and which took the 'individual' the 'family' and 'society' as given rather than thinking about how they came to take the form which they did. We will see later in this chapter how subsequent psychologists developed discourses which were much more radical.

Multi-culturalism

The attacks on the assimilationist approach led to the development of a recognition of difference and multi-culturalism (Parekh, 2000). The principal drawback, however, was that multi-culturalism disregarded the crucial notion of power.

Emphasis on celebration of diversity led to the avoidance of acknowledging racism and societal responsibility for dealing with it. Multi-culturalist policies construct cultures as static, historic and in their' essence' mutually exclusive of other cultures, especially that of the 'host society'. Moreover, 'culture' in the mainstream discourse is often collapsed into religion, with religious holidays becoming the signification of cultural differentiation within 'multi-cultural' school curricula.

Gilroy (1982) argued that by bringing data about the daily lives of black communities in Britain into the public domain researchers were wittingly or unwittingly colluding with racism. By using qualitative methods they were portraying children, young people and families as 'different' and 'exotic' and thereby confirming racial stereotypes. Quantitative methods were also criticised for simply providing accounts for example of crime and educational performance and failing to develop understanding of complex social processes. Bourne (1980) called for an explicitly anti-racist agenda to prevent the reinforcing in research of 'otherness'. Debates raged throughout the decade and the Institute for Race Relations was severely criticised by black researchers who saw its work as dominated by white liberals. Research by white researchers was criticised for producing 'cultural strangers'. For example, Shaw (1988) undertook an ethnographic study of the Pakistani community in Oxford, and discussed in detail the issues of her role as a researcher, noting that, 'Rather than entering into the debate on whether or not "assimilation" is a good thing, I am concerned to portray the Pakistani Community from its own terms and to show the continuity of tradition' (Shaw, 1988: 7). Shaw gave a detailed account of the lives of the children and their families and spent time in Oxford and Pakistan to portray their lives.

In their book, *Black Youth in Crisis* (1982) Cashmore and Troyna recognised the issues for them as follows:

> the social gulf which lies between white academic researchers and young blacks is precarious. The reader may feel, even at this point that the book *Black Youth in Crisis* is plummeting to the bottom of an abyss. Young blacks did not write this work...this book is a collection of guesswork. Systematic, informed and well articulated guesswork, but guesswork nevertheless...Knowledge is a form of control, and really social scientists who challenge their world by seeking out new ways of understanding it are increasing the sophistication of control, albeit inadvertently. (1982: 13–14)

Cashmore and Troyna's work was also severely criticised by black researchers. They wrote at a time when black youth was being seen as a social problem. The race riots of the early 1980s led to increasing concern about the circumstances of young black and minority ethnic people in Britain. This was a period of intense debate in the media and a range of views were expressed, some being explicitly racist. For example, the Honeyford episode, when a Bradford City headmaster publicly denounced Muslim immigrant children as inferior and as having a 'purdah mentality'. His views were very much shared by the Right in British and French politics. The mobilisation of parents in Bradford against Honeyford resulted in his retirement, after a long struggle. But the debacle underlined a new, heightened sense of racism within the community of Bradford.

The growing debates within sociology about value freedom, influenced by the work of Becker (1967), were reflected in the arguments between researchers during this period. Becker's famous essay 'Whose side are we on?' recognised that in research, as in other areas of life, it is the powerful who have the capacity to define reality. Social scientists can either challenge or accept this view. Within the study of deviance Becker argued for the importance of adopting the view of subordinate groups and his work influenced studies by black researchers who argued for an approach which privileged the views of discriminated people. There was sustained criticism of white researchers who were seen as perpetuating racist assumptions in their work (Bruar, 1992). Becker, however, argued that 'Whatever side we are on we must use our techniques impartially enough that a belief to which we are especially sympathetic could be proved elsewhere' (Becker, 1967: 246). The validity of methods employed in educational research with children and young people have been debated seriously, and often between black and white researchers. For example, Hammersley and Gomm's (1993) critique of Mac an Ghaill's (1988) research into pupil and teacher perceptions centred on the suggestion that by adopting an openly anti-racist stance the researcher collected biased data which privileged the views of the students to the relative exclusion of the teachers.

Education has been a central theme in research with black and minority ethnic children and young people throughout the last 30 years. In the late 1970s, Fuller researched young black and Asian women in their last year at school. Her account records the girls' own thoughts and words about their situation, for example, 'I think people trust you more when you're a boy, they say you're more reliable, more trustworthy. Because my dad always says that, he says you can take a boy and show him a trade, but you can take a girl and the next minute their heads are filled up with boys, that she just doesn't want to know. So I'm going to show him, you see!' (Fuller, 1982: 94). In her study Fuller argued that the girls' exam success can be partly attributed to the support from their culture and she concludes that it is in some ways surprising that the double exclusion of race and sexual domination should give rise to a positive sense of self-worth.

A later study found that for most (Pakistani) Muslim girls little or nothing at school reflected the girls' life experiences at home: the implicit content of what they learned in history, literature and geography placed them very much at the margins of realities. The curriculum was firmly enclosed in an assumed uniformity of white British Protestant experience, which was postulated as the norm and rendered everything else 'different'.

Anti-racism

Within race relations during the 1980s there was a major challenge from anti-racism to the rather cosy view of society as multi-cultural. The alternative which was put forward focused on the structures of power and the institutions and social practices which produce racial oppression. There has been increasing recognition of the structures of racism and discrimination within education, however, the risk here is that they become reductive and lead to the conclusion that racist processes are the only or primary cause of all the unequal outcomes and exclusions which black and minority ethnic children and young people experience. Class and gender inequalities are equally important and are intertwined with racism and as a result are often underplayed.

Given this history it is not surprising that 'researching race' has become another arena in which the anti-racist struggle needs to take place. Identifying or developing an anti-racist epistemology needs to be based in the real life experience of black people and have relevance and meaning and not be simply a philosophical discourse that replicates the power imbalance we are struggling to eradicate. The exclusion of white researchers from research into black people as subjects, according to Rhodes (1994) assumes 'a congruence of interests between black researchers and subjects which disguises internal conflicts and suggests an artificial harmony. The only significant dimension of exploitation is assumed to be that between white investigator and black subject; other dimensions of social inequality may often be more significant to participants' (1994: 99). However, there is an increasing coming together of black researchers to form coherent research communities, for example the South Asian researchers and in Scotland the Scottish Association of Black Researchers (SABRE).

Within this complex set of debated terms and constantly evolving recognition and discussion of race we turn to explore current areas of research.

An area which has received relatively little attention, is the health and welfare of black and minority ethnic children. People's good health is directly related to the quality of their economic, social and political environment. For black and minority ethnic people racism and poverty have a critical impact on their health. The health and well-being of children is clearly a very important issue for parents. A survey, conducted in Edinburgh, found that black and minority ethnic children appeared to suffer from common cold, asthma, sleep disorders and bed-wetting to a much greater extent than the general child population in Scotland. There were causal factors that affected the children's health, the most significant being racial harassment. Most parents interviewed claimed that their children's health problems were related to fear, stress, anxiety and depression. The children were reluctant to go out and play in the open (Bibi, Egan and Lee, 1996).

Research has often ignored the socio-economic and environmental causes of ill health and concentrated instead on over-generalised and stereotyped socio-ethnic factors. Simplistic explanations based on cultural differences might in some case divert attention from real explanations, to be found in the inadequacy of service provision to the Asian community.

The role of social work with black children and their families has been the subject of limited research but much controversy. For some years now social work training has required social workers to be sensitive to issues of inequality and racism; however, research quoted by Owusu-Bempah and Howitt (2000) suggests that there is room for considerable improvement. The Report of the National Commission of Inquiry into the Prevention of Child Abuse (Mostyn, 1996), found that most of the research which has been undertaken in respect of child protection has failed to address race adequately. Some studies have addressed issues for black and minority ethnic community families. Thus, Farmer and Owen (1995) reported that black families found the process as stressful as white families, and that the difficulties 'were compounded by language problems, in addition to differences in cultural value base and a high number of investigations ended in uncertainty'.

Farmer and Owen discussed the particular implications of talking to children about stressful matters:

> In all 15 children were interviewed during the course of the research. Particular attention was paid to ensuring that those who talked to us did not feel pressured to do so and that they were sufficiently in control of the interviews to tell us if they did not want to answer any of our questions, or if they wanted to stop the interview. We practised with children how to refuse to answer our questions using the rehearsal technique developed by Marjorie Smith at the Institute of Child Health. (1995: 28)

More recent research, for example by Humphreys, Atkar and Baldwin (1999), has examined child protection practice by talking to Asian families and their social workers. Humphreys et al. concluded that there was little evidence that individual social workers discriminated against the Asian children and their families with whom they worked. 'However the effects of their work when interpreting services fell short, when children could not be accommodated in culturally sensitive placements, or when child protection procedures focussed on incidents of abuse with little attention to context, these were to provide an experience of oppression for Asian children and their families.' (1999: 291)

Within research in education fierce debates continued about the nature of valid research. For example, a study by Foster, Gomm and Hammersley (1996) concluded that there was no convincing evidence currently available for any sustained role on the part of schools in generating inequality in educational outcomes between social class, gender or ethnic group. The authors were criticised by Gillborn (1998) for a depoliticised image of scientific neutrality which adopted a particular definition of racism which resulted in accounts by the students being interpreted in a way which minimised racist aspects of their experience.

Research into the areas of education and young people from minority ethnic communities has employed various methods and quantitative data has been deployed to examine school exclusion and racism. In England, studies have shown that African-Caribbean children, particularly boys, are six times more likely than others to be excluded. Of 16 per cent of permanently excluded children from ethnic minority communities (DfEE, 1991), about 8 per cent of these were African-Caribbean, yet African-Caribbean pupils only made up about 2 per cent of the general school population (Searle, 1994). These studies highlight the value of quantitative research, which can demonstrate broad trends: this would be much more difficult in a qualitative study. However, their disadvantage is twofold: they could be used as 'evidence' of racist assumptions that black young men are inherently more disruptive, and they do not tell us the 'meanings' attached to their behaviour by either staff or students. One study of exclusion (Connolly and Troyna, 1998) looked at students' experience of exclusion and at the report cards completed by teachers. The careful reading of documentary evidence by the researchers found that African-Caribbean boys were excluded for less serious reasons than Asian or white boys and, furthermore, that some of the report cards contained openly racist statements by teachers about the boys. This illustrates the value of research which adopts two or more methods to examine the data.

Triangulation (Guba and Lincoln, 1989) in research methods has various meanings but in summary the term is often used to describe the validation of findings by comparing data collected by a variety of methods, or from a variety of sources, researchers or theoretical perspectives. This approach has increasingly been criticised as positivistic and mechanistic and Richardson (1994: 522) argued that in 'post modern mixed-genre texts we do not triangulate; we crystallise'. In other words this reflects the different value positions of researchers. One of the complexities of researching racial issues is establishing a working definition of racism which can be operationalised. The increasing popularity of ethnographic research approaches has been accompanied by debates about how racism can be defined and proved. Rhodes (1994) has argued for a reconsidering of ethnography and its function in research with black and minority ethnic people.

There have often been complaints in the media about a disproportionate level of crime among and anti-social behaviour of African-Caribbean young people. The stakes concerning this relationship were raised considerably following a widely published letter from Sir Paul Condon, Commissioner of the Metropolitan Police, to leaders of the black community expressing concerns about the rise in crimes of violence against people in the context of reductions in crimes reported to the police in London: 'It is a fact that very many of the perpetrators of muggings are very young black people, who have been excluded from school and/or are unemployed' *(The Guardian,* 24th October 1995). This letter provoked debate but also served to perpetuate the stigma attached to young black men in London. The actual research base of this view is uncertain. As discussed earlier, reliance upon statistics to reach specific conclusions about causes or effects is fraught with difficulty and has been a matter of concern in research with black and minority ethnic young people. We do have evidence to suggest that young people of African-Caribbean descent are over-represented about eightfold in the prison population of England and, despite the complexity of the patterns revealed, the available evidence suggests that they are also more likely to be stopped, arrested and charged than their white counterparts. Statistics are the end result of a series of decisions by victims, the police and the courts and as such are socially constructed. However, if we look at other statistics which have been gathered in respect of those who control crime we can see that, in 1999, 1.8 per cent of the police in England and Wales were from minority ethnic communities, as were only 0.3 per cent of judges and 0.2 per cent of senior barristers. However, we cannot rely solely on the gathering of statistics. Rather, we need an interpretive approach to understanding the complexity of influences of power and racism in society.

Research methods

So far in this chapter we have seen how both qualitative and quantitative methods have been deployed to examine different aspects of the lives of black young people. As can be seen from the preceding paragraph, quantitative data can tell us about the differential experiences of young people, for example within education and the criminal justice system. But, like all statistics, they have to be used with care. Much social research still fails to incorporate an adequate race dimension, mainly because social research (in the UK) is usually conducted within predominantly Euro-centric, white conceptual frameworks. Inherent within such approaches is the lack of insight or understanding of black experiences and perceptions. It is true to say that commissioned research, in general, expects researchers to inquire about the 'needs' of black communities rather than to examine aspects of human rights and social justice.

Despite pressure from black researchers (for example, Gilroy and Solomos) for appropriate methodological and theoretical frameworks for race research, those who influence, determine and, to some extent, control the research agendas have been slow to respond to the changes that are required. Researchers have either tended to ignore population differences or to generalise for all on the basis of the majority white population group. Funders continue to encourage separate and exclusive research projects for black and white communities. Black and white communities are rarely considered together as part of the same research. A recent example of missed opportunities in a major study can be seen in a study of school breakfast clubs (Shemilt et al., 2003) which involved a postal survey of 6,500 parents. Although the article reported socio-economic factors and ethnicity there was no specific discussion of the needs of parents or children from minority ethnic communities.

Within psychology in America from the 1980s onwards, black radical discourses were developed relating to conceptualising the process of identity formation (see Phinney, 1990 for a review). The experience in Britain has been less coherent and is discussed by Owusu-Bempah and Howitt (2000) who warn that the greatest care is needed when applying, cross-culturally, concepts originating in any culture, Western or otherwise.

Recent research examples have sought to understand and express the narratives of young people. There has been a growing recognition of the scope of ethnographic methods. For example, Cross (2002) in her research with children in Jamaica and Scotland noted that:

> Consideration [of ethics and methods] began with the awareness that constructs of children and constructs of colonised cultures have been used in Western discourse

to mutually define both as inferior, conflating them into a development paradigm...Feminist research has pointed out that the greater the power imbalance between researcher and researched, the greater the danger that the imbalance will affect the communication exchanged...The power imbalance a child feels, sitting in a classroom confronted with some grammatical structure that makes no apparent sense, is quite different when for instance, they perceive the researcher futilely using up an entire box of matches attempting to burn her damp trash, they are then in a position to offer to start the fire for the visiting foreigner, and, using the drippings from a melting polythene bag, manage to do so in one attempt. (2002: 8)

Atkin, Ahmad and Jones (2001) in their research with deaf Asian young people describe how they used interviews and focus groups with their participants. For young people who had minimal language skills in either BSL (British Sign Language) or spoken language the researchers used photographs, show cards and drawings and the participants drew or wrote on the drawings issues which were important to them, chose and rated the cards, and discussed the photographs in relation to ethnicity, deafness and gender. This enabled the researchers to introduce complex and abstract ideas about identity in terms that the young people could relate to. They concluded that 'the narratives of young people informed our discussions with other family members and enabled the researchers to recognise that the barriers faced by the young people lay in the inability of the wider society to recognise that difference and diversity is at the heart of the problems they face' (2001: 44).

Another example of a narrative approach with young people is that adopted by Wright, Weekes, McGlaughlin and Webb (1998) who looked at the experiences of young males of African-Caribbean origins in terms of their expression of their black male identity. The background to their study was the increasing numbers of young men excluded from school and the differences in educational achievement between African-Caribbean girls and boys. The underachievement of boys has stereotypically been attributed to pathological aspects of Caribbean culture and family life. The authors note that these explanations overlook the structural basis of racism and the individual ways in which black males and females respond to education. They challenge the notion that black masculinities in schools are restricted to confrontation and aggression and conclude that 'To suggest that black identities are constructed out of negativity because they have failed to achieve whiteness renders meaningless the attempts of young male excludees to challenge the differential treatment to which they are subjected generating damaging stereotypes of black male pupils as threatening, overtly stylistic and confrontational' (1998: 247).

This research, which looked in depth at the 'meanings' of the young men, has contributed to understanding their experiences of what happens to them in the school context. Nevertheless there is still relatively little research which tells us about the experiences of racism among young black and minority ethnic children, or the power differentials between children of different groups. Connolly's (2000) study of South Asian girls aged five and six years considers these issues and discusses also the ethical and gender issues involved in the study.

Conclusion

In this chapter we have considered the complexity of the issues in research with black and minority ethnic children and young people. We have not offered a blueprint of how to do research in this area, but have sought to raise the issues with which researchers have struggled. Some of the issues, for example debates about the relative merits of quantitative and qualitative methods, can be found in many areas of research and arise in different chapters within this text. However, as we have discussed, assuming that 'value free' methods will result in meaningful research neglects the power relations within society. When research is disseminated these power relations can lead to the research stereotyping and compounding racist assumptions. Effective research with black and minority ethnic children and young people has to remember the lessons of earlier research and take into account the constantly evolving and changing discourses, discourses which underpin the racialisation of any given group of people.

As Gilroy has noted: 'there can be no neat and tidy pluralistic separation of racial groups in this country. We must be aware of the use of ethnicity to wrap a spurious cloak of legitimacy around the speaker who evokes it. Culture, even the culture which defines the groups we know as racist is never fixed, finished or final' (1999: 246).

References

Atkin, K., Ahmad, W.I.U. and Jones, L. (2001) 'Young South Asian deaf people and their families: Negotiating relationships and identities', *Sociology of Health and Illness,* 24(1): 21-45.

Becker, H. (1967) 'Whose side are we on?' *Social Problems,* 14: 239-247.

Bhopal, K. (1997) *Gender, 'Racism' and Patriarchy – A Study of South Asian Women,* Aldershot, Ashgate.

Bhopal, R. (1998) 'Racism in the Twentieth Century', in M. Bulmer and J. Solomos (eds), *Racism Oxford Reader,* Oxford, Oxford University Press.

Bourne, J. (1980) 'Cheerleaders and ombudsman: the sociology of race relations in Britain', *Race and Class,* 21: 331-335.

Bourne, J. (2001) 'Notes on race', *Race and Class,* 43: 43-51.

Boxill, M. (ed.) (2000) *Racism, A Reader,* Oxford, Oxford University Press.

Braham, P., Rattansi, A. and Skellington, R. (1992) *Race and Racism,* London, Sage.

Bruar, H.S. (1992) 'Unasked questions, impossible answers, the ethical problems of researching race and education in Leicester', in M. Leicester and M. Taylor, (eds), *Ethics, Ethnicity and Education,* London, Kogan Page.

Bulmer, M. and Solomos, J. (eds) (1999) *Racism*, Oxford, Oxford University Press.

Cashmore, E. and Troyna, B. (1982) *Black Youth in Crisis*, London, George Allen and Unwin.

Cheetham, J. (1972) *Social Work with Immigrants*, London, Allen and Unwin.

Coard, B. (1971) *How the West Indian Child is made Educationally Subnormal in the British School System*, London, New Beacon Books, The Caribbean Education and Community Workers Association.

Connolly, P. (2000) 'Racism and young girls' peer group relations – the experience of South Asian girls, *Sociology*, 43: 46–57.

Connolly, P. and Troyna, B. (eds) (1998) *Researching Race in Education: Politics, Theory and Practice*, Buckingham, Open University Press.

Cross, B. (2002) '*Children's stories negotiated identities: Bakhtim and complexity in upper primary classrooms in Jamaica and Scotland*', Edinburgh University PhD.

DfEE (Department for Education and Employment) (1991) *Census Data 1991*, London. DfEE.

Dominelli, L. (1997) *Anti – Racist Social Work*, Basingstoke, Macmillan.

Farmer, E. and Owen, M. (1995) *Child Protection Practice: Private Risks and Public Remedies*, London, HMSO.

Foster, P., Gomm, R. and Hammersley, M. (1996) *An Assessment of Research on School Processes*, London, Falmer.

Fuller, M. (1982) *Dimensions of Gender in School*, University of Bristol PhD thesis.

Gillborn, D. (1998) 'Racism and the politics of qualitative research learning from controversy and critique', in P. Connolly and B. Troyna (eds), *Researching Race in Education: Politics, Theory and Practice*, Buckingham, Open University Press.

Gilroy, P. (1982) *The Empire Strikes Back*, London, Hutchinson.

Gilroy, P. (1999) 'The end of anti-racism', in M. Bulmer and J. Solomos, (eds), *Racism*, Oxford, Oxford University Press.

Guba, E.G. and Lincoln, Y. (1989) *Fourth Generation Evaluation*, Newbury Park, CA, Sage.

Hammersley, M. and Gomm, R. (1993) 'A reply to Gillborn and Drew on "race", class and school effects', *New Community*, 19(2): 348–353.

Humphreys, C., Atkar, S. and Baldwin, N. (1999) 'Discrimination in child protection work: recurring themes in work with Asian families', *Child and Family Social Work*, 20: 283–291.

Kardiner, A. and Ovesey, L. (1972) *The Mark of Oppression*, New York, Norton Books.

Lobo, E. (1978) *The Children of Immigrants to Britain: Their Health and Social Problems*, London, Allen and Unwin.

Mac an Ghaill, M. (1988) *Young, Gifted and Black*, London, Routledge.

Macpherson, Lord (1999) *Inquiry into the Death of Stephen Lawrence*, London, HMSO.

Mama, A. (1995) *Beyond the Masks: Race, Gender and Subjectivity*, London, Routledge.

Modood, T., Berthoud, R., Lakey, J., Nazroo, J., Smith, P., Virdee, S. and Beishon, S. (1997) *Ethnic Minorities in Britain: Diversity and Disadvantage*, London, Policy Studies Institute.

Modood, T., Berthoud, J. and Nazroo, J. (2002) ' "Race", racism and ethnicity: a response to Ken Smith', *Sociology*, 36(4): 57–66.

Mostyn, W. (1996) *Childhood Matters: Report of the National Commission of Inquiry into the Prevention of Child Abuse*, London, The Stationery Office.

Owusu-Bempah, K. and Howitt, D. (2000) *Psychology Beyond Western Perspectives*, Leicester, BPS Books.

Parekh, B. (2000) *Rethinking Multiculturalism*, London, Routledge.

Phinney, J.S. (1990) 'Ethnic identity in adolescents and adults, review of research', *Psychology Bulletin*, 108(3): 499–514.

Race Relations Act (1976) London, HMSO.

Rex, J. and Moore, R. (1967) *Race, Community and Conflict: A Study of Sparkbrook*, London, Institute of Race Relations/Oxford University Press.

Rex, J. and Tomlinson, S. (1979) *Colonial Immigrants in a British City: A Class Analysis*, London, Routledge.

Rhodes, P.J. (1994) 'Race and interviewer effect in qualitative research: a brief comment', *Sociology*, 28(2): 97–100.

Richardson, L. (1994) 'Writing a method of inquiry', in N. Denzin and Y. Lincoln (eds), *Handbook of Qualitative Research*, Thousand Oaks, CA, Sage.

Robinson, C., Maniam, M., Docherty, M. and Singh, S. (2001) *Putting Racsim Back on the Agenda: Social Work for a New Scotland*, Glasgow, Glasgow Caledonian Unversity.

Searle, C. (1994) 'The culture of exculsion', in J. Bourne, L. Bridges and C. Searle (eds), *Outcast England: How Schools Exclude Black Children*, London, Institute of Race Relations.

Shemilt, I., O'Brien, M., Thorburn, J., Harry, I., Balderson, P., Robinson, J. and Camma, M. (2003) 'School breakfast clubs, children and family support', *Children and Society*, 17: 37–52.

Singh, S. (2002) 'Assessing Asian families in Scotland: a discussion in *Shaping childcare practice in Scotland*, ed. M. Hill, BAAF publications. Originally published in *Adoption and Fostering Quarterly*, Spring 1997, and reprinted in *Signposts in Fostering*, (ed.) M. Hill, BAAF publications, 1999.

Singh S., Patel, V. and Falconer, P. (2000) 'Confusions and conceptions: social work perceptions regarding Black children in Scotland', in M. Hill and I. Dorota (eds), *Child Welfare Policy and Practice*, Basingstoke, Jessica Kingsley Publications.

Singh, S., Macfadyen, S. and Gillies, A. (2002) 'To attach and belong: family placement needs of Black children in Scotland', in D. Sachdev and A. van Meeuwen (eds), *Are we Listening yet?* Barkingside, Barnardo's.

Smith, K. (2002) 'Some critical observations on the use of the concept of ethnicity in Modood et al., *Ethnic minorities in Britain*', *Sociology*, 36(2): 97–101.

Taylor, J.H. (1973) 'Newcastle-upon-Tyne: Asian pupils do better than whites', *British Journal of Sociology*, 24(4): 167–181.

Wright, C., Weekes, D., McGlaughlin, A. and Webb, D. (1998) 'Masculine discourses enter education and the construction of Black male identities amongst African Carribbean youth', *British Journal of Sociology*, 49(2): 241–260.

SECTION 4 RELEVANCE, EVALUATION AND DISSEMINATION

16 Health and Social Care
HELEN ROBERTS

'... where something of interest to students does come up, the teachers and parents listen sympathetically to what the students have to say, then go on and do exactly what they want...It's no surprise to me that smart kids do not want to get involved. It is no fun. Why not spend the time doing sports, going to parties, shopping or at the movies?' (Henry, 19-year-old student from Germany in Woollcombe, 1998: 238–239)

'Well, quite honestly, I said I hope this research is worth it. I said to my Mum I've got this lady coming to see me this morning. She said, what about? I said I hope it's not a load of old rubbish. Because there's been so much research on such rubbishy things I feel money's been wasted. So she said, oh, it probably is....Well it's a bit indulgent isn't it, really, just talking about yourself all the time?' (Oakley, 1979: 309)

When I was asked to write this chapter, I recalled two pieces of work. One was Ann Oakley's *Becoming a Mother*, where her final chapter, an endnote on being researched, begins with the comment above, where a young mother ponders the usefulness of research. The second was a chapter called 'Putting the show on the road: the dissemination of research findings', which I wrote 10 years ago for a book which Colin Bell and I edited on politics, problems and practice in social research (Roberts, 1994). Since those two pieces were written, there has been a huge burgeoning of work both on 'being researched' and on dissemination and implementation. At one level – though a cynic might say that this is at the level of rhetoric – the 'subject', or endpoint user, or consumer of research has moved to, or at least closer to, centre stage. The links between research, policy and practice do not need to be so fiercely argued. Indeed, some believe that the pendulum has swung so far in the other direction that fundamental research in the social sciences is at risk. Certainly, there are pressures, some of which are described below, to develop and strengthen policy and implementation links. Despite all this, there remain practical, ethical and political problems not just in listening to children and young people, but going one step further and that ensuring their voices are heard, and that those in a position to do so respond.

The 'is it worth it?' 'what will happen to this research?' question is a reasonable response from those with whom we research to the demands made by researchers on their time. And since time is one of the resources over which children (at least in the UK) have some control, it is a legitimate concern. A good deal of research with children is heavily informed by understandings from feminist social science of a generation ago (Mayall, 2002). We are largely working with people much less powerful than ourselves; we are drawing on their resources. In this context, the relationship between research and researched presents a whole range of challenges.

This chapter addresses one end of the research process – the question of what happens to research studies when they have been completed. It looks at the extent to which this kind of research can make a difference to policy, practice and children's lives. The concluding section reflects on the ways in which health and social welfare research is evaluated in respect of dissemination and implementation. The examples on which I draw are largely from research that my colleagues and I have been working on in the Child Health Research and Policy Unit at City University, and before that, in Barnardo's, the childcare charity. The chapter describes some of the mechanisms for getting research into practice, as well as some of the obstacles to this happening. It describes the policy and practice contexts for 'involving' children, and it explores the extent to which it may or may not be appropriate for researchers to become engaged in the process of policy and practice development themselves.

Getting the messages out: levers and obstacles

Three of the drivers for research dissemination and implementation come from very different starting points. The first is the children's rights agenda, the second the agenda of the Research Assessment Exercise (RAE) within the UK university system, and the third the agenda of funding bodies.

The Convention on the Rights of the Child treaty spells out the basic human rights that children everywhere – without discrimination – have: the right to survival, the right to develop their fullest potential, the right to protection from harmful influences, abuse and exploitation; and the right to participate fully in family, cultural and social life (Ivan-Smith, 1998). The Children's Rights Information Network (http://www.crin.org last accessed 01/09/03) points out that since its adoption in 1989 after more than 60 years of advocacy, the United Nations Convention on the Rights of the Child has been ratified more quickly and by more governments (all except Somalia and the USA) than any other human rights instrument.

The research agenda with (as opposed to for, or on) children and young people is also a participation agenda. Governmental and non-governmental organisations are aware of the dangers of policies and practices which do not include the experiences and voices of those most closely affected. Articles 12, 13 and 17 are particularly relevant to this discussion. Article 12 outlines the right of freedom of expression for children capable of forming a view, and due weight being given to those views. Article 13 concerns the child's right to obtain and make known information and Article 17 promotes the accessibility to children of information from a range of sources, and the encouragement of mass media dissemination of information which is of social and cultural benefit to the child. Allied to this rights agenda has been a commitment from UK government initiatives – the Children's National Service Framework (NSF) in health; and in social care the work of the Children and Young People's Unit (CYPU) for instance, which aims to encourage children's participation. The Department of Health publication *Listening, Hearing and Responding* (Department of Health, 2002) presents an action plan for involving children and young people. The children's NSF meanwhile outlined publicly from the start a clear commitment to the participation of children and parents whose lives are affected by health service delivery. In this context, since the NSF includes the healthy child, this means all children and families. The consultation document from the Children and Young People's Unit meanwhile has a range of core principles relating to participation (http://www.cypu.gov.uk/corporate/about/further-coreprinciples.cfm last accessed 01/09/03) and a document, *Learning to Listen*, which was published in 2001 (http://www.cypu.gov.uk/corporate/downloads/LearningtoListen2.pdf, last accessed on 27/05/03). All of this means that there is a solid policy infrastructure to support consulting with children, and to encourage decisions which are informed by this consultation.

Despite all of this activity, there is a long way to go in the implementation of a children's rights agenda in the UK. As the Children's Rights Alliance for England makes clear in a recent report (CRAE, 2003) (http://www.crights.org.uk/pdfs/CaseforaCRCforEngland.pdf last accessed on 27/05/03), while children in Wales already have a Commissioner, and Scotland and Northern Ireland are in the process of establishing independent bodies to monitor, promote and protect children's human rights, no such arrangement is yet in place in England.

The second major driver, the Research Assessment Exercise (RAE) attempts to assess the quality of research in the UK. Funding is distributed to universities on the basis of this assessment. The last exercise, in 2001, included 'user' members on some panels. The core of the assessment was scientific excellence, largely assessed through publications. It is likely, however, that for the majority of panels, direct 'usefulness' or use by endpoint users was not a major factor in assessing research outputs. Indeed, many would have been alarmed had direct 'use' been given too great a weight. Without the scientific capital provided by basic research, scholarship would be in a poor way. And we frequently do not know at the time that it is produced which research is going to be genuinely useful (as opposed to influential or fashionable). In terms of work impacting on the agenda for children and young people, it is likely that the kinds of publications most likely to have a broad 'reach' – websites, articles in broadsheet newspapers or trade journals such as *Community Care* or *Pulse*, or magazines aimed at children and young people – would not carry very much weight in terms of scholarship. And what would be good dissemination in terms of getting heard, and having influence – similar or the same message frequently repeated, little and often, reminders and so on – might not carry much weight in terms of academic excellence. Even a glance at relatively recent history shows that the best-disseminated work is not necessarily the best work. Professional lobbyists, advocacy experts and salesmen and women can get research into the public domain. Whether it makes a difference to endpoint users, and preferably encourages an interest in the desired direction, is a different matter.

Thirdly, research funders, both the research councils and others, have made 'user' involvement a more important part of applications for funding and final reports in recent years. Research funding proposals will frequently go to user referees, and finished research reports will go to user organisations. These will usually be mid-point rather than endpoint users – children's charities and children's organisations for instance, rather than children and young people themselves. When I was head of R&D in a user organisation, my colleagues and I would brace ourselves just before the final date for a research council call for bids for an email inbox full of requests that we sign up as potential 'users' of whatever research had been applied for. Of course, things don't work that way, even when the quality of the research is good. As any sociologist of organisations can tell you, for research to get embedded into an organisation, you are more likely to have success when that organisation and the stakeholders within it are involved upstream, rather than banged over the head with a ready-completed application or a heavy book of research findings once the research is completed.

The Carnegie Young People's Initiative (http://www.carnegie-youth.org.uk/ last accessed on 27/05/03) promotes the involvement of young people aged 10–25 in decision making. Guidance for the Joseph Rowntree Foundation's programme on work with children and young people included advice on dissemination and the involvement of participants in the work, and the work included in the programme involved research on young people and urban regeneration, young people and the political process, and disabled young people's access to leisure. All of these included young people in the process. The ESRC programme on children 6–16 also addressed a whole range of research issues relating to children and a good deal of innovative methodological work. All of these programmes have involved active dissemination programmes alongside the research funding.

Some organisations, such as Consumers in NHS research (http://www.conres.co.uk last accessed on 27/05/03) have as strategic objectives the development of alliances to promote greater user involvement in research and empowering consumers to become more involved in NHS R&D. They also monitor and evaluate the effects of consumer involvement in NHS public health and social care R&D. They have a clear strategy for ensuring that endpoint users are involved in every point in research work, from the decision making on what constitutes a research question, through funding applications, the conduct of the research, research dissemination and research implementation. This organisation regularly has items in its newsletter about work involving children and young people.

Pressure groups

The part played by special interest groups in getting research on to wider agendas (or preventing it getting on to anyone's agenda) is widely discussed in relation to commercial and political interests. In an article on intimidation of researchers by special interest groups, the authors describe how the lead industry undermined the work of those working on the risks of low-level lead (Needleman et al., 1979, 1992 in Deyo et al., 1997). Deyo et al. also refer to pressure put on funding agencies by the National Rifle Association and its allies following work on the risks posed to families by guns in the home (Kassirer, 1995). These may be extreme examples affecting the health and well-being of children and young people in important areas involving big players. They are also in a different socio-cultural context – in this case the United States. But we should be under no illusions that pressure to hide or disseminate research is a uniquely non-British activity. An interviewee I spoke to in connection with a study commissioned by the Joseph Rowntree Foundation on getting research into practice (Barnardo's R&D, 2000) described the consequences of an effectiveness review of anti-depressants.

> ...after it was published in the *BMJ*, their shares dropped and the *Financial Times* carried it in a column. It is interesting that financial markets incorporated our research *immediately*. Doctors, *years later*. It was fascinating. [Company name] bought 500 copies of the *Bulletin*, as they were prescribing the drug that did better, so they loved it. For these guys, this stuff was really important. One of the other companies spent thousands of pounds in producing counter propaganda to rubbish our study. They produced something, put it in lovely glossy covers and sent it to every GP. That's how we knew that we were having some impact. Someone takes you seriously and it's quite frightening. We're not used to anyone paying attention to research.

Nor is the (ab)use of research by special interest groups confined to the commercial sector. New report from X organisation shows young people need more X (which our organisation happens to provide), or new report from Y organisation shows that the UK is the worst in Europe for [insert whatever the current campaigning issue is] will not always withstand methodological scrutiny.

Sometimes, on the other hand, ambivalence about sensitive issues can stand in the way of publication. Sometimes, adults can be ambivalent about the ability of children and young people to tell the truth. And of course the literal truth is always elusive, for adults and children alike. We all construct our own true stories of our lives, our experiences and our histories. A colleague (not in my own organisation) recently described some interviews he had carried out in a large UK city. He had done an interview with a young woman in which she described her experiences in detail. He then went to her file, from which he deduced that none of the things she described had happened. There are a number of plausible explanations for this. Not all young people (or adults) speak the truth the whole time. Not all accounts (or file records) are complete. It may well be that the young woman told an interviewer, who was undoubtedly kind and approachable, what she felt he wanted to hear. It may be that what she described was a metaphor for the literal truth. It may be that her account was accurate and the records were at fault. This incident exemplifies why good research – with a good sample size and a good sampling procedure, with triangulation of one set of data against another, and with proper informed consent for respondents, and a clear understanding from both researcher and researched of what is going on, and what will become of the research – is important.

Some examples: dissemination, communication and knowledge transfer

What follow are three examples of work done which involved children and young people, each of which raises issues for dissemination, communication and knowledge transfer. These projects were a consultation with children and young people about their health services in central London, research on sexual exploitation (sometimes called child prostitution) in south London, and public health research on a central London housing estate which included group interviews with children in a local primary school.

All of these were projects which had a link (potential or achieved) to policy and, in some cases, practice development.

Healthy Futures

In 2001, the then Camden and Islington Health Authority commissioned Barnardo's and City University to carry out a consultation to ask children and young people locally what they thought about health services. The project – Healthy Futures (Liabo et al., 2002) – ran from June 2001 to March 2002 and included direct consultation with around 140 children and young people aged 4–18 living in or using health services in Camden and Islington. Additional contacts with children and young people were made through the Healthy Futures' website (www.healthyfutures.org.uk last accessed 01.09.03). The consultation drew on children and young people's understanding of health services, and who provides what kind(s) of care; their positive experiences of health care; and issues which have been less positive.

The consultation aimed to be an enjoyable experience for the children and to ensure that children and young people fed into all stages of the project. Both the commissioners and the researchers had from the outset a commitment to ensuring that this was not one more tick-box piece of work – we've done the consultation with children, let's put it in the filing cabinet. But even with the best of intentions, the path between commissioning and implementation is uneven. In our case, between commissioning and completion, all the local organisations changed. The health authority which had commissioned the work disappeared to be replaced by a strategic health authority, the four local primary care groups were replaced by two primary care trusts, the local director of public health who had been pivotal to the work moved to a different kind of post. Meanwhile, the two local community health councils (CHCs) were also in the process of change. This work was not at the top of anyone's agenda, and was a considerable way down some.

In order to fulfil our obligations to the children and young people, whose views we had promised to deliver to decision makers, we put effort into dissemination nationally, locally and back to the children and young people themselves. We tried to ask ourselves who the groups were that we needed to influence, and how this might be done. This meant that dissemination was done locally with small groups of senior nurses in the trusts, the local community health councils, the commissioners (including parent – but no young people – representatives), and stakeholders involved in strategic decision making on the future of children's services.

We wrote back to the children and young people we had spoken to, or their organisations, and gave them a link to our website, which summarises the findings and asks for feedback on priorities. What seemed to move matters on in this case was when our press officer along with our link in the (now reorganised) organisation which had commissioned the research put out a release to local papers asking for feedback from young people on the priorities. Shortly after this had been agreed, a letter went out to trusts and other stakeholders from the strategic health authority, asking whether they were able to address any of the issues children and young people had raised. Meanwhile, after our talk to the CHCs, one of their officers had written to local trusts inviting feedback on some of these issues. Nationally, my colleagues Katherine Curtis and Kristin Liabo spoke at NHS Consumers in Research meetings, Public Health meetings, and Medical Sociology meetings. For all of us, these large scientific meetings are a way not just of disseminating, but of learning from others' experiences. In this particular case, local stakeholders became more interested in the work as they saw that it was attracting some attention beyond the local area.

The outcomes remain to be seen. We hope that as a minimum, one of the local trust estate managers might pick up on the access issues for disabled children in hospital, or a practice manager of an outpatient clinic might do something about the gap between books for small children and women's magazines in waiting rooms. Where changes are made, they will be signalled on the website. We think it is likely that if the young people with whom we worked can see they have made a difference, it will encourage them to participate more generally, and not just in relation to health services.

SexEx (Sexual Exploitation of Children and Young People in Lambeth, Southwark and Lewisham)

Some years ago, Barnardo's initiated a project for vulnerable young women. The Streets & Lanes Project in a northern English city identified children vulnerable to sexual exploitation and developed a model of the way in which children may be ensnared in prostitution. A girl may well consider the pimp who controls her to be her boyfriend and remain loyal to him despite the fact that he forces her to engage in sexual activity with 'punters' whom Barnardo's view as sexual abusers. Similarly, boys abused through prostitution rarely see themselves as victims of abusive sexual behaviour. As a result of learning from this practice base, services, research and development and campaigning have developed. As Barnardo's and other children's charities have pointed out, young people do not make their own decisions to 'sell sex'. They are coerced. The abuse of children and young people through prostitution is not new but the extent is largely unknown.

A London Health Action Zone (HAZ) commissioned Barnardo's to carry out work to consider the nature and extent of sexual exploitation in south London. The report produced (Liabo et al., 2000) was also made available by the HAZ on the Internet. Although no peer-reviewed journal articles derived from that particular piece of research, it was one of a range of reports which had some influence in policy development in this area (Department of Health and Home Office, 2001) as well as influencing local policy and practice development. This was achieved not through wide dissemination of the report, but through the use of a professional reference group, ranging from police officers and voluntary sector workers, to teachers, social workers and nurses, who worked with us to steer the project, bringing their own expertise, but drawing on the expertise of others, and in that sense involved from the start in the development of policy and practice recommendations.

Prevalence of working smoke alarms in local authority inner city housing

This heading sounds rather unpromising for a chapter on dissemination and implementation in relation to research with children. Read on. Injuries are the main cause of death in children in the UK, with a very steep social class gradient. Sixteen times more children in the poorest households than in the best-off households die in a house fire (Roberts, 1997). Providing and installing free smoke alarms to poor, urban households seems a straightforward intervention, and one likely to reduce deaths. However, not everything that looks sensible on paper works in real world conditions. A group of researchers from the London School of Hygiene and Tropical Medicine and the Institute of Child Health ran two trials to look at this. Our research group at City was involved in qualitative work in the second trial, talking to children and families about levers and barriers to smoke alarm use.

It turned out (Rowland et al., 2002) from the trials that smoke alarm distribution does not reduce fire-related injuries and may be a waste of resources. The editor's choice section of the *British Medical Journal* the week the article was printed suggests: 'Sometimes the problem is acting on the evidence gathering rather than acting on the results' (Editor's choice, 2002: 979).

Of all academic journals, the *British Medical Journal* (*BMJ*) is probably the most outstanding in terms of its commitment to, and influence on, dissemination and implementation, and the requirement to provide an evidence basis for claims. Boxed sections of the articles give a summary both of what is already known, and what the new study adds. We felt, on publication, that the editor's remarks, and a favourable editorial (Pless, 2002) indicated that our findings might have a decent 'reach' into policy and practice. Indeed, new housing guidelines were issued. However, a letter to the online version of BMJ about the article is instructive on a certain ambivalence of some to issues of process and implementation in scientific journals.

> When I was a student – admittedly 50 years ago – the *BMJ* was a prestigious publication whose articles I read with interest and some profit. What is then one to make of six pages devoted to the hardly surprising fact that feckless families do not bother to use smoke alarms. Not only that but the Editor gives the articles headline status on the front page! The Journal is not what it used to be. (http://bmj.com/cgi/eletters/325/7371/979#26666 last accessed on 27.05.03)

A response from the *BMJ* editor Richard Smith suggests the writer 'tries living for a few months on a very low income in one unheated room with several children in a rough and dangerous area of London. He might discover that "feckless" is a highly loaded word' (http://bmj.com/cgi/eletters/325/7371/979#26694 last accessed on 27.05.03).

All of this indicates that getting information out to those who might be able to use it is less straightforward than it may seem. It was clear to us in interviewing children resident on the estate that there were a number of practical issues to be addressed. Just as adults often see car alarms as a nuisance rather than a warning, a number of the children had a similar (and potentially life-threatening) view of smoke alarms:

> When the smoke alarm goes off, I have to turn up the television 'cos I can't hear it (8-year-old boy)

Unexpected issues were also identified. A bright child from an asylum-seeking family described what he would do if the alarm went off:

Are dissemination programmes evaluated? (n=51)

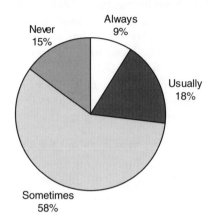

Figure 16.1

Boy: I take a 50p and then I just put the 50p in the phone box and then call the fire engine.
Interviewer: You don't need money to call the fire engine. You just dial 999. It's free.
Boy: But if you don't have money you can't call.
Interviewer: You can still call if you don't have any money.
Boy: 'Cos if you don't have money and you need to pay, that means you can't call the 999. You have to go by yourself to the fire station.

Talking to children may raise issues that do not arise with adults, and that call for different dissemination and implementation strategies.

Evaluating dissemination activities

Knowing whether one's research has made a difference is difficult. Despite the importance attached to dissemination, a Barnardo's study (Barnardo's R&D, 2000) found that only just over a quarter of respondents from a range of health and social care organisations said they 'always' or 'usually' evaluated their own dissemination programmes (Figure 16.1).

One centre suggested that evaluation should address three levels of dissemination objectives: immediate, intermediate and ultimate. The immediate objectives are concerned with the extent to which the materials are read. The intermediate stage is when there is evidence that the research is being referred to: in proposals about new services, for example. The ultimate objective is concerned with using the research to make an impact for children and families.

There is little evidence that research organisations (our own included) have developed sophisticated measures of success in meeting these objectives.

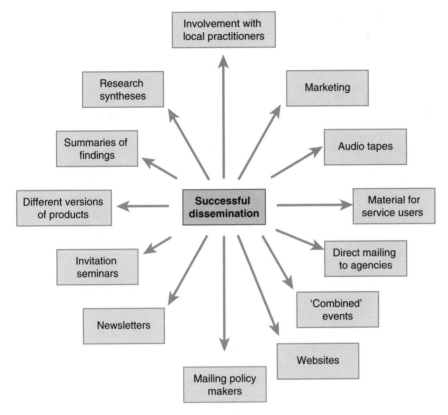

Figure 16.2

On the whole, most respondents in the Barnardo's study relied on making judgements about their success according to factors such as being asked back to do more work, and observational evidence that people were making use of the products of the research. For example,

'Not only did the [department] fund the research, but they also funded a very major dissemination programme after the research was completed... They bought a lot of copies, and gave a lot of copies away free. They put on a whole series of training seminars which they invited us to attend, they funded us to work with children and young people, they purchased a copy of this for every young person in care. So it was the fact that they actually purchased a major dissemination programme which is again evidence that they thought it would be useful to them. And the fact that subsequently we've been asked to do further work for the [department] is also evidence of the fact that they found this research useful, and influenced what happened.' (Barnardo's R&D, 2000)

Respondents highlighted a number of factors which contribute to successful dissemination (Figure 16.2).

What can researchers do to maximise policy/practice interest ?

Research lies somewhere within this plethora of influences on decision making. The Barnardo's study on getting research into practice (Barnardos R&D, 2000) found that respondents confirmed that research alone rarely influences decisions. Rather it tends to be one of a complicated mix of factors:

> 'I think for each decision reached there are factors to deal with: what is the hierarchy's powerful message at the moment; what are the factors within the social work team; what is the level of experience. I think research is one of a number of factors, probably not always one of the more powerful ones.'

> '...One piece of research wouldn't inform a decision. There is a whole range of activities which would involve being aware of what is out there in the field in terms of current research or government reports or aspects of the external environment. Actually talking to people, listening to what service users are telling us, a whole range of things that all fit together of which a piece of research might only be one part. So I actually don't see that very close link between research and decision making.'

The role of research underpins many policies and procedures and may lie behind the way people approach a decision, without the links being explicitly made. Government policies such as Quality Protects and the move towards family support were cited as research based without practitioners necessarily being aware of the research findings themselves:

> 'Maybe social services or the caring professions are not explicit about how much we do use research. Government policies are informed by the research...I mean they always talk about the move towards family support coming out of the Messages from Research...We have always wanted to move towards family support but when you haven't got the policy and the bucket of money and the hierarchy who believe in it, you are pretty stumped...So maybe we are not as explicit about the research but we are actually moving in a certain direction because we have been informed by research.'

Research organisations have become increasingly aware of the need to get research messages into policy and practice. There is some evidence that we have got better at this – certainly as far as policy makers are concerned. There is a push to use research evidence to inform (or justify) policy intentions. The relationship between policy and research is not always a happy one. There can be a mismatch between what policy makers want and what research can deliver. Policy makers tend to need messages that are timely, unequivocal and relevant to current and near-future issues. Research is often retrospective, and when it is prospective, the horizons explored may seem distant to policy makers. It is frequently 'messy', and nuanced, with findings that are contradictory and difficult to package in simple messages. Nevertheless, research organisations have made important moves to make research more useful to policy makers both in the way findings are communicated and in consulting research user organisations when planning programmes of research. Of course, there are risks in pursuing policy-relevant research, with implications not just for dissemination strategies but for the type of research carried out and methods used. The desire for a fast turn-around encourages studies which can report findings quickly but may act as a disincentive to invest in research which takes a longer-term view.

The relationship between research and practice is even more problematic. This has been recognised for some time and whilst there are some important initiatives to forge a more meaningful link between researchers and practitioners, there are still concerns that research does not inform practice to the extent that it should. If it is to do so, the messages from research need to be presented in accessible ways and be relevant to practitioners' current concerns. But that is only one half of the equation. Research-mindedness is not, on the whole, an essential criterion for a career in social care. There is no strong expectation placed upon practitioners to keep up to date with current developments in research. There is also a lack of critical appraisal training within social care professions so that research messages which find their way into practice are largely undifferentiated. It is perhaps not surprising, then, that recent SSI (Social Services Inspectorate) inspections have found it difficult to ascertain the basis on which many decisions are made.

Dissemination and implementation, like consent to research, are processes rather than events. This chapter describes some of the things we have tried, with more or less success, in user engagement, dissemination and implementation. These range from engaging users in the development of research questions through to advice from young users on the design and structure of websites. Web dissemination is a particular democratisation of the research process. And while not all children and young people, or others who may want to use research with them, will have access to the Internet, we can be pretty sure that more of them will access it than will access academic journals. The use of newspapers, direct feedback to respondents, feedback through local newsletters and local events (not much RAE kudos there) may also ensure that findings are put into the hands of those most directly affected.

Conclusions

Not all research is directed towards practitioners or policy makers, and researchers are not always the best people to communicate their results to endpoint users or other stakeholders. It may well be argued that this is not necessarily a job for researchers, any more than selling widgets is the job of engineering researchers, or ensuring that GPs prescribe particular drugs is the job of those carrying out R&D in the pharmaceutical industry. The Director of R&D in a big pharmaceutical firm is not the same person who goes round GP surgeries, or who writes up the findings for trade journals.

However, as researchers, we have a duty to deliver on promises made to respondents and to funders. If we claim that a piece of work is policy or practice relevant to get the funds, then the end report either needs to demonstrate how it was relevant, or (as will sometimes be the case in any scientific endeavour), put our hands up if early promise of policy or practice relevance comes to nothing.

The related question on whether 'relevance' or insertion into policy and practice should be one of the criteria by which health and social welfare research is assessed, already touched on in the section on the Research Assessment Exercise, is a problem. How would we measure success? Policy and practice change? Impact? The number of column inches of coverage?

Sometimes, it is more important to keep things *out* of policy and practice than to get them in. Particularly in terms of interventions in children's lives, the pressure to innovate, to change, to 'save' children, however well meaning, has not always had good results.

We need to be clear about what is being communicated and why. In an information-rich society, not every message can be taken in. This points to a need to focus. What are the things that will make the *biggest* difference to children and young people? Sometimes they will be able to guide us on this, but sometimes they will not. But it is not always self-evident where priorities might lie. A decade or so ago, school bullying, by and large, was seen as a relatively low-level form of abuse, even though its impact on some children could be very great. Even more recently, children under 16 involved in selling sex were given cautions by the police, while their 'customers' were not treated as the child abusers they are. Children in hospitals would rarely be asked for their own consent to treatment, or to research. While it is important for children to have good experiences in the here and now, the longer view is also crucial. We will sometimes not know the results of our good intentions for many years. This should tell us two things: one is to do the soundest and most rigorous research we possibly can; the other is to stop, look and listen before we try to bring about policy and practice change.

Acknowledgements

I am grateful to my former colleagues in the Barnardo's R&D team for permission to draw on work we did together (Barnardo's R&D, 2000). My colleagues in the Child Health Research and Policy Unit at City University, in particular Katherine Curtis and Kristin Liabo, are a rich source of constructive criticism, and I am grateful to them for reading the chapter, and for allowing me to draw on studies in which they were involved.

References

Barnardo's R&D (2000) *Making Connections: What Works in Getting Research into Practice*, Barkingside, Barnardo's.

CRAE (2003) *The Case for a Children's Rights Commissioner for England*, London. CRAE.

Department of Health and Home Office (2001) *National Plan for Safeguarding Children from Commercial Sexual Exploitation*, London, Department of Health.

Department of Health (2002) *Listening, Hearing and Responding: Core Principles for the Involvement of Children and Young People*, London, Department of Health.

Department of Transport, Local Government and the Regions (2002) *Housing and Housing Policy. Smoke Alarms in Local Authority Housing.* http://www.housing.dtlr.gov.uk/information/fire

Deyo, R., Psaty, B., Simon, G., Wagner, E. and Omenn, G. (1997) 'The messenger under attack – intimidation of researchers by special interest groups', *New England Journal of Medicine*, 336(16): 1176–1179.

Editor's choice (2002) 'When to act on evidence?' *British Medical Journal*, 2 November; 325(7371): 979.

Ivan-Smith, E. (1998) Appendix 3: 'The United Nations Convention on the Rights of the Child – history and background', in Victoria Johnson, Edda Ivan-Smith, Gill Gordon, Pat Pridmore and Patta Scott (eds), *Stepping Forward: Children and Young People's Participation in the Development Process*, pp. 310–312, London, Intermediate Technology Publications.

Kassirer, J.P. (1995) 'A partisan assault on science – the threat to the CDC', *New England Journal of Medicine*, 333: 793–794.

Liabo, K., Bolton, A., Copperman, J., Curtis, K., Downie, A., Palmer, T. and Roberts, H. (2000) *The Sexual Exploitation of Children and Young People in Lambeth, Southwark and Lewisham*, London, Barnardo's/LSL HAZ. http://www.lho.org.uk/pubs/haz/pdf/sex_exp_yp.pdf

Liabo, K., Curtis, K., Jenkins, N., Roberts, H., Jaguz, S. and McNeish, D. (2002) *Healthy Futures: a Consultation with Children and Young People in Camden and Islington about their Health Services*, London, Camden and Islington Health Authority.

Mayall, B. (2002) *Towards a Sociology for Childhood: Thinking from Children's Lives*, Buckingham, Open University Press.

Needleman, H.L. (1992) 'Salem comes to the National Institutes of Health: notes from inside the crucible of scientific integrity', *Pediatrics*, 90: 977–981.

Needleman, H.L., Gunnoe, C., Leviton, A. et al. (1979) 'Deficits in psychologic and classroom performance of children with elevated dentine lead levels', *New England Journal of Medicine*, 300: 689–695. [Erratum, *New England Journal of Medicine*, 1994; 331: 616.]

Oakley, A. (1979) *Becoming a Mother*, Oxford, Martin Robertson.

Pless, B. (2002) 'Smoke detectors and house fires', *British Medical Journal*, 2 November; 325(7371): 979–980.

Roberts, H. (1994) 'Putting the show on the road: the dissemination of research findings', in C. Bell and H. Roberts (eds), *Social Researching: Politics, Problems, Practice*, London, Routledge & Kegan Paul.

Roberts, I. (1997) 'Cause specific social class mortality differentials for child injury and poisoning in England and Wales', *Journal of Epidemiology and Community Health*, 51: 334–335.

Rowland, D.C., DiGiuseppi, I., Roberts, K., Curtis, H., Roberts, L., Ginnelly, M., Sculpher, M. and Wade, A. (2002) 'Prevalence of working smoke alarms in local authority inner city housing: randomised controlled trial', *British Medical Journal*, 2 November; 325(7371): 998–1001.

Woollcombe, D. (1998) 'Children's conferences and councils', in *Stepping Forward: Children and Young People's Participation in the Development Process*, ed. Victoria Johnson, Edda Ivan-Smith, Gill Gordon, Pat Pridmore and Patta Scott, London, Intermediate Technology Publications.

17 Education
ANNE EDWARDS

If any group of researchers should understand how knowledge is evaluated and used it ought to be educational researchers. For many of us, our life's work is centred on studying and making suggestions about how people can become proficient producers and users of socially relevant knowledge. Those of us who are educators as well as researchers plan our teaching sessions carefully to construct learning opportunities by clarifying key constructs, modelling associated skills, designing tasks and manipulating the environment so that learners can engage with what we intend to share with them. Their engagement is not a matter of passively acquiring the knowledge presented to them. Rather, when we teach we try to be aware of what learners are bringing to settings, what is relevant for them and how we can build on their everyday knowledge to enable them to act in and on their worlds in more informed ways.

However, there is not an exact parallel between the practices of teaching and learning and those of researching and using research. Despite a shared intention to empower the learner or practitioner as a user of knowledge, there are at least two differences. Firstly, researchers are usually producing new knowledge, or at least insights, and are therefore not inducting learners into established bodies of knowledge. Secondly, the users of research are often expert practitioners and have knowledge of what is going on in and around practice that researchers need if the research is to do justice to the complex and changing field that is education.

The pedagogic demands on educational researchers are therefore considerable if they are to plan for and manage interactions between research and practice. I am stressing the planning needed to enable these interactions, because I shall be arguing that relationships between users and producers of research-based knowledge should start even before a research project begins. I shall also be suggesting that research design should pay attention to how users' knowledge is managed into research studies, as well as to how research knowledge is shared with users. If these issues are tackled only at the end of the research process, the main method of knowledge sharing is likely to be restricted to the dissemination of research findings. The term 'dissemination' does not do justice to the complex relationships between educational research and the practices of research users that I intend to explore.

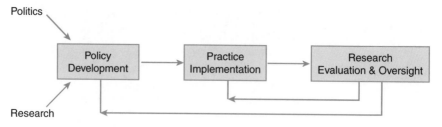

Figure 17.1 *Implementation of policy (OECD, 2002)*

We certainly don't seem to have got those relationships right yet. If we rely on simple linear links between research, policy and practice we find that they are not clear-cut or effective. This has led to a tendency to attack the quality of research. For example, David Hargreaves has proposed that the quality of educational research is to blame for poor connections between educational research and practice (Hargreaves, 2000). Mary Kennedy has been more measured and has suggested that we have all expected too much from educational research (Kennedy, 1997). Alan Schoenfeld's conclusion is that research and its applications should not be seen in binary opposition (Schoenfeld, 1999). I'm with Schoenfeld. The relationship between research, policy and practice is not simply a matter of what Zanussi used to call 'the appliance of science'. The separations of research and practice, knowledge and action, theory and practice are unnecessary and unhelpful.

But let us start with a linear view of how educational research impacts on practice (Figure 17.1). It comes from the 2002 review of educational research and development in England undertaken by the Organisation for Economic Co-operation and Development (OECD).

This model has its virtues. It suggests that research will inform policy development and what practices are implemented. But its seductive simplicity underplays the range of ways in which policy and practice relationships with research might operate. A major concern is that the model appears to be based on the belief that making the outcomes of research robust and easy to understand will lead to it being applied in practice. However, we already know that the appliance of science versions of the research, policy and practice linkages have had limited success. If policy and practice are to be informed by research we need to explore other connections. These will include ensuring that the questions addressed by research are regarded as relevant or valid in the fields in which the research is to be used and that we take seriously how research-based knowledge is fed into policy and practice communities.

I am therefore proposing that the relationship between research, policy and practice should be that of a two- or three-way knowledge exchange so that research, policy and practice are constantly mutually informing. In Figure 17.2 we can see that the dynamic between the elements is ongoing and shifting; different communities may take the lead and argue for their priorities at different times.

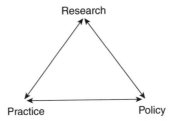

Figure 17.2 *The mutual informing of educational research, policy and practice*

I suggest that we should see the dynamic as something that goes on throughout the entire research process, from the first stages of problem identification through to the sharing of research outcomes, though the balance of the relationships will change as the research proceeds. It is a challenging model, which demands considerable mutual trust and a willingness to learn among members of all three communities.

What counts as knowledge?

The models of the relationship between research knowledge and its users shown in Figures 17.1 and 17.2 are based on two different views of scientific knowledge, how it is generated and put into use. Scientific knowledge is a complex concept, but researchers do need to reflect on how they view knowledge from the moment they start to articulate the aims of their research and formulate their research questions. Charles Taylor is helpful if one is thinking about research associated with enhancing learning. Talking about psychology, he makes a useful distinction between two models of science: 'one of brute data versus one that admits of interpretation' (Taylor, 1985: 124). He goes on to propose that interpretative research is of most use if we are trying to understand processes as complex as human learning and how it is supported. Arguably the OECD analysis belongs to Taylor's brute data category and the alternative offered in Figure 17.2 to his interpretative category. But, as always, categorisations can oversimplify.

Taylor was not suggesting that one approach to knowledge was more valuable than the other. Instead he was disappointed by the oppositional stance taken by proponents of each. He called their interaction a 'dialogue of the deaf' (p. 124). This lack of connection is unfortunate, as the polarisation of the versions of science is unhelpful, particularly if it inhibits how field-based knowledge both informs and is informed by research. Like Taylor, I will not be disregarding brute data evidence. Indeed the well-planned trials that brute data researchers undertake should be based on careful theorising, model building and sound exploratory trials all of which should be sensitive to features of the field of inquiry. Furthermore, the trials should only lead to claims for external validity within the populations sampled. Their work therefore has something to say to the broader practice communities in which they have gathered their evidence.

But I am arguing that their evidence is only part of the story. If we are to take the production and sharing of research-based knowledge seriously we need to shift our focus from worrying about why it is so difficult to apply brute data knowledge in classrooms. Instead we should think more about how knowledge is managed in and out of policy, practice and research communities.

The notion of a community, such as early education or post-compulsory education, which has shared social and discourse practices and both generates and uses knowledge is useful even if this is only because it challenges us to think about how knowledge moves between communities and is transformed in the process. It again reminds us that knowledge sharing is not simply a matter of making research findings accessible and available as commodities, so that they can be applied unchanged, rather like paint to a wall. Let us therefore explore a little more how knowledge is used and produced within discrete communities.

How knowledge is generated and used in communities

The analysis of how we produce and use knowledge is rooted in a socio-cultural approach to learning. In brief, that approach finds evidence of learning in learners' abilities to interpret aspects of their world in increasingly informed ways and to know how to, and be able to, respond to those interpretations. For example, after conversations with a mentor or a session on pupil behaviour with a tutor, a student teacher may change her interpretation of a pupil she has been experiencing as difficult to handle. She may move on from a view of the pupil as troublesome and instead see her as troubled. The student teacher would then respond differently to the pupil to the extent that the practices of the school allowed her to do so. In socio-cultural theory, this change in interpretation, which has allowed the student teacher to see the pupil in more complex ways, is called 'expanding the object' (Engeström et al., 1999). In these terms the pupil is the object who is seen in a new and more informed way thanks to the ideas (or intellectual tools) that the student teacher now applies to her.

This definition of learning captures how knowledge provides the lens through which we interpret events and how contexts and the social practices embedded in them enable or prevent forms of practice. Let us look in turn at knowledge as a set of intellectual tools, and then at how context can shape interpretations and actions.

Socio-cultural approaches to learning categorise knowledge either as everyday concepts or as more powerful scientific concepts which allow a sharing of meaning across contexts and which enable practitioners to deal with unfamiliar events. Everyday concepts are limited because their currency is heavily located within a specific community. For example, the everyday concepts in use in childcare routines in a day care centre, or in ways of giving feedback to pupils in classroom question and answer sessions are frequently specific in their nuanced detail to a particular nursery or school. They have grown out of the history of the organisation, expectations held of the children and what is valued as good practice among colleagues and they are often difficult to articulate and rarely questioned.

Scientific concepts, on the other hand, empower users by allowing conceptualisations that can transcend at least some contextual boundaries. For example, the idea that encouraging responsive eye contact between parents and their infants will enhance children's capacities for conversational turn taking is clearly articulated and has value across contexts. An advantage of scientific concepts is that they allow practitioners to work creatively with the resources available to them in order to respond to learners' needs. In a study of learning in nursery provision that I carried out with Angela Anning we found that the same scientific concept was incorporated into practices in very different ways in different pre-school settings. In one setting the concept of eye contact and turn taking led to a song book which built on the cultural strengths of the community served by the nursery and in another to a structured programme of remediation with parents of two-year-olds who had difficulty in interacting with their children (Anning and Edwards, 1999).

There is, of course, a difference between organisations which encourage enriched interpretations, the valuing of scientific concepts and the changes in practice that may result and those which prefer to work unquestioningly with the custom and practice of everyday concepts. Knowledge-generating organisations, whether they are schools, community nurseries or research teams, are places where prevailing social practices value evidence, examine it for relevance, explore, question and test it. The understandings that are generated during those processes then transform how events are interpreted and responses made. The field of practice is therefore susceptible to constant change if only because practitioners in knowledge-generating organisations are changing the field and their actions in and on it through changing their interpretations and responses to it. Researchers need to know what the field looks like to participants in it if their work is to be relevant and inform the questioning and development of practice. We see here the virtuous circle of knowledge use and production which can benefit both practice and research and which is reflected in Figure 17.2

It is, therefore, not enough to disseminate research-based information. Systems, such as schools, need to be able to evaluate research, examine its relevance and incorporate knowledge into their practices and their reflections on them and their contexts. But we shall return to that issue in more detail a little later.

Knowledge management in participatory research

Knowledge management is not yet well understood, but lies at the core of studies of the learning society (OECD, 2000) or learning organisations (Wenger, 1998). One lesson from these analyses is that simple forms of knowledge application do not work. Instead what appears to be happening is that knowledge that is neatly codified as public knowledge (i.e. scientific concepts) is transformed and recodified when it comes into contact with the tacit knowledge (i.e. everyday concepts) of practitioners (Lundvall, 2000). The result, Lundvall argues, is a hybrid but enriched form of local knowledge which is held within an organisation or networks of organisations and which works for them.

Figure 17.2 offers a way of thinking about how research might be informed by local transformations and in turn inform them. So let us tease out what the Figure 17.2 framework might mean for the design of a research project. In doing so I'll simply point towards implications for the formulation of the research aims and questions and the ongoing research process, as these phases of research are addressed elsewhere in this volume. My focus for the moment will be primarily on how knowledge is managed into policy and practice communities so that it has some effect on practices and the experiences of children and young people.

Educational research, as I have argued elsewhere (Edwards, 2001, 2002a), is an engaged social science. It is usually close to practice and charged with the moral imperative of improving the life chances of learners. It needs to be sensitive to the field and changes within it. Research questions, if they are to lead to research which addresses this particular imperative, need to be informed by the field as much as by the theoretical frameworks of researchers and their preferred approaches to research. Educational research is therefore likely to benefit from the participation of users in formulating research questions. In the UK this concept has recently been clearly acknowledged in the emphasis placed by a number of major research funders on user involvement throughout the research process.

Equally, research commissioned by policy communities and aimed at enhancing practices is likely to benefit from researcher involvement before the actual research questions are posed (Furlong and White, 2001; Edwards, T., 2003). Researcher engagement at this early stage would ensure that existing, close to the field, research knowledge could inform the aims and questions set by the policy communities.

Once the research questions have been agreed, attention turns to research design. If knowledge management is important researchers need to identify in their research designs the points in the research process when research findings can be shared with user-participants, for what purposes and how, and how field-based knowledge is fed into the research project. Let us take an example of a one-year evaluation of an intervention aimed at developing home–school–community links for children aged five to seven to improve their literacy. Planning for knowledge sharing might involve answering the following questions.

- Who would like to know what? (A stakeholder analysis)
- How could the stakeholder groups inform the development of the research? (Could they help to check the validity of the ongoing analysis? Can they be encouraged to post opinions on the project website? How can feedback from children be captured?)
- Would we expect or want any of the stakeholders to act on the knowledge we are sharing? (To what extent is the study designed to assist in the development of the practices it is examining? How is feedback to be gathered?)
- When will the study be able to offer findings that would be useful to practitioners other than those directly involved in the study? (How might the practitioners involved in the study be involved in the knowledge sharing?)

Once these questions have been answered the research plan needs to be designed accordingly and the relationships with stakeholders negotiated. This negotiation is crucial and beginning researchers should be careful to offer only what they can deliver and to ask very clearly for what they will want. In complex studies it may be advisable to draw up a knowledge management plan alongside the research plan and discuss it with the project steering group. Of course, new and developing information and communication technologies present an increasing range of possibilities for sustained user engagement that need careful planning. For example, feedback from practitioners might be gathered on-line during a one-day time limited conference or chat space. Time limitation is important as the postings would need to be filtered by a researcher before becoming public.

I am beginning to describe here a form of participatory research, which is not simply aiming at ensuring that the voices of participants are heard in the account of the intervention. Instead I am assuming that the research impacts on the field it is examining as part of the research process and at the same time the field impacts on the focus of the research and the analyses of evidence. The relationship between research and the field of practice may be seen as a constant spiralling of knowledge in and of the field to the benefit of the research study and children and young people. Some of the stakeholders in the intervention may become immediate users of research knowledge. For example, practitioners may be encouraged to reflect on and question their practices and the contexts which shape those practices through examining the evidence and ongoing analyses offered by researchers. Ideally in doing so they develop a capacity for continuous reflection and questioning.

Engaging practitioners with research

However, the primary purpose of this chapter is to examine what happens at the end of a study. For example, what claims for relevance can be made? How might the outcomes inform professional practice and improve the life chances of children or young people? Making claims for relevance, in one sense, returns us to questions about the nature of knowledge and the extent to which it is possible to claim that the findings from one study can be applied in another setting. Another approach to relevance is simply to consider its usefulness for users. Is it timely and will it present practitioners with helpful ideas which will provoke a questioning of their own practices and contexts?

The processes of participatory research indicated in the previous section certainly help to support claims for immediate relevance to practitioners. Findings are likely to be grounded in recent experiences so they should resonate with the preoccupations of potential users. However, as I have already indicated, the sites of practice are constantly changing. These changes come about through shifts in policy and as a result of the development in practices that occur in learning organisations. Consequently research which turns its outcomes into sets of mechanistic tips for practitioners will become out of date before the research report is published. Researchers therefore need to share with users the scientific concepts that shaped and are developed in their studies as well as sharing their findings. This sharing will ensure that the ideas as well as the tips feed into the hybrid discourses to be found when research-based knowledge meets tacit professional knowledge. The scientific concepts empower practitioners to then work with and question their own practices and contexts and to work with the findings of the study.

I am not proposing the simple application of knowledge by a more subtle route. Instead I am suggesting that the scientific concepts of research-based knowledge are most likely to influence practice when they become incorporated in what Benhabib (1992) has described as the processes of discursive or interactive rationality. Discursive rationality is a process of knowledge testing and knowledge building in interaction with others in conversations which are driven by a sense of social responsibility. It takes us away from a simplistic view of knowledge as a commodity which can simply be applied in a uniform way. But it does not accept a view that all knowledge is relative and no actions are likely to be more worthwhile than others (Edwards et al., 2002). Here our concern is the discursive knowledge building of education professionals. Educators who test and build knowledge drawing on evidence and ideas from research can be seen as responsible professionals capable of making informed decisions about what is needed in often ambiguous and shifting settings. Importantly, their decisions are informed by the intellectual tools (or good ideas) they have at their disposal. They will nonetheless transform those ideas to connect them with local resources and the specific events they face.

An example of the power of a good idea is found in the meta-analysis of formative assessment undertaken by Black and Wiliam (1998) and their subsequent follow-up work with teachers. The meta-analysis was not a piece of participatory research, but an analysis of existing analyses of the impact of formative assessment on pupils' learning. It was based on a hypothesis that formative assessment enables pupils as learners. The methodology belongs more to Taylor's brute data knowledge category than to the interpretative. After publishing the report of the study, the research team worked with teachers in order to answer the research question that their brute data meta-analysis had not managed to deal with.

The question was 'Is there evidence of how to improve formative assessment?'. This is more of an interpretative question, as teachers will work in different ways in different contexts. As a result of this work the researchers became aware that the teachers needed and wanted to build models of how pupils learn so that they could work responsively with them when giving formative feedback. The team concluded that the key good idea to be grasped in relation to feedback was ' to find ways to help pupils restructure their knowledge to build in new and more powerful ideas' (Black et al., 2002: 14). The original hypothesis about formative assessment came from a social constructivist perspective on learning and in the end the researchers shared not only their findings, but also their theoretical frameworks with their research users. Also in the process the research team learned a great deal about how formative assessment could be incorporated into practice.

The meta-analysis satisfied policy communities that it was sufficiently robust to be taken seriously and the work has also been extremely influential in schools. When communicating with both these communities, Black and Wiliam have not pulled any theoretical punches. They have very skilfully presented their findings in ways that immediately engaged hardpressed policy makers and practitioners with their relevance in talks and publications.

Here I am making a distinction between research outcomes and research outputs. The outcome that formative assessment improves pupil performance can be shared in research outputs as varied as detailed research reports, articles in refereed journals, books for student teachers and short paper and web-based research reviews aimed at practitioners and at policy communities. The educational research community is certainly becoming more adept at translating research outcomes into research outputs that aim to empower teachers and other professionals as decision makers in their workplaces. The British Educational Research Association (BERA), for example, is currently publishing a series of reviews, each based on extensive research studies, which is aimed at a practitioner readership. The series is being developed with the help of practitioners who act as critical readers prior to publication. The developing methodology will also be published by BERA.

Improving research–user interfaces

There are at least two ways forward. The first way focuses on the educational system and argues that spaces for conversations between researchers and users should be set up and practitioners should be encouraged to seek research-based solutions to problems they identify in practice and provision. This argument tries to incorporate both versions of knowledge by suggesting (a) that research from large scale studies can be applied and (b) that practitioners might benefit from engaging in participatory research either as researchers or research partners. The second way forward belongs to a socio-cultural approach to learning and knowledge production and calls for a rethinking of the relationship between research-based knowledge and those who use it by recognising that knowledge is transformed *de facto* when it moves from the research to the practice or policy communities.

The first approach is exemplified by the Commonwealth Department of Education, Training and Youth Affairs in Australia report of five studies of the impact of educational research (Commonwealth DETYA, 2001). It argues for policies which encourage a system that is able to connect researchers and education professionals.

> There is a subtle, complex and productive relationship between researcher and educator developed through a wide range of education processes, both formal and informal. This fragile relationship depends on policies and structures that provide incentives and strengthen the capacity for communication. Governments, universities and schools have roles in that regard. (Commonwealth DETYA, 2001 as cited in Edwards, 2002a: 162)

These subtle relationships are discussed in the report as a 'connecting web' the nodes of which are both formal and informal. The authors note that if teachers are to enter the web, they must want to seek a solution for a professional problem. Teachers must therefore be in a position to move beyond the everyday concepts and customs and practices of their workplaces and be able to question and problematise practices. This suggestion calls for a focus on schools as learning organisations which encourage such questioning and wide-ranging systemic changes (Edwards, 2002b). The aim is laudable and should be supported by the research community. Nonetheless it has to be a long term aim.

The second approach is perhaps more likely to succeed in the short term. The premise is that once research-based knowledge is managed into a practice community it is transformed by that community to meet its needs. Therefore there should be a sustained iterative relationship between producers and users of research which is mutually informing. The impact of new intellectual tools on a practice community may be that its discourse practices are enriched by the scientific concepts that are being introduced into it. But what is produced is a form of local hybridity, rather than a clear and replicable application of that knowledge in the practices of the professionals.

Furthermore, that hybridity in turn impacts on researchers' evaluations of the relevance of their work.

A nice example of this continuous shifting in meaning for both users and researchers comes from an analysis of product design which examines how designed objects are used once they leave the workshop and how they are developed in interaction with users (Hyysalo, 2002). The example is of a wristband that operates as an alarm that can be set off by patients in long term care settings to summon help. Two phenomena were observed during the development of the band. Firstly that users adapted its use to meet their local needs and therefore brought to the attention of the designers new ways in which it might be used. Secondly the expertise of the research team developed over the time they responded to its use in practice, with the result that the band was improved so that it was better able to adapt to the needs of the users.

Hyysalo's work resonates with that of Victor and Boynton, who have analysed the forms of knowledge in use in a range of business settings (Victor and Boynton, 1998) and have argued for increased interactivity at the product–user interface. While the language of business does always not fit well with educational discourses, the concept of 'co-configuration' which they employ to describe the ongoing shaping of product in interaction with those who use it is perhaps a useful one. Here I am drawing a parallel between the product of a design process and the intellectual tools used in and refined by a research study. They talk of co-configuration in the following way.

> the customer becomes, in a sense, a real partner with the producer. And that partnership can endure for as long as the product or service platform can continue to grow and adapt to the customers' needs. All three "partners" share the co-configuration work. (Victor and Boynton, 1998: 199)

To some extent, the BERA methodology for shaping the outputs of research so that they have immediate relevance for practitioners is a step in this direction. But the Hyysalo and Victor and Boynton arguments point towards the need to ensure an ongoing relationship between users and producers of research knowledge, which keeps research close to practice and to how practice changes when new research-based knowledge is fed into existing stocks of professional knowledge. The relationship outlined in Figure 17.2 therefore needs to extend beyond the production of research outcomes. It needs to give attention to the refining of those outcomes and the generation of further research questions. We have already seen one example of this process in this chapter in the work that Black and his colleagues carried out with teachers once their meta-analysis had been completed (Black et al., 2002).

Research projects, according to this argument, need to be designed to include a post-findings stage, which is not simply a matter of dissemination. Instead, the stage should focus on examining how the ideas are used in practice, how practice develops as a consequence and what further research questions are then raised. Networks of practitioners supported by researchers are one obvious way forward and are indeed being encouraged by several funders. However, they are usually presented as a way of disseminating research findings and not in terms of a dynamic that might generate further questions. The problem comes from thinking of dissemination as something that occurs only at the end of the research process in order to apply the knowledge produced. If networks are set up alongside a project they can both inform and be informed by the project as it develops.

The argument being made here is that participatory interpretative research should (or at least, could) be a continuous and cyclical process. There are at least two advantages of this way forward over the DETYA solution. Firstly co-configuration can be built into the design of individual educational research studies and does not rely on system-wide change. Secondly a focus on the development of specific intellectual tools is sustained over time. Co-configuration therefore should not be seen in instrumental terms. Instead the process can provide the context in which the practical rationality of practitioners and their moral commitment to enhancing the life experiences of children and young people can be woven into a research process.

But so far I've talked mainly about practitioners. The research process also has implications for the involvement of children and young people. It can provide a framework for engaging children and young people by encouraging researchers to examine with them how they use, for example, the services they are offered. In a current project we are involving children aged between 5 and 13 as research partners as, together with practitioners, we explore with them their experiences of a range of services aimed at social inclusion in their communities. This is not simply a matter of ensuring that children's voices are heard in the data. Rather they engage, as informed participants, in a research process and both inform the process and are informed by it as we all work towards enhancing their life experiences.

Like Chaiklin I am suggesting that the

> goal is to continue building our tools for understanding individuals engaged in meaningful practices in a way that acknowledges and builds the human values contained in those practices, and with a view for these ideas to be potentially incorporated as a part of the practice. (Chaiklin, 1993: 398)

As those processes are under way further questions will arise and shape research. But perhaps more importantly, ideas from research will feed into the discursive rationality of practitioners and inform their thoughtful decision making in professional contexts which are often complex and frequently ambiguous.

The future development of research on, for and with children and young people

Co-configuration

One of the attractions of co-configuration as a concept as part of a knowledge management process is that it enhances the capacities of the users of research to work critically and questioningly with the products of research. At the same time it ensures that the research process remains in touch with changes in the field. I have argued elsewhere (Edwards, 2001, 2002a) that educational research as an engaged social science needs to remain in close contact with the field. This contact is crucial if only to ensure that interpretative educational research remains sensitive to nuances and changes in the field and is able to question and inform the assumptions on which the work of the brute data scientists is built.

Participation of children and young people

Children and young people are as much the users of research and part of the field as are the professionals who work with them and their families. They too need to be involved in identifying the research questions and evaluating the relevance of research findings for enhancing their life experiences. Participatory research processes focusing on eliciting children's opinions and engaging them as researchers are already well advanced (Lewis and Lindsay, 1999). The next stage is to include them as partners in co-configuration work to ensure that they too contribute to questioning assumptions and to the shaping of opportunities that are being informed by educational research.

Interventionist research

Childhood is so fleeting an experience, and so important, that research on, for and with children and young people should endeavour to improve the conditions of their lives as rapidly as possible. I would certainly argue that interpretative research should, as part of the design process, responsibly examine possibilities for frequent feedback loops from the research to stakeholders in the sites of the research. These loops should not simply share findings, but also share the ideas that are being used and refined in the exploration of the field. In doing so researchers can explore with practitioners the contradictions and tensions that these ideas reveal in order to inform both practice and research (see Chaiklin, 1993 for a discussion of a dialectical approach to social science research and practice).

Interdisciplinarity

Throughout this chapter I've focused on educational research as a discrete community or set of communities. However, educational research is of interest to a wide range of policy communities, to practitioners offering joined up services and to other social scientists. Consequently we need to develop our capacity for interdisciplinary work to support interprofessional needs.

A corollary of my argument for hybridity in practice communities is a similar enrichment of the discourses of research communities. I've been arguing that educational research communities need to be aware of the languages and concerns of practice. However, I would stress that researchers need to enrich their scientific concepts (or good ideas) rather than move towards the everyday conceptualisations of situated practice. Instead, at a time of interagency collaboration for the benefit of children and their families, we need to strive for interdisciplinary collaboration with other social scientists and demand that our organisations enable our interactions. Researchers also benefit from enriching their stocks of knowledge.

References

Anning, A. and Edwards, A. (1999) *Promoting Learning from Birth to Five: Developing the Early Years' Practitioner*, Buckingham, Open University Press.

Benhabib, S. (1992) *Situating the Self: Gender, Community and Postmodernism in Contemporary Ethics*, London, Routledge.

Black, P. and Wiliam, D. (1998) 'Inside the black box', *Phi Delta Kappan*, 80(2): 139–148.

Black, P., Harrison, C., Lee, C., Marshall. B. and Wiliam, D. (2002) *Working Inside the Black Box: Assessment for Learning in the Classroom*, London, Department of Education and Professional Studies, King's College.

Bullock, H., Mountford, J. and Stanley, R. (2001) *Better Policy Making, Centre for Management and Policy Making*, London: Cabinet Office.

Chaiklin, S. (1993) 'Understanding the social science practice of Understanding Practice', in J. Lave and S. Chaiklin (eds), *Understanding Practice: Perspectives on Activity and Context*, Cambridge, Cambridge University Press.

Commonwealth Department of Education, Training and Youth Affairs (DETYA) (2001) *The Impact of Educational Research*, Canberra, Commonwealth Department of Education, Training and Youth Affairs.

Edwards, A. (2001) 'Researching pedagogy: a sociocultural agenda', *Pedagogy, Culture and Society*, 9(2): 161–186.

Edwards, A. (2002a) 'Responsible research: ways of being a researcher', *British Educational Research Journal*, 28(2): 157–168.

Edwards, A. (2002b) 'The role of research and scientifically-based knowledge in teacher education', in P-O. Erixon, G-M. Frånberg and D. Kallos (eds), *The Role of Graduate and Postgraduate Studies and Research in Teacher Education Reform*

Policies in the European Union, pp. 19–32, Umeå, The Faculty Board for Teacher Education.

Edwards, A., Gilroy, P. and Hartley, D. (2002) *Rethinking Teacher Education: Collaborative Responses to Uncertainty*, London, Falmer.

Edwards, T. (2003) *Educational Policy and Research across the UK: Report of a BERA Colloquium November 2002*, http://www.bera.ac.uk.

Engeström, Y., Miettinen, R. and Punamäki, R-L. (eds) (1999) *Perspectives on Activity Theory*, Cambridge, Cambridge University Press.

Furlong, J. and White, P. (2001) *Educational Research Capacity in Wales: a Review*, Cardiff, Cardiff University School of Social Sciences.

Hargreaves, D. (2000) '*How to implement a revolution in teacher education: some lessons from England*'. Paper presented at the 1st ENTEP Conference on Teacher Education Policies in the European Union and Quality of Lifelong Learning, Loule, Portugal.

Hyysalo, S. (2002) 'Transforming the object in product design', *Outlines: Critical Social Studies*, 4(1): 59–83.

Kennedy, M. (1997) 'The connection between research and practice', *Educational Researcher*, 26(7): 9–17.

Lewis, A. and Lindsay, G. (eds) (1999) *Research with Children: Perspectives and Practices*, Buckingham, Open University Press.

Lundvall, B-Å. (2000) 'The learning economy: some implications for the knowledge base of health and education systems', in OECD (ed.), *Knowledge Management in the Learning Society*, Paris, OECD.

Organisation for Economic Co-operation and Development (OECD) (ed.) (2000) *Knowledge Management in the Learning Society*, Paris, OECD.

Organisation for Economic Co-operation and Development (OECD) (2002) *Educational Research in England: Examiners' Report*, Paris, OECD.

Schoenfeld, A. (1999) 'Looking towards the 21st century: challenges of educational theory and practice', *Educational Researcher*, 28(7): 4–14.

Taylor, C. (1985) *Human Agency and Language*, Cambridge, Cambridge University Press.

Victor, B. and Boynton, A. (1998) *Invented Here*, Boston, MA, Harvard Business School Press.

Wagner, J. (1997) 'The unavoidable intervention of educational research: a framework for reconsidering researcher–practitioner cooperation', *Educational Researcher*, 26(7): 13–22.

Wenger, E. (1998) *Communities of Practice: Learning, Meaning and Identity*, Cambridge, Cambridge University Press.

18   Childhood Studies
JIM McKECHNIE AND SANDY HOBBS

Since the early 1990s there has been a flourishing of research on childhood. The period has also seen the emergence of a new paradigm for such research, under the name New Sociology of Childhood (for which see James and Prout, 1997, but also Hobbs, 2002). In the face of this activity it is reasonable to ask questions about its impact, in particular to consider the relationship between the research findings and the actual social policy decisions adopted. It may be too early to attempt a definitive assessment of programmes such as the ESRC's Children 5–16: Growing into the 21st Century. However, it is appropriate to explore some of the factors influencing how childhood research impacts on policy.

In discussing this relationship we shall address a number of issues. These include debates on the usefulness of the social sciences, the emergence of specific areas of childhood research, the dissemination of research findings and the wider impact of research. We shall focus on two areas of contemporary research – bullying and child employment – drawing specific examples from these fields. However, before looking at recent research in these areas we shall look back to an earlier research programme, that of Bowlby on maternal deprivation. This work is well known across a number of disciplines concerned with childhood. Turning the clock back in this way gives us the advantage of adopting an historical perspective which is difficult to achieve when dealing with more recent work. By examining the impact of Bowlby's research we hope to elucidate some of the complex relationships between research and policy.

An historical perspective

John Bowlby (1907–90) spent most of his professional life researching a phenomenon known as 'maternal deprivation'. Put simply, the concept implies that healthy psychological development depends on satisfactory bonding between the individual and a mother figure in the early years of life. Trained as a psychoanalyst, Bowlby worked at a child guidance clinic and made a comparison of the backgrounds of samples of delinquent and non-delinquent children. In 1951, he published a report sponsored by the World Health Organisation (WHO) on the psychological condition of children without families. An abridged version *Child Care and the Growth of Love* was published by Penguin Books (Bowlby, 1953).

Reactions were sometimes hostile. Fellow psychoanalysts were critical because, in contrast to their emphasis on fantasy life, Bowlby was studying the child's 'real life' (Ainsworth and Bowlby, 1991: 333). Bowlby concluded that psychoanalysis had an 'out of date' nineteenth-century underpinning (Dinnage, 1979: 325) and turned to ethology, the study of behaviour by zoologists, as a more satisfactory conceptual framework.

To understand why the WHO accepted Bowlby more readily than his fellow psychoanalysts, we should look to the historical circumstances. During the Second World War, many thousands of children were orphaned or separated from their families. Since he was arguing that separation from a mother could have serious emotional repercussions, Bowlby was well placed to be asked by WHO to collate the views of researchers and others dealing with children without families.

Child Care and the Growth of Love had a wide readership. Reaction may be treated under three different headings. First, there is the question of children in institutions. This includes children living relatively permanently in homes and children temporarily staying in hospital. Some see his influence here as profound and beneficial. Bowlby's ideas 'have so permeated social practice with children that we are scarcely aware of it' (Dinnage, 1979: 323). However, Bowlby himself emphasised not his own writing but a film by his colleague, James Robertson, *A two-year old Goes to Hospital*. It was Robertson who campaigned for more caring treatment of children separated from their families. Bowlby supported Robertson but 'refused to be drawn away from an emphasis on research and theory' (Ainsworth and Bowlby, 1991: 335). Would the policy changes which Dinnage attributed to Bowlby have come about without Robertson's efforts?

Then there is the question of mother–child bonding in the family, in particular, the issue of working mothers. One mother said:

> He said mothers should never leave their children and I used to feel guilty whenever I went to the cinema. (quoted in Dinnage, 1979: 324)

Whilst this may be an exaggerated response, there were many who certainly regarded Bowlby's findings as meaning that the mothers of young children should not go out to work. Note the particular historical context. During the Second World War many women had been encouraged to take jobs vacated by men in the armed forces. When the war was over, the authorities urged women to return to their homes and shut day nurseries which had been opened for working mothers in wartime. Later feminist writers saw Bowlby as a conservative figure encouraging women to stick to their traditional roles as homemakers. However, how significant was Bowlby's voice compared to the other forces operating at the time? One feminist writer points out that in *Child Care and the Growth of Love*, Bowlby does not say that mothers should never leave their children. Nevertheless, she sums up the content of a pamphlet Bowlby wrote in 1958, *Can I Leave My Baby?* as having the literal answer 'Yes' but 'the real answer implied is No' (Riley, 1983: 101). Bowlby's writings are subject to differing interpretations. We may also note that the existence of this pamphlet shows that Bowlby did not devote himself entirely to research and theory.

Thirdly, there is the academic reaction to Bowlby's work. Many research studies were undertaken to throw further light on maternal deprivation. Rutter (1981: 217) says that 'Bowlby's...original arguments...have been amply confirmed' in so far as they were that deprivation and disadvantage are important factors in psychological development. However, Rutter also concludes: 'It is now very clear that deprivation involves a most hetero-geneous group of adversities, which operate through several quite different psychological mechanisms' (1981: 213).

It is possible to view such an outcome as being both favourable and unfavourable to Bowlby. His research had a big impact but further investi-gations indicated his original formulation was too simple. Bowlby himself says that he continued to carry out research because he was aware of 'the multiplicity of the variables that influence the effect of separation' (Ainsworth and Bowlby, 1991: 335).

Clearly Bowlby's work had a significant impact on practitioners and influenced policy makers at a number of levels. However, this example also suggests that research, and its use, will be influenced by context. Research findings will be qualified over time and we should be cautious of thinking that research is uncovering unchangeable 'truths' that will not be contested. From this example it is also evident that the process by which research impacts on policy and practice may be a complex one.

Possibilities for influence

According to Platt (1991), common criticisms of social science include that it relies on jargon, its material is abstract, it is 'soft' science, is ideologically driven, it reaches no definitive conclusions and it is not applicable. Such complaints do need to be treated seriously for some of them have major implications for any decision making.

The criticism that social scientists fail to reach agreement on important issues overlooks the fact that knowledge may be advanced through debate. Even when agreement cannot be achieved, debate may lead to a clarifica-tion of differences. Recently international discussion of what constitutes 'labour' by children has resulted in greater clarity in the use of concepts, as reflected in the International Labour Organisation's (ILO) attempt to specify tolerable and intolerable forms of labour (ILO, 2002). Disagreements are therefore resolvable and the closer one gets to policy implementation the more such issues are likely to be resolved. Platt (1991) is surely correct to argue that disagreement amongst social scientists is greatly exaggerated.

The 'lack of applicability' criticism is also open to question. If certain research findings are not immediately translated into changed policies, that is not necessarily the fault of the researchers. Policy makers may only be willing to draw on research which supports their existing views. At the practitioner level the non-implementation of research may derive from the different agendas of researcher and practitioner. Practitioners may focus on making specific decisions within a tight time frame. Researchers may stress the complexity of relationships between variables. In addition, practitioners and researchers do not always mix in the same worlds. Recent attempts at improving the use of research in policy making have identified the need to encourage contact between practitioners and researchers (Nutley et al., 2002).

Models of the influence of research have been proposed by Bulmer (1982) and more recently by Weiss (1998). For Weiss the question is: how might decision makers use research evidence? She identifies four forms of use:

- *Instrumental use*: Research feeds directly into policy and practice.
- *Conceptual use*: Research evidence influences ideas, allowing new ways of thinking about issues to emerge.
- *Mobilising support*: Research evidence is used to persuade others regarding a course of action.
- *Wider influence* (also referred to as 'enlightenment' by Bulmer, 1982): Research exerts an influence on the wider community and may ultimately influence policy paradigms.

It might appear that it is the first type of influence which most researchers would aim for. However, it has been argued that in reality this type of utilisation of research is quite rare (Nutley et al., 2002). Underlying Weiss's typology is the belief that there is more than one use for research in the policy and practice arenas. It is also possible that any one piece of research may be used in a number of different ways by different bodies. We will draw upon these models later. For the moment we shall address a fundamental question: how are problems identified?

There are two questions to ask about the fact that 'childhood' has become an area of special interest in the last 15 years. Firstly, why the interest in 'childhood' and, secondly, why are some aspects of childhood studied and others are not? At the international level the United Nations Convention on the Rights of the Child (UNCRC) has had a major impact, placing children's rights on the research and policy agenda (Boyden, 1997). Many non-governmental organisations (NGOs) have been encouraged by UNCRC to undertake and disseminate research. The UNCRC also requires governments to submit regular monitoring reports on progress towards its targets. This requires governments to support basic research and also stimulates NGOs to focus their research on areas which challenge government assumptions.

This means that research is focused on social problems of childhood, but why are some areas researched? Hulley and Clarke (1991) pose a series of questions: What conditions come to be defined as social problems? How are they defined and explained, and by whom? What are the social consequences of these definitions? These questions undoubtedly apply to research on childhood. For example, child abuse only emerged as a 'problem' worthy of research in the late twentieth century (Corby, 2002). Abuse of children had existed before then but had not been deemed problematic. Hulley and Clarke reached the conclusion that social problems are socially constructed.

Such a conclusion leads us to acknowledge that society is not static. One need only think of the changing nature of family structures to realise why the impact of divorce on children's development is now a significant research area. Changes in normative patterns in society have an impact on research areas as well as on policy and practice. Research should therefore not be thought of as providing static 'truths' but as reflecting our best understanding at a particular time. Our earlier example of Bowlby's work makes it evident that our understanding of attachment and mother–child relations has developed over time.

Two contemporary cases

We shall now turn our attention to two contemporary examples of research in the childhood area: bullying and child employment. Whilst we do not have the benefit of historical perspective which the case of Bowlby gave us, these do provide contrasting illustrations of research–policy relationships.

Bullying

Research in Britain on bullying amongst children has expanded dramatically since the late 1980s, having previously been largely neglected as a topic. Initial research indicated the nature and extent of bullying in British schools. Partly in response to publicity in the mass media, Smith (2000) suggests, the Department for Education sought appropriate intervention strategies by funding the Sheffield Anti-bullying Project (Smith and Sharp, 1994). From this came a pack of materials for use in schools. In addition to central government, NGOs initiated research at different stages. NGOs such as the Gulbenkian Foundation and Kidscape supported the development of anti-bullying material for use in schools.

The mass media had another contribution to make. In 1992 an adolescent girl who had been bullied committed suicide. Media attention once again brought the topic of bullying to wider public attention. As a result, the government faced increased scrutiny through questions in Parliament.

Their response was to issue all schools in England and Wales with an action pack on tackling bullying. A similar process took place in Scotland, where anti-bullying packs developed by the Scottish Council for Research in Education were supplied to all schools.

In 1999 the Scottish Executive established the Anti-Bullying Network which grew out of an earlier organisation founded in 1992. It has been charged with taking a lead role in the dissemination of good practice in tackling bullying. In England and Wales the government has required all schools to have an anti-bullying policy.

Internationally the topic of bullying also gained a high research profile throughout the 1990s. The work of Olweus in Scandinavia in the early 1980s clearly acted as a catalyst, helping to spark work in Britain (Olweus, 1993). Furthermore, as Smith and Brain (2000) demonstrate, bullying has been taken up as a research and policy issue across Europe, North America, Japan and Australasia.

It is apparent that clear links now exist between research, policy and practice. In Britain, anti-bullying initiatives have been evaluated and have had a direct influence on the ways in which schools are required to address this behaviour. Research findings have required policy makers to ensure that appropriate responses are in place. Parents and school students have a heightened awareness of their responsibility. In Scotland in 2001 newspapers reported that 11 legal cases had been started by school students against education authorities for failing to protect them from bullying at school (Lawson, 2001). Against this backdrop it can be argued that bullying research has had a substantial impact on policy. Let us turn to the topic of child employment, where a rather different picture of the research–policy relationship emerges.

Child employment

Research into child employment in contemporary Britain was sporadic until the 1990s, when two reports (Lavalette et al., 1991; Pond and Searle, 1991) demonstrated its nature and extent. Many young people under the age of 16 were found to combine full-time education with part-time employment. Amongst policy makers and in society generally it had previously been assumed that few children were working, that if they did work it was in appropriate 'children's jobs'; and that the legislation which was in place protected and monitored what they did (Hobbs et al., 1992).

The research evidence which emerged clearly refuted all of these assumptions. It was apparent that the majority of children had experience of paid employment outside of the home, that they worked in a wide range of jobs and that legislation was ineffective (Hobbs and McKechnie, 1997; Lavalette, 1999; Mizen et al., 2001).

From a policy perspective, a major issue was the ineffectiveness of the existing legislation. A number of local authorities responded by commissioning research to assess the scale of the problem within their area of responsibility. The issue gained further prominence in 1994 when the European Union introduced a directive which aimed to harmonise legislation across member states on this issue. Britain negotiated a temporary opt- out of the Directive, denying that child employment was an issue and insisting that present legislation was adequate.

A number of non-governmental organisations became involved in this area, including the Low Pay Network and Save the Children Fund. The latter funded some research emphasising the need to listen to children's views about their employment (Pettitt, 1998; Leonard, 1999). As with bullying, the media focused on certain aspects of this research. They picked up on the atypical extreme examples relating to exploitative pay levels, inappropriate jobs and serious accidents at work. Questions were also raised in Parliament (Cornwell et al., 1999).

In 1997–98 Chris Pond MP introduced a Private Member's Bill on the Employment of Children, aiming to improve and update the existing legislation. Pond drew heavily on the research findings to justify the need for action. The government's reaction was to offer to set up a review of this area if the Bill was withdrawn. This indicated that policy makers recognised the need to react to the growing body of evidence. Some attempts had already been made to 'improve' the legislation by issuing guidelines to local authorities regarding the updating of local bylaws. However, there was little evidence that this had been effective.

The report of the government was delivered to ministers in the late 1990s. At the time of writing this chapter the report has not been made public and no major action has been taken. In effect child employment has slipped off the policy agenda. One might be surprised by this if it was not for the fact that this is a case of history repeating itself. At least twice in the twentieth century child employment attracted attention and action seemed about to be taken (Stack and McKechnie, 2002). For example, in 1973 Parliament went so far as to put new legislation on the statute book but failed to make provision for the legislation to be enacted (Cornwell et al., 1999).

In contrast to the limited impact on British policy makers, internationally child employment research has had a more significant effect. Throughout the 1990s research across a range of countries, in both the so-called developed and underdeveloped economies, has analysed and compared child employment in these different settings. Research has emphasised the need to listen to the views of child workers and to recognise that such employment has both positive and negative outcomes (Boyden et al., 1998; McKechnie and Hobbs, 2002).

This research has influenced organisations active in this field. The ILO had originally adopted the view that all such work should be banned. The most recent ILO publication now acknowledges the need to target 'intolerable' forms of work and that policy initiatives need to attend to the realities of children's lives and their views (ILO, 2002).

Contrasting effects of research

It is apparent that research in these two areas has had different impacts on policy and practice. In Britain, the contrast is quite stark. Bullying research has been very influential, but child employment research so far has not. How might we explain such variation?

One possible approach would be to compare the amount of research undertaken and the methodologies adopted in these areas. However, we believe that such an approach will at best only partially explain the differential impact. An alternative strategy is to consider what factors influence whether research is used in policy and practice. We might follow the lead of Weiss (1998) when she outlines the way that evaluation exercises may or may not be utilised by decision makers. It has been argued that Weiss's analysis can be applied more generally to explain when research evidence is likely to impact on policy (Nutley et al., 2002).

Following Weiss, we suggest that policy makers will incorporate research findings if:

- the implications are non-controversial and conflict can be avoided;
- changes can be accommodated without major disruption;
- there is relative stability in the environment, no changes to leadership or budget issues;
- change is more likely if there is a 'crisis' situation and action is needed.

Can we apply these ideas to explain the impact of bullying and child employment research? It could be argued that the proposed responses to bullying are non-controversial. In a society where the 'protection of children' is a dominant theme the reaction to bullying fits well. In contrast some child employment research raises complex questions about the nature of childhood, the relationship between work and education and societal expectations of children's role. Compared to bullying, consensus on child employment seems less likely.

Both bullying and child employment responses involve costs. The acceptability of such costs may play a role in deciding the extent to which action is taken. For example in 1973 enactment of the new child employment legislation was delayed explicitly because of cost considerations (Cornwell et al., 1999). However, other factors also influence ease of accommodation. In the case of bullying the responses to research have been channelled through the school system. Schools take responsibility for developing codes of practice and responding on a day to day basis. Child employment legislation is formulated in terms of local authority responsibilities, leaving the schools' role unclear. No pressure groups support bullying but employers' organisations may oppose restrictions on child employment.

Instability within the environment may also explain the different responses to these two areas of research. In 1997 a Conservative administration was replaced by a Labour one. The bullying research had already started to have an impact on policy and practice in the early 1990s and the momentum was maintained after the change. The Conservative government had only started to respond to child employment research when it lost office. The New Labour administration was soon forced to react to Pond's Bill. However, the lack of subsequent action may reflect changing political priorities.

The nature of a 'crisis' as described by Weiss is open to interpretation. We will extend the concept to include the idea of an issue's profile and scrutiny. Smith and Sharp (1994) note that the media coverage of bully-related suicide could be viewed as creating pressure on bodies who needed to be seen to be responding. In contrast the 'crisis' which attracts attention to child labour is at the international level rather than the domestic one. The 'problem' is not on our doorstep but on that of 'less-developed economies'.

This analysis has offered a brief overview of some of the reasons which explain the complex nature of the impact of research on policy and practice. Some alternative explanations are more difficult to pin down. For example, Smith (2000) refers to his initial foray into researching bullying as being 'at the right time'. Similarly he talks of bullying research having 'taken off' in an historical epoch when concerns about human rights are to the fore.

General issues

We shall now move on to consider some more general issues concerned with the dissemination and impact of research, illustrating them with further points about bullying and child employment.

Process of influence

We suggested earlier that, of the four forms of influence proposed by Weiss, the instrumental model, while appearing to be the most rational, was also the least likely to occur. In interpreting this rather pessimistic view of the role of research, it may be helpful to note the distinction between *evidence based* and *evidence determined* policy (Nutley et al., 2000). In the latter, policy decisions would conform to the instrumental rational model. The former implies that research evidence is only one element in determining policy. In such cases it is recognised that all decision making is a matter of political judgement, which in turn is subject to many influences.

The influence of research on decision makers may sometimes be pervasive. Bowlby's work had an impact on how issues such as working mothers and institution management were conceptualised. Boyden (1997) notes that Piaget's views have had a major influence on the idea of child development that different policy makers work with. Such views have permeated international debates about childhood and children. Problems arise, however, if policy makers are unaware of the dynamic nature of research. Theories are constantly being modified. Furthermore, the complexity of research findings may cause problems for policy makers.

An example of the latter can be found in the bullying research. Recent work by Sutton (2001) has questioned the traditional 'deficit' model in which the bully is assumed to lack social skills and understanding. How one develops practice would depend on whether one accepts or rejects the 'deficit' model. Sutton argues that 'empathy training', which some have regarded as an appropriate way of handling this 'deficit', may actually enhance bullies' understanding of their power. Clearly this would be counterproductive. Sutton's position implies that practitioners need to modify strategies which were based on previous research.

Multiple channels of dissemination

Researchers in academic institutions have typically been encouraged to publish their findings through academic channels such as conferences and journals. Too much emphasis on these outlets might mean that academics talk to each other and dissemination takes place within a closed circle, with policy makers and practitioners left on the outside. Nowadays the process of dissemination has become more sophisticated. Many academic conferences have their own press officers whose job it is to 'advertise' the research to relevant sections of the media. Many NGOs are well schooled in the need to address dissemination since they specialise in advocating policy changes and require support for their positions. The Joseph Rowntree Foundation has produced guidelines for researchers to follow when they come to disseminate their findings.

Two issues are worth noting regarding dissemination. First, the same research findings will need to be reported in different ways to different audiences. Let us draw upon our own research to provide an example. We recently completed a study of senior school students' employment (McKechnie et al., 2002). The dissemination to date has consisted of a formal project report to the research funders, an oral presentation to head teachers, a poster display in each school and an oral presentation for senior students in each school. These have preceded the preparation of a report suitable for an academic journal. Since the research was funded by an education authority, which hoped that our research would have an immediate impact, we gave priority to their needs over our intention to convey our findings to colleagues in the academic research community.

Secondly, there are multiple channels of communication. Researchers are not the sole disseminators of their work. There are numerous NGOs who act as advocates for children. Organisations such as Barnardo's, Save the Children Fund and UNICEF act at the interface between research and policy and practice. They rely upon research to identify key issues, propose solutions and mobilise support for their campaigns. Such organisations can be thought of as both consumers and producers of research. As consumers of research they often deal with the media to target wider audiences and influence public opinion.

The mass media have their own agenda. While we have noted that the media played a positive role in the case of bullying, this is not necessarily always the case. Research findings are typically complex, yet the media seek brief, unambiguous statements. The same studies may be reported in different ways in different newspapers. Such variations may depend on what journalists believe will interest their readers or reflect the underlying ideology of the paper.

In recent years the dissemination of research findings has been viewed as an important part of the overall process of conducting research. This may be seen, for example, in the establishment of the ESRC's Evidence Network. Implicit in the drive to disseminate is the assumption that some-one will attend to the information that is being provided. In the policy arena attention will be driven by the decision makers' agenda and values. In the practice arena, the issue is whether practitioners can access the mater-ial that they might find useful. Dissemination of research is therefore not only about 'sending material out', it is also about ensuring that relevant groups can gain access to material when they need it.

Funding research

The sources of funding for research on childhood are many and varied. In our examples of bullying and child employment research funding and sup-port came from central and local government and numerous NGOs. It is common to find funders of research programmes not only identifying the research questions they wish to see addressed but also influencing the methodology adopted. One significant feature of the ESRC Children 5–16 project is that it was driven by a distinctive style of research adopting the 'new sociology of childhood' perspective. Whether this sort of biasing in research methodology by funders is a good thing is open to debate.

Recently some academics have raised concerns over changes in the fund-ing of research. Walters (2003) draws attention to the increasing commer-cialisation of research in criminology. For Walters the pressures on academics not only to carry out research but also to generate research income has a number of implications.

One consequence is that carrying out research for a specific funder will involve contractual relationships. Such contracts may also impact on the dis-semination process. As Walters notes, it is not uncommon to find some fun-ders specifying how and in what form research findings can be released. Issues clearly arise when the research findings do not sit comfortably with the fun-ders' aims. In such cases legal pressures may be brought to bear to ensure that research findings are not released. In effect the dissemination process becomes selective. Many of the themes Walters identifies regarding the funding of criminological research resonate within wider academic circles.

The influence of childhood research

In this concluding section we shall follow up a suggestion made by both Bulmer (1982) and Weiss (1998), namely that research has a wider influence, beyond the obvious links between specific findings and specific policy or practice. They argue that research has another impact on policy makers in that it influences the way in which they conceptualise issues. We would argue that childhood research generally has had a clear impact of this sort.

Children as social actors

It could be argued that one of the most significant effects of the recent research on childhood has been the emphasis on children as social actors. In Britain writers from the 'new sociology of childhood' perspective have claimed that traditional research has tended to view children as passive and emphasised their potential as adults rather than their experience as children. This neglects the active role children play in constructing their childhood. Based on this argument, an increasing weight has been placed on 'listening to children's voices' in the belief that in this way both researchers and policy makers will gain a fuller understanding of childhood. This emphasis is important in that it charges researchers and policy makers to address the opinions and views of this marginalised group. Not only is this in the spirit of the UNCRC but we also gain insights into otherwise neglected aspects of childhood.

An example from the field of child labour demonstrates the potential value of 'children's voices'. Strategies which aim to ban child labour may involve pressurising employers to remove children from their labour force. In one case a TV programme highlighted the presence of child workers in a garment factory in Morocco. As a result these girls lost their jobs. Research aimed at discovering the experiences of these child employees demonstrated the negative consequences. Losing their jobs had resulted in greater problems for the children. They had to find other forms of work, most of which had poorer pay and worse conditions. Their new jobs were also less likely to lead to the attainment of skills that would be of value in their adult lives (Zalami et al., 1998).

This example demonstrates the potency of 'children's voices' by showing a consequence of not listening to them. In Britain there are now a number of NGOs that emphasise the input of children to their policy processes.

Some bodies such as Article 12 are organised by and for young people and campaign on issues which they perceive as important. Both the Welsh Assembly and the Scottish Parliament have taken steps to create Commissioners for Children and Young People, who will ensure a place for the voices of youth in decision making.

Research is only one amongst a number of factors leading to this change of emphasis. We should also note that the idea of 'children's voices' is not unproblematic. Roberts (2000) points to an important distinction between listening to the voices of children and providing for genuine participation in decision making. Other problems include the question of how to prioritise children's views amongst all the other views on policy and how we determine whether the children's voices we hear are representative (Lavalette and Cunningham, 2002; McKechnie, 2002).

Research methodology

The emphasis placed on children's interpretation of their experience means that childhood studies has stressed the usefulness of qualitative research approaches. The debates about qualitative and quantitative approaches to research have been long running (McKechnie, 2002). Childhood research has facilitated an acceptance of the qualitative approach amongst decision makers. However, a potential problem emerges if this approach is perceived as always the most appropriate one for all childhood research.

Nutley and her colleagues (2002) argue that there is a need to recognise that policy and practice questions may be addressed in a number of different ways. According to them the emphasis should be upon methodological pluralism rather than debates between different research paradigms. Childhood research needs to remain open to the fullest range of techniques available to researchers if it is to be able to address the range of future policy questions.

Social constructionism

The re-emergence of childhood research has been strongly linked to the position of social construction. According to this view there is a need to accept that childhood is a socially constructed concept. As Lavalette and Cunningham (2002) point out, social constructionism is appealing in that it draws attention to the dynamic of human relations. In doing so it undermines a number of commonsense notions about key relationships in society, for example, 'women have always stayed at home to look after the children'. By arguing that these social relationships are constructed by society and showing alternatives in different settings, we can question the 'necessity' of such relationships.

The danger which arises from this approach is its recourse to cultural relativism, where we cannot make statements of universal application. This has implications for the research process and its links to policy and practice. The logic of the social constructionist position is that any research and its conclusions are only valid within the context of that original study. While it is important to acknowledge the need to attend to 'local solutions for local problems', do we really need to address every problem as 'new', defined by its specific context? Such a position would limit any attempt to generalise research findings and create major problems for policy makers. The reality is that while constructionism warns us against taking for granted the generalisability of findings, we must at some level still make general statements. There is a need to identify areas of commonality across different contexts to justify any general statement, and there also needs to be an acceptance that this is possible (Weiss, 1998).

In concluding this chapter it can be said that the new wave of childhood research has had an impact at both the specific and the general level. The emergence of a strong research base on childhood-related issues, against the backdrop of the UNCRC, has resulted in decision makers and practitioners recognising the value of drawing upon this material. In this chapter we have considered different ways in which research and policy may be linked. We would also hope that such linkages are not taken for granted. Relationships between researchers and policy makers are not straightforward. For example, we should be aware that research and its dissemination do not take place in a vacuum. Understanding what happens after the research is finished requires us to attend to the process of dissemination and the numerous forces which may ultimately influence the interpretation and impact of any research project.

References

Ainsworth, M.D.S. and Bowlby, J. (1991) 'An ethological approach to personality development', *American Psychologist*, 46: 333–341.

Bowlby, J. (1953) *Child Care and the Growth of Love*, Harmondsworth, Penguin Books.

Boyden, J. (1997) 'Childhood and the policy makers: a comparative perspective on the globalization of childhood', in A. James and A. Prout (eds), *Constructing and Reconstructing Childhood: Contemporary Issues in the Sociological Study of Childhood*, 2nd edn, London, Falmer Press.

Boyden, J., Ling, B. and Myers, W. (1998) *What Works for Working Children*, Smedjebacken, UNICEF and Save the Children.

Bulmer, M. (1982) *The Uses of Social Research: Social Investigation in Public Policy-making*, London, Allen and Unwin.

Corby, B. (2002) 'Child abuse and child protection', in B. Goldson, M. Lavalette and J. McKechnie (eds), *Children, Welfare and the State*, London, Sage.

Cornwell, D., Graham, K. and Hobbs, S. (1999) 'Honoured in the breach: child employment law in Britain', in M. Lavalette (ed.), *A Thing of the Past?: Child Labour in Britain in the Nineteenth and Twentieth Centuries*, Liverpool, Liverpool University Press.

Dinnage, R. (1979) 'John Bowlby', *New Society*, 10 May: 323–325.

Hobbs, S. (2002) 'New sociology and old psychology', in B. Goldson, M. Lavalette and J. McKechnie (eds), *Children, Welfare and the State*, London, Sage.

Hobbs, S. and McKechnie, J. (1997) *Child Employment in Britain: A Social and Psychological Analysis*, Edinburgh, The Stationery Office.

Hobbs, S., Lavalette, M. and McKechnie, J. (1992) 'The emerging problem of child labour', *Critical Social Policy*, 12: 93–105.

Hulley, T. and Clarke, J. (1991) 'Social problems: social construction and social causation', in M. Loney et al. (eds), *The State or the Market: Politics and Welfare in Contemporary Britain*, 2nd edn, London, Sage.

International Labour Organisation (2002) *A future without Child Labour*, Geneva, International Labour Organisation.

James, A. and Prout, A. (eds) (1997) *Constructing and Reconstructing Childhood: Contemporary Issues in the Sociological Study of Childhood*, 2nd edn, London, Falmer Press.

Lavalette, M. (ed.) (1999) *A Thing of the Past? Child Labour in Britain in the Nineteenth and Twentieth Centuries*, Liverpool, Liverpool University Press.

Lavalette, M. and Cunningham, S. (2002) 'The sociology of childhood', in B. Goldson, M. Lavalette and J. McKechnie (eds), *Children, Welfare and the State*, London, Sage.

Lavalette, M., McKechnie, J. and Hobbs, S. (1991) *The Forgotten Workforce: Scottish Children at Work*, Glasgow, Scottish Low Pay Unit.

Lawson, T. (2001) 'Bullying court claims soar', *The Scotsman*, 25 October: 4.

Leonard, M. (1999) *Play Fair with Working Children: A Report on Working Children in Belfast*, Belfast, Save the Children.

McKechnie, J. (2002) 'Children's voices and researching childhood', in B. Goldson, M. Lavalette and J. McKechnie (eds), *Children, Welfare and the State*, London, Sage.

McKechnie, J. and Hobbs, S. (2002) 'Work by the young: the economic activity of school-aged children', in M. Tienda and W.J. Wilson (eds), *Youth in Cities: A cross-national Perspective*, New York, Cambridge University Press.

McKechnie, J., Hill, S. and Hobbs, S. (2002) *Work and School: Part-time Employment amongst Senior School Students*, Paisley, University of Paisley.

Mizen, P., Pole, C. and Bolton, A. (eds) (2001) *Hidden Hands: International Perspectives on Children's Work and Labour*, London, Routledge Falmer.

Nutley, S., Davies, H. and Tilley, N. (2000) 'Getting research into practice', *Public Money and Management*, October–December: 3–6.

Nutley, S., Davies, H. and Walter, I. (2002) *Evidence-based Policy and Practice: Cross sector Lessons from the UK*. ESRC UK Centre for Evidence Based Policy and Practice, Queen Mary, University of London http://www.evidencenetwork.org/ Document/wp9.pdf (accessed 31 January, 2003).

Olweus, D. (1993) *Bullying at School: What We Know and What We Can Do*, Oxford, Blackwell.

Pettitt, B. (ed.) (1998) *Children and Work in the UK*, London, Child Poverty Action Group.

Platt, J. (1991) 'The contribution of social science', in M. Loney et al. (eds), *The state or the Market: Politics and Welfare in Contemporary Britain*, 2nd edn, London, Sage.

Pond, C. and Searle, A. (1991) *The Hidden Army: Children at Work in the 1990s*, London, Low Pay Unit.

Riley, D. (1983) *War in the Nursery: Theories of the Child and Mother*, London, Virago.

Roberts, H. (2000) 'Listening to children: and hearing them', in P. Christensen and A. James (eds), *Research with Children: Perspectives and Practice*, London, Falmer Press.

Rutter, M. (1981) *Maternal Deprivation Reassessed*, 2nd edn, London, Penguin Books.

Smith, P.K. (2000) 'Why I study...Bullying in schools', *The Psychologist*, 13: 348–349.

Smith, P.K. and Brain, P. (2000) 'Bullying in schools: lessons from two decades of research', *Aggressive Behavior*, 26: 1–9.

Smith, P.K. and Sharp, S. (1994) *School Bullying: Insights and Perspectives*, London, Routledge.

Stack, N. and McKechnie, J. (2002) 'Working children', in B. Goldson, M. Lavalette and J. McKechnie (eds), *Children, Welfare and the State*, London, Sage.

Sutton, J. (2001) 'Bullies: thugs or thinkers', *The Psychologist*, 14: 530–534.

Walters, R. (2003) 'New modes of governance and the commodification of criminological knowledge', *Social and Legal Studies*, 12: 5–26.

Weiss, C. (1998) 'Have we learned anything new about the use of evaluation?' *American Journal of Evaluation*, 19: 21–33.

Zalami, F.B., Reddy, N., Lynch, M.A. and Feinstein, C. (1998) *Forgotten on the Pyjama Trail: A Case Study of Young Garment Workers in Meknes Morocco Dismissed from their jobs Following Foreign Media Attention*, Amsterdam, Defence for Children International.

Index